Purchasing to improve health systems performance

D1420025

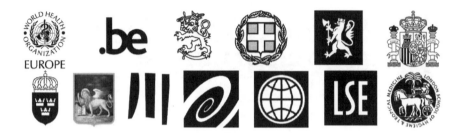

The European Observatory on Health Systems and Policies is a partnership between the World Health Organization Regional Office for Europe, the Governments of Belgium, Finland, Greece, Norway, Spain and Sweden, the Veneto Region, the European Investment Bank, the Open Society Institute, the World Bank, the London School of Economics and Political Science, and the London School of Hygiene and Tropical Medicine.

European Observatory on Health Systems and Policies Series

Edited by Josep Figueras, Martin McKee, Elias Mossialos and Richard B. Saltman

Purchasing to improve health systems performance

Edited by

**Josep Figueras,
Ray Robinson and
Elke Jakubowski**

Open University Press

Open University Press
McGraw-Hill Education
McGraw-Hill House
Shoppenhangers Road
Maidenhead
Berkshire
England
SL6 2QL

email: enquiries@openup.co.uk
world wide web: www.openup.co.uk

and Two Penn Plaza, New York, NY 10121–2289, USA

First published 2005

A catalogue record of this book is available from the British Library

ISBN 0335 21367 7 (pb) 0335 21368 5 (hb)

Library of Congress Cataloging-in-Publication Data
CIP data applied for

Typeset by RefineCatch Limited, Bungay, Suffolk
Printed in the UK by Bell and Bain Ltd, Glasgow

European Observatory on Health Systems and Policies Series

The European Observatory on Health Systems and Policies is a unique project that builds on the commitment of all its partners to improving health care systems:

- World Health Organization Regional Office for Europe
- Government of Belgium
- Government of Finland
- Government of Greece
- Government of Norway
- Government of Spain
- Government of Sweden
- Veneto Region
- European Investment Bank
- Open Society Institute
- World Bank
- London School of Economics and Political Science
- London School of Hygiene and Tropical Medicine

The series

The volumes in this series focus on key issues for health policy making in Europe. Each study explores the conceptual background, outcomes and lessons learned about the development of more equitable, more efficient and more effective health systems in Europe. With this focus, the series seeks to contribute to the evolution of a more evidence-based approach to policy formulation in the health sector.

These studies will be important to all those involved in formulating or evaluating national health care policies and, in particular, will be of use to health policy makers and advisers, who are under increasing pressure to rationalize the structure and funding of their health systems. Academics and students in the field of health policy will also find this series valuable in seeking to understand better the complex choices that confront the health systems of Europe.

The Observatory supports and promotes evidence-based health policy making through comprehensive and rigorous analysis of the dynamics of health care systems in Europe.

Series Editors

Josep Figueras is Head of the Secretariat and Research Director of the European Observatory on Health Systems and Policies and Head of the European Centre for Health Policy, World Health Organization Regional Office for Europe.

Martin McKee is Research Director of the European Observatory on Health Systems and Policies and Professor of European Public Health at the London School of Hygiene and Tropical Medicine as well as a co-director of the School's European Centre on Health of Societies in Transition.

Elias Mossialos is Research Director of the European Observatory on Health Systems and Policies and Brian Abel-Smith Reader in Health Policy, Department of Social Policy, London School of Economics and Political Science and Co-Director of LSE Health and Social Care.

Richard B. Saltman is Research Director of the European Observatory on Health Systems and Policies and Professor of Health Policy and Management at the Rollins School of Public Health, Emory University in Atlanta, Georgia.

European Observatory on Health Systems and Policies Series

Series Editors: Josep Figueras, Martin McKee, Elias Mossialos and Richard B. Saltman

Published titles

Health policy and European Union enlargement
Martin McKee, Laura MacLehose and Ellen Nolte (eds)

Regulating entrepreneurial behaviour in European health care systems
Richard B. Saltman, Reinhard Busse and Elias Mossialos (eds)

Social health insurance systems in Western Europe
Richard B. Saltman, Reinhard Busse and Josep Figueras (eds)

Health care in Central Asia
Martin McKee, Judith Healy and Jane Falkingham (eds)

Hospitals in a changing Europe
Martin McKee and Judith Healy (eds)

Funding health care: options for Europe
Elias Mossialos, Anna Dixon, Josep Figueras and Joe Kutzin (eds)

Regulating pharmaceuticals in Europe: striving for efficiency, equity and quality
Elias Mossialos, Monique Mrazek and Tom Walley (eds)

Forthcoming titles

Mental health policy and practice across Europe
Martin Knapp, David McDaid, Elias Mossialos and Graham Thornicroft (eds)

Primary care in the driver's seat
Richard B. Saltman, Ana Rico and Wienke Boerma (eds)

Contents

List of tables

List of boxes

List of figures

List of contributors

Toni Ashton is an Associate Professor in Health Economics and Director of the Centre for Health Services Research and Policy at the University of Auckland, New Zealand.

Philip Berman is Director of the European Health Management Association.

Michael Borowitz is Director of the Public Health Programme, Open Society Institute, New York.

Helmut Brand is Director of the Institute of Public Health in North-Rhine-Westphalia, Germany.

Reinhard Busse is Professor of Health Care Management at the University of Technology Berlin and Associate Research Director of the European Observatory on Health Systems and Policies.

Andrea Donatini is Chief of the Health Economics Unit at the Regional Health Agency of Emilia-Romagna, Bologna, Italy.

Antonio Duran is Director of the consulting firm Tecnicas de Salud and a lecturer at the Andalusian School of Public Health, Spain.

Tamas Evetovits is an Assistant Professor at Semmelweis University Health Services Management Training Centre, Budapest, Hungary.

Andre P. den Exter is an Assistant Professor of Health Law at the Erasmus University Rotterdam, the Netherlands.

Josep Figueras is Head of the Secretariat and Research Director of the European Observatory on Health Systems and Policies.

Julian Forder is Researcher at the Social Services Research Unit of the London School of Economics and Political Sciences, London, United Kingdom.

Péter Gaál is a lecturer in health policy at the Health Services Management Training Centre, Semmelweis University, Budapest.

Chris Ham is Professor of Health Policy and Management at the Health Services Management Centre at the University of Birmingham, United Kingdom. Between 2000 and 2004 he worked on secondment to the Department of Health where he was Director of the Strategy Unit.

Brian Hardy is a Principal Research Fellow at the Nuffield Institute for Health, University of Leeds, United Kingdom.

Petr Hava is Researcher at the Faculty of Social Sciences at the Institute of Sociological Studies, Charles University, Prague, Czech Republic.

David J. Hunter is Professor of Health Policy and Management in the School for Health and Wolfson Research Institute at the University of Durham, United Kingdom, and is Chair of the UK Public Health Association.

Danguole Jankauskiene is a lecturer at the Social Medical Centre, Vilnius University, Lithuania.

Elke Jakubowski is acting Regional Adviser, Futures Fora, at the WHO Regional Office for Europe, and a research associate of the European Observatory on Health Systems and Policies.

Maris Jesse is a health policy and finance analyst, PRAXIS Center for Policy Studies and part-time lecturer at Tartu University, Estonia. She has been Director of Estonian Health Insurance Fund.

Ninel Kadyrova works at the Mandatory Health Insurance Fund, Ministry of Health in Kyrgyzstan.

Joe Kutzin is Regional Adviser, Health Systems Financing, WHO Regional Office for Europe.

John C. Langenbrunner is a senior health economist, Europe and Central Asia Region, World Bank, Washington, D.C.

Donald W. Light is a fellow at the Center for Bioethics at the University of Pennsylvania and a professor of comparative health systems at the University of Medicine and Dentistry of New Jersey, United States.

Hans Maarse is Professor in Health Care Policy Analysis at the Faculty of Health Sciences, University of Maastricht, the Netherlands.

Nicholas Mays is Professor of Health Policy at the London School of Hygiene and Tropical Medicine.

Martin McKee is Professor of European Public Health at the London School of Hygiene and Tropical Medicine and a research director in the European Observatory on Health Systems and Policies.

Eva Orosz works at the Health Policy Unit of the Organisation of Economic Co-operation and Development (OECD) in Paris, France.

John Øvretveit is Director of Research, The Karolinska Institute Medical Management Centre, Stockholm, and Professor of Health Policy and Management, The Nordic School of Public Health, Gothenburg, and Bergen University Faculty of Medicine, Norway.

Dominique Polton is Director of CREDES, Paris, France.

Alexander S. Preker is Lead Economist at the World Bank, Washington, D.C.

Thomas A. Rathwell is Professor and Director of the School of Health Services Administration and Head, PAHO/WHO Collaborating Centre for Health Care Systems Research and Development, Dalhousie University, Halifax, Canada.

Sabine Richard works at the Allgemeine Ortskrankenkasse (AOK) Berlin, Germany.

Igor Sheiman is Professor of Health Economics at the Moscow High School of Economics and Project Leader of the presidential administration health reform group.

Ray Robinson is Professor of Health Policy at LSE Health and Social Care, London School of Economics and Political Science, United Kingdom.

Constantino Sakellarides is Professor at the Escola Nacional de Saude Publica, Lisbon, Portugal.

Markus Schneider is Director of the Beratungsgesellschaft für Angewandte Systemforschung (BASYS), Augsburg, Germany.

Sergey Shishkin is Professor at the Institute for the Economy in Transition in Moscow, Russian Federation.

Peter C. Smith is Professor of Economics in the Centre for Health Economics at the University of York, United Kingdom.

Francesco Taroni is Head of the Regional Health Agency of the Emilia-Romagna Region, Bologna, Italy.

Marcial Velasco-Garrido is Research Fellow at the Health Care Management Department at the University of Technology Berlin, Germany.

Miriam M. Wiley is Professor and Head of the Health Policy Research Centre at the Economic and Social Research Institute, Dublin, Ireland.

Series editors' introduction

European national policy makers broadly agree on the core objectives that their health care systems should pursue. The list is strikingly straightforward: universal access for all citizens, effective care for better health outcomes, efficient use of resources, high-quality services and responsiveness to patient concerns. It is a formula that resonates across the political spectrum and which, in various, sometimes inventive, configurations, has played a role in most recent European national election campaigns.

Yet this clear consensus can only be observed at the abstract policy level. Once decision makers seek to translate their objectives into the nuts and bolts of health system organization, common principles rapidly devolve into divergent, occasionally contradictory, approaches. This is, of course, not a new phenomenon in the health sector. Different nations, with different histories, cultures and political experiences, have long since constructed quite different institutional arrangements for funding and delivering health care services.

The diversity of health system configurations that has developed in response to broadly common objectives leads quite naturally to questions about the advantages and disadvantages inherent in different arrangements, and which approach is 'better' or even 'best' given a particular context and set of policy priorities. These concerns have intensified over the last decade as policy makers have sought to improve health system performance through what has become a Europe-wide wave of health system reforms. The search for comparative advantage has triggered – in health policy as in clinical medicine – increased attention to its knowledge base, and to the possibility of overcoming at least part of existing institutional divergence through more evidence-based health policy making.

The volumes published in the European Observatory on Health Systems and Policies series are intended to provide precisely this kind of cross-national health policy analysis. Drawing on an extensive network of experts and policy makers working in a variety of academic and administrative capacities, these studies seek to synthesize the available evidence on key health sector topics using a systematic methodology. Each volume explores the conceptual background, outcomes and lessons learned about the development of more equitable, more efficient and more effective health care systems in Europe. With this focus, the series seeks to contribute to the evolution of a more evidence-based approach to policy formulation in the health sector. While remaining sensitive to cultural, social and normative differences among countries, the studies explore a range of policy alternatives available for future decision making. By examining closely both the advantages and disadvantages of different policy approaches, these volumes fulfil central mandates of the Observatory: to serve as a bridge between pure academic research and the needs of policy makers, and to stimulate the development of strategic responses suited to the real political world in which health sector reform must be implemented.

The European Observatory on Health Systems and Policies is a partnership that brings together three international agencies, six national governments, a region of Italy, two research institutions and an international non-governmental organization. The partners are as follows: the World Health Organization Regional Office for Europe, which provides the Observatory secretariat; the governments of Belgium, Finland, Greece, Norway, Spain and Sweden; the Veneto Region; the European Investment Bank; the Open Society Institute; the World Bank; the London School of Hygiene and Tropical Medicine and the London School of Economics and Political Science.

In addition to the analytical and cross-national comparative studies published in this Open University Press series, the Observatory produces Health Care Systems in Transition (HiTs) profiles for the countries of Europe, the journal *EuroHealth* and the newsletter *EuroObserver*. Further information about Observatory publications and activities can be found on its Web site, www.observatory.dk.

Josep Figueras, Martin McKee, Elias Mossialos and Richard B. Saltman

Foreword

Countries across the whole European region are constantly searching for ways to improve health systems performance. Many see purchasing mechanisms as the key to making health services deliver better quality care. They also believe the contracts, which are central to purchasing, can push health care providers into taking account of the wider issues, like prevention, which have such a huge impact on the health of Europe's citizens.

Clearly if policy makers really want contracts to lever better performance they need to do more than simply reimburse providers for the costs of products and services. They need to insist on a more sophisticated approach that delivers efficiency and quality. Just as crucially, or perhaps more crucially, they need to line up purchasing tools with the health needs of society. Surely if we, as the leaders of health systems, buy care we should be able to ensure that what we buy matches the aims and values of society. We must be able to see that the money we spend leads to the most cost effective and the fairest provision of services possible. And we absolutely must bring public health into the picture. European policy makers are well aware of all this but they do not always have the evidence they need to implement purchasing.

This study will help fill the evidence gap. It provides a comprehensive review of purchasing across Europe and demonstrates that it does have the potential to improve the health and wellbeing of our populations. The volume identifies those areas where the potential of purchasing could be further realized and suggests ways of making it more effective. It is full of rich lessons drawn from practical experience. Two of these are particularly important and are very much at the heart of WHO policy.

First, the analysis shows that without strong stewardship purchasing will not manage to properly reflect population health needs or even the wishes of individual citizens. It analyses how and why some health system stewards are better at translating health policy commitments into spending decisions. Second, the study shows how important evidence must be in determining purchasing needs. Evidence can really drive change, and provided we look not only at cost but also at the effectiveness of interventions we can achieve a shift in how resources are used that benefits people.

The study will help bring evidence to bear on practice. As with all other volumes of the Observatory series it cannot tell policy makers what to do or provide a magic bullet. There are no simple single solutions that can be applied across the richness and variety of our Region. Rather the Observatory tries to present a comprehensive synthesis of the evidence accessibly and clearly so that policy makers can use it, together with other tools, to strive for better health and better health systems. On behalf of all the Partners of the Observatory therefore, it is a pleasure for me to introduce this volume. I am confident it will contribute to better policy making in all our countries.

Marc Danzon
WHO Regional Director for Europe

Acknowledgements

This volume is one of a series of books produced by the European Observatory on Health Systems and Policies. We are very grateful to all our authors, who responded promptly both in producing and later amending their chapters in the light of ongoing discussions.

In addition to the work of the authors, this volume draws heavily on a series of twelve country case studies provided by Andrea Donatini (Italy), Tamas Evetovis and Peter Gaal (Hungary), Andre den Exter (Netherlands), Petr Hava (Czech Republic), Dangole Jankauskiene (Lithuania), Maris Jesse (Estonia), Ninel Kadyrova (Kyrgyzistan), Dominique Polton (France), Sabine Richard (Germany), Ana Rico (Spain), Ray Robinson (United Kingdom), Igor Sheiman and Sergey Shishkin (Russian Federation). These case studies will be published in a forth-coming volume of the Observatory.

We appreciate the valuable comments of those reviewers who participated at various stages in the process. These included the Observatory's steering commit-tee members who commented on the original proposal and the various versions of this manuscript. They also included those who participated in a workshop to discuss a draft of the volume in Venice. These were in addition to the case study writers and the authors who helpfully commented on each others' chapters, Luigi Berttinato, Chris Ham, Charles Normand, Constantino Sakellarides and Franco Toniolo. We are particularly grateful for the contributions of our reviewers Toni Ashton, Phillip Berman, Reinhard Busse, Antonio Duran, Suszy Lessof, Hans Maarse, Nicholas Mays and Mathias Wismar.

Finally we are especially grateful to the Veneto Region Department of Health, which generously hosted the workshop in Venice. Particular thanks go to Luigi Berttinato and Franco Toniolo for the leadership and support to the workshop.

part one

chapter one

Introduction

Ray Robinson, Elke Jakubowski and Josep Figueras

Context

European health care systems have faced major challenges in recent years. These have included drives for more effective cost containment, particularly in the public sector; the quest for greater efficiency in the use of scarce resources; increasing pressures to become more responsive to the needs and preferences of patients and the public; increased emphasis on health outcomes and population health gain; and renewed scrutiny of the roles of government in health (Saltman *et al.*, 1998). Of course, not all countries have faced these challenges to the same extent. Variations in emphasis have been apparent between, for example, Beveridge and Bismarckian systems, and between Eastern and Western Europe. Despite this diversity, what has been in many ways more remarkable is the emergence of certain common trends in health sector reform. Among these, there has been a move from hierarchical, often highly integrated forms of service delivery and finance, towards devolved models based upon the separation of the responsibility for purchasing services from the responsibility for providing them. The distinct role of purchasing has been established as part of these changes.

Recognizing the potential of this approach, the *World Health Report 2000* put forward strategic purchasing as a major option for improving performance of health systems. It argues that where a purchaser model exists, countries should move from passive purchasing – whereby a predetermined budget is followed or bills are simply reimbursed retrospectively – to strategic forms of purchasing in which proactive decisions are made about which health care services should be purchased, how and from whom (WHO, 2000).

In fact, a number of countries in both Eastern and Western Europe have already moved from integrated command-and-control models of publicly operated health care services towards some form of purchasing-based model. In these models, public, or quasi-public, third-party payers are kept organizationally separate from health service providers. The rationale for this purchaser–provider split can be summarized in terms of five main objectives. First, services may be improved by linking plans and priorities to resource allocation, for instance, shifting resources to more cost-effective interventions and across care boundaries (such as from inpatient to outpatient care). Purchasing can thus be regarded as an alternative way to take some of the measures that have been traditionally pursued via planning. Second, population health needs and consumer expectations may be met by building them into purchasing decisions. Third, providers' performance can be improved by giving purchasers levers such as financial incentives or monitoring tools, which can be used to increase provider responsiveness and efficiency. Fourth, the separation of functions within publicly operated health systems can reduce administrative rigidities generated by hierarchically structured command-and-control models. Management can be decentralized and decision making devolved by allowing providers to focus on efficiently producing the services determined by the purchaser. Finally, the separation of functions can be used to introduce competition or contestability among public as well as private providers and thereby use market mechanisms to increase efficiency (Savas *et al.*, 1998).

Countries that have introduced some form of purchasing within the public sector include Sweden (beginning in several county councils in 1990), Finland (1993) and the United Kingdom (1991). Southern Europe also has several examples. For instance, in Spain a number of regions such as the Basque country and Catalonia have adopted a system of purchasing. In Italy, purchasing relationships exist but are limited to teaching hospitals with trust status in certain regions and the degree of implementation varies greatly between them. In Portugal, special agencies with the responsibility to contract with health care providers were established in every regional health administration in 1998. The scope for purchasing is still limited, but more recently in 2003 legislation has been passed to create a new form of self-governing public hospital trust and purchasing is set to expand rapidly.

The separation of functions and provision of services through contractual relationships has, of course, been part of the Bismarck-style, social-insurance-based health systems of continental Europe since their inception. Until recently, however, purchasing was a passive exercise that involved the reimbursement of expenses to providers with only some financial incentives and overall budget ceilings to ensure cost containment. Contracts did not focus on price or efficiency, nor were they understood to be contestable. For instance, in social health insurance countries such as Germany or the Netherlands, sickness funds traditionally had the legal obligation to enter into uniform and collective contracts with each physician established in their working area.

In recent years, however, countries such as Austria, Germany, Israel and the Netherlands have sought to transform insurers from being relatively passive payers to become more discriminating and prudent purchasers. These countries are progressively introducing more selective forms of purchasing according to performance criteria. A triggering factor has been the introduction of insurance competition in many of these countries, allowing individual citizens to choose among statutory insurers and purchasers. This reform, first discussed in Europe by the Dekker Commission in the Netherlands, suggests that introducing market incentives for insurers will lead to better administration of collection, more innovative practices and more cost-effective purchasing. However, as discussed later in this volume, many of these countries are facing substantial difficulties in implementing selective contracting among providers.

In many countries of Eastern Europe, the introduction of social health insurance systems has separated functions between insurance funds responsible for purchasing and financially autonomous hospitals responsible for service provision. Countries moving in this direction include Armenia, the Czech Republic, Estonia, Georgia, Hungary, Latvia, Lithuania, Poland, Romania, the Russian Federation, Slovakia and Slovenia.

Taken overall, however, the move towards strategic purchasing has been variable in practice. Some countries have embraced the general principle of strategic purchasing in their health care reforms. In others, the approach has been confined to local experimentation. Passive purchasing still dominates in many countries. The variability of purchasing arrangements is compounded because countries differ in the nature of the purchasing agent; its political and technical accountability including the composition of the purchasing boards or the degree of political direction; the population group covered; and the range of purchaser responsibilities. Similarly, the financial, contractual and regulatory mechanisms available to these purchasing organizations to steer provider performance differ substantially. The question of determining the appropriate purchasing agent – that is, what configuration buys health services more cost-effectively and according to the needs and wants of the population it represents – has yet to be answered.

Rationale and objectives

Despite the inclusion of strategic purchasing in many European countries' health care reforms, there is at present no comprehensive account of the ways in which the health purchasing function has been developed, let alone evidence on their impact. In the light of this gap, this book provides an overview of the existing evidence on purchaser organizational and functional arrangements, evidence on alternative approaches to purchasing and policy lessons on introducing and reforming arrangements for purchasing health services. It is aimed primarily at policy makers, technical experts designing and putting in place purchasing structures and health policy analysts in general.

The book comprises a series of chapters written by international experts on the key components of the purchasing process as well as on the published literature, grey literature and informal intelligence gathered on health care purchasing, together with material provided through case studies undertaken in selected European countries by national experts (Figueras *et al.*, forthcoming).

In sum, the book aims to provide:

- a systematic overview of the theory and practice of purchasing for health services in Europe;
- an up-to-date descriptive analysis of recent experience with purchasing arrangements in Western Europe, the countries of Central and Eastern Europe

(CEE) and the former Soviet Republics that are more loosely linked to the Commonwealth of Independent States (CIS).

- a review of the evidence on purchasing and a distillation of the lessons that can assist policy makers in the formulation of more effective purchasing strategies.

Conceptual framework

The first dilemma when aiming to assess purchasing experience is to define the concept of purchasing itself. Most approaches, such as that of the *World Health Report 2000*, start from the separating of health system functions. Purchasing together with revenue collection and pooling of resources are three inter-related components of the health system's financing function, the three other core functions of the health system being resource generation, provision and stewardship.

Purchasing is often linked to resource allocation. This approach departs from the fact that the function of health service provision requires the mobilization and effective use of financial resources. Purchasing is thus regarded as a mechanism by which those who hold financial resources allocate them to those who produce health services (Perrot, 2002).

Øvretveit (1995) argues that purchasing needs to be differentiated from other functions such as commissioning and contracting. In his approach, health services purchasing is narrower than commissioning. Commissioning is oriented towards maximizing population health and equity by purchasing health services and influencing other organizations to create conditions which enhance people's health. Commissioning is a government or public sector function that involves the development of a national health strategy and its implementation through a wide range of public health functions including health services, health prevention and intersectoral strategies. Purchasing, on the other hand, is mainly concerned with buying health services from health care facilities such as ambulatory visits, diagnostic tests, surgery, hospitalization and so forth. Contracting is, then, more narrowly defined as the negotiated agreement between purchasers and providers about services they will provide in return for payment. It includes service specification, tendering, monitoring and reviewing contract performance.

This volume provides a wider view of purchasing than just the allocation of funds to provider organizations. As noted earlier, and in line with the proposition contained in the *World Health Report 2000*, we argue that purchasing can play a key role in improving the performance of the health system, particularly when we move from passive forms of purchasing – the mere reimbursement of providers – to more proactive and strategic forms of purchasing that consider *which* interventions should be purchased, *how* they should be purchased and *from whom*. As all health systems exercise some form of purchasing, the key question therefore becomes how to move along a continuum towards more strategic purchasing so we achieve a cost-effective allocation of available resources and maximize population health gain.

In seeking to understand the various components of strategic purchasing and the organizational environment within which it operates, this book has adopted a principal–agent theoretical perspective. This has provided a framework within which the relationships between different actors may be examined. In fact, in this context, we have adopted a triple principal–agent framework that identifies: (i) the relationship between consumers/users and third-party purchasers, (ii) the relationship between purchasers and providers and (iii) the relationship between the government and the purchaser.

The first set of agency relationships take place between the consumer (the *principal*) and the third-party purchaser (a health authority, local government, sickness fund), which acts as the consumers' *agent* in the purchase of health care services on their behalf. Key questions here concern the extent to which the agent reflects the needs and preferences of users and the public. In a second set of agency relationships the third-party purchaser, as the *principal*, employs a series of financial, contractual, regulatory and monitoring mechanisms to ensure that the provider (such as a hospital), as its *agent*, will deliver the appropriate mix of health care, of acceptable quality, at an agreed price. In this relationship the forms of contract that are used and the mechanisms through which providers are paid are important considerations. Moreover, the organizational environment within which the provider functions (for example, monopoly or competitive, for-profit or not-for-profit), and the provider's internal management mechanisms (for example, effective or non-effective combination of financial and clinical management) can also be expected to impact upon this principal–agent relationship. In the third agency relationship the purchaser acts as agent for the government or state. In this instance, the government as *principal* will seek to ensure that national health priorities are met. This relationship introduces the role of the government as a steward of the health system, a role recently highlighted as 'arguably the most important' health system function.

This framework and the insights provided by theory are used throughout the book in seeking to understand better how purchasers behave and ways in which their performance could be improved. However, a word of clarification about the use of the principal–agent framework needs to be made at the outset. The theory has been developed by economists and can become rather arcane in some theoretical discussions. Our interest, on the other hand, is multidisciplinary and primarily applied. We are interested in how purchasing works in practice and how policy learning can be encouraged. We use economic theory as a tool, not as an end in itself. For this reason, we take due account of political, administrative, legal and other factors that can be expected to influence the principal–agent relationship.

Structure

The book is divided into two main parts.

Part One contains three chapters, including this introduction. It draws on literature reviews and intelligence, specially commissioned case studies and, most importantly, material presented in the individual chapters in Part Two.

Chapter 2 presents a review of the organization of purchasing as it presently exists in the countries of Western and Eastern Europe; and a taxonomy of the main components of the purchasing process, including institutional arrangements, functional analysis, market environments, accountability mechanisms, incentives, and decision-making mechanisms. Chapter 3 contains a review of the available evidence on the performance of different purchaser arrangements and presents a summary of the lessons from international experience that are available to policy makers. The aim of these two chapters is to provide a broad description of the main approaches and developments in purchasing as well as a synthesis of the main lessons for policy making derived from the study. They are aimed at those readers who wish to have a broad and integrated overview of the field.

Part Two, by contrast, provides a more in-depth analysis of the various components of purchasing, ranging from a detailed discussion of the theories underpinning purchasing to a thorough analysis of some of the main tools for purchasing such as contracting or payment systems. These dimensions are presented following the triple agency perspective as set out in our conceptual framework. Part Two contains nine chapters prepared by collaborating teams of multicountry experts.

The first chapter in Part Two, Chapter 4, focuses on theories of purchasing. It covers a number of recent developments in the new institutional economics or economics of organization, and applies these to purchaser organizations. These include discussion of alternative methods of economic organization, including the respective merits of hierarchies, markets and networks, and the role of the new public management in understanding organizational behaviour. The chapter shows how the economics of organization – although a rather amorphous set of theories – provides a framework for comparing governance arrangements according to the net costs of undertaking transactions. Its relevance to policy analysis is in drawing relationships between choice of governance structure and outcomes, mediated by the features of the transaction and the principal–agent configurations involved.

Building on the theoretical perspective set out in Chapter 4, Chapter 5 concentrates on one important aspect of the organization of purchasing, namely the role of markets and competition in purchasing. In the last decade a number of European countries have experimented with the introduction of different degrees of market mechanisms in health care sectors. This chapter reviews these developments – in relation to purchasing – and discusses the advantages and disadvantages of market-based approaches. It argues that, if properly implemented, a market in purchasing may increase responsiveness to citizens, act as a spur to innovation and lead a drive for better information. On the other hand, it can increase administrative complexity and bureaucratic costs, threaten equity between patients and lead to instability and market failure.

Chapter 6 deals with consumer participation and accountability. It takes the perspective of the purchaser as the public's agent. It discusses various mechanisms drawing on public participation. These may take the form of 'voice' mechanisms, such as public consultation exercises, advocacy group activity, formal representation of public and patients on purchaser committees, and the rapidly evolving patients' rights movement. Alternatively, user influence may be exerted through 'exit' mechanisms; that is, the classic market response whereby consumers are free to shop around and exit from choices that do not suit their preferences.

Chapter 7 focuses on purchasing to promote the population's health. It assesses the extent to which different purchasing arrangements take account of the public health perspective both in theory and in practice. The chapter covers this dimension in the framework of each of the three principal–agency perspectives. First, with regard to the public–purchaser relationship, the chapter looks at whether purchasing organizations have access to public health skills, take a wide population-based health-needs assessment perspective and reflect public health priorities in their purchasing plans. Second, it considers the extent to which national health priorities are reflected in purchasing priorities. Third, the chapter looks at the strengths of mechanisms available to purchasers to ensure that public health priorities are taken up and implemented by providers.

Stewardship is the focus of Chapter 8. It offers a conceptual framework for analysing this function; demonstrates the core tasks of stewardship in relation to purchasing with empirical examples drawn from case studies; discusses the nature of good stewardship; and distils practical lessons. In doing so, it draws on the concept of stewardship as developed in the WHO's *World Health Report 2000* to explore three defined tasks of stewardship in the context of purchasing: (i) formulating health policy – defining the vision and direction; (ii) exerting influence – including approaches to regulation; and (iii) collecting and using intelligence.

Chapter 9 is devoted to an analysis of contracts as a tool for purchasers to influence provider behaviour. Through the contractual relationship, purchasers have the potential to ensure that an appropriate mix of services is supplied on specified terms and conditions (for example, in terms of cost, quantity and quality). However, as the chapter shows, the concept of a 'contract' is understood in different ways in different European countries. This chapter reviews the legal status of contracts, their content, the use of quality standards and information and monitoring activities. It also discusses the relative performance of different modes of contracting.

Chapter 10 adds the critical dimension of quality to the framework on health purchasing. Whereas previous chapters discuss the theoretical underpinnings for separating the purchaser from the provider and the introduction of contracting, Chapter 10 examines whether, and by which mechanisms, the introduction of purchasing increases the quality of health care. The chapter presents a concept of quality of care from the perspective of the purchaser, as the principal of the health care provider. The chapter then explores the mechanisms applied across Europe to link the purchasing process with quality improvement.

The ways in which purchasers reimburse providers are also an important aspect of the purchaser–provider, principal–agent relationship. This is the subject of Chapter 11. The chapter starts with an overview of payment systems, as it is well known that different payment systems offer different forms of incentive structure. It not only examines payment and reward patterns but also seeks to provide an assessment of their effects in Western and Eastern European countries.

The last chapter, Chapter 12, deals with provider organizations and their responses to the new demands of purchasing. The chapter offers illustrations from a number of European countries, about how the success of newly established purchaser organizations in achieving their objectives will depend crucially on key aspects of provider organizations. For example, the ability of providers to respond to purchasers' objectives will depend on factors such as their form of ownership, their scope for decision making and the structure of the market within which they operate. The chapter provides an analysis of the typology and variety of hospital provider organizations in Europe, examines types of organizational responses to purchasers and the factors influencing these responses – the latter will be subject to policy adaptations in countries wishing to take the introduction or development of a purchasing function in their health care systems a step further.

Thus, taken overall, this book aims to provide insights for the further development of strategic purchasing in European health care systems.

References

Figueras, J., Robinson, R. and Jakubowski, E., eds. (forthcoming) *Purchasing to improve health systems performance: Case studies in European countries*. Copenhagen, European Observatory on Health Systems and Policies, World Health Organization.

Øvretveit, J. (1995) Purchasing for Health. *In*: Øvretveit, J., *Purchasing for health*. Buckingham, Open University Press.

Perrot, J. (2002) Health financing technical brief. Analysis of allocation of financial resources within health systems. Conceptual paper. Geneva, World Health Organization.

Saltman, R.B., Figueras, J. and Sakellarides, C., eds. (1998) *Critical challenges for health care reform in Europe*. Buckingham, Open University Press.

Savas, S., Sheiman, I., Tragakes, E. and Maarse, H. (1998) Contracting models and provider competition. *In*: Saltman, R.B., Figueras, J. and Sakellarides, C., eds. *Critical challenges for health care reform in Europe*. Buckingham, Open University Press.

WHO (2000) *The world health report 2000. Health systems: improving performance*. Geneva, World Health Organization.

chapter two

Organization of purchasing in Europe

Ray Robinson, Elke Jakubowski and Josep Figueras

Introduction

Strategic purchasing has been identified as a key component for the improvement of health systems performance. In its ideal form it brings together a range of separate functions with the potential to improve efficiency, effectiveness and responsiveness. It can also make a major contribution to the achievement of public health goals and wider social objectives of equity within the health care system. In practice, however, the extent to which individual countries have attained this ideal varies enormously. In this chapter we assemble empirical evidence on the present state of purchasing in a range of Eastern and Western European countries.

The aim of the chapter is to provide a descriptive analysis of purchasing in different countries and thereby to enable comparison of experiences and identification of international trends. After a discussion of the ways in which purchasing is organized in different countries, the chapter describes the key components of strategic purchasing. Each of these components is discussed in more depth in the individual chapters in Part Two of the book. Evidence about the impact of these purchasing strategies is summarized in Chapter 3, together with the main lessons for policy makers.

Chapter 2 draws heavily on a series of case studies of the purchasing arrangements in 11 countries prepared specifically for this project (Figueras *et al.*, forthcoming) together with additional material drawn from the European Observatory Health Systems in Transition profiles and other Observatory work (www.observatory.dk). This material provides the basis both for the text and for illustrative examples of different aspects of purchasing presented in the tables in this chapter. Our analysis also draws extensively upon material presented by individual authors in the chapters in Part Two of this book.

After a brief description of the organization of purchasing in European countries, the chapter reviews the main components of the triple principal–agent relationship outlined in Chapter 1. This focuses on the relationships between purchaser organizations and:

- the public and patients on behalf of whom they purchase services;
- the provider organizations from whom they purchase services;
- the government, which acts as a steward of the overall health care system, including purchaser organizations.

Organization of purchasing

European health care systems display considerable diversity in terms of the organizations that carry out purchasing. Countries differ in terms of the types of organizations that act as purchasers (for example, central government, regional government, municipalities, health insurance funds), the numbers of organizations that carry out this function (that is, market concentration) and the ways in which they interact with each other, in particular whether there is competition between purchasers. They also vary in terms of their funding sources (for example, social insurance versus tax-based), and jurisdictions (for example, geographical, occupational, religious affiliations). This diversity derives from a complex interplay of social, economic, cultural and historical factors. Different mixes of public–private ownership, scope and level of population coverage, forms of management and systems of accountability are some of the other dimensions on which there is substantial variation.

Within this complexity, however, we believe that two important dimensions are of particular interest. These are the dimensions of *vertical* and *horizontal* organization, which can be expected to exert profound influences on purchaser behaviours.

On the vertical dimension, a key consideration is often national–local relationships and, in particular, the degree of autonomy possessed by local managers and decision takers. On the horizontal dimension, the number of purchasing organizations, their market shares and the extent of competition between different purchasers are all factors that will exert an impact upon performance.

Vertical organization

Purchasing functions may take place at the *macro* (central), *meso* (regional) and *micro* (local) levels, but these are not watertight categories. Often there are elements of more than one level in any particular country. Secondary and tertiary care may be purchased at a more aggregate level than primary care. In many countries, services involving advanced technologies are often purchased centrally, whatever the arrangements for other services. Complications such as these can make deciding whether a system is more accurately described as macro, meso or micro problematic. Nonetheless, the tripartite categorization does permit the identification of some broad features of purchasing behaviour. In particular, where central government or its agencies are responsible through a central health insurance fund (that is, the macro level) there is often little autonomy for local organizations such as regional branches of the funds, and little decentralized decision making. However, administration of contracting and reimbursement can still be decentralized, such as in the case of Hungary (Box 2.1). At the meso and micro levels, autonomy tends to be greater but this can vary according to particular national arrangements. The size of a country will also be a relevant consideration. The following discussion sets out to highlight differences in autonomy between levels of purchasing and also some important variations between countries at the same level.

Macro-level purchasing

Good examples of centralized macro-level purchasing are provided by countries such as Hungary and Lithuania (Box 2.1). In these countries there is a single health insurance fund. Although these funds have a network of regional offices, they have very limited autonomy on purchasing matters. On the other hand, some countries have sought to break away from centralized systems, by introducing devolved purchasing, only to return to strong central control in the face of failings in the devolved system. Estonia is one such example.

Meso-level purchasing

The majority of European countries assign responsibility for purchasing to some form of meso-level organization. These may be regional governments or health funds with regional affiliations. The meso level is not necessarily territorial. It can also cover employment-based health funds with similar numbers of insured. In essence, the term 'meso' is reserved for those arrangements where devolved purchasing responsibilities are assigned to organizations catering for around 100 000 to 500 000 people. Typically, these organizations operate within an overall structure where certain functions reside at the macro level (for example, revenue raising) and others at the micro level (for example, service provision), but the meso level usually has primary responsibility for major purchasing decisions.

The meso-level purchasing countries can be divided into three main categories. First, there are countries that have national health services for the funding and delivery of services, such as those of Italy and Spain where general taxation raised by central government is transferred to regional governments with general purchasing responsibilities (Box 2.2). It is, however, relevant to note that in both Italy and Spain the extent of the regional purchasing function varies within the country. Regions such as Lombardy in Italy and Catalonia in Spain have developed quite strong strategic purchasing approaches, whereas other regions – such as the Veneto region in Italy – have less distinct purchasing systems.

Box 2.1 Macro-level central purchasing

Hungary

In Hungary a compulsory social insurance scheme operates through a National Health Insurance Fund. The funding system remains centralized with central government control. The National Health Insurance Fund Administration (NHIFA) is a single, national purchaser. The central purchaser buys a range of health care services on behalf of the whole population. The NHIFA is a not-for-profit organization that is closely supervised by the Ministry of Health and has a decentralized set of branches around the country, which contract with local health care providers and reimburse service costs. The decentralization of administration does not mean, however, that there has been much devolution of power. This is still closely managed from the centre.

Lithuania

In Lithuania there is also a single statutory health insurance fund covering about 90% of public expenditure on health. This was introduced in 1997. The insurance scheme makes annual allocations to the central state sickness fund. Although the fund has ten regional branches, decisions about the allocation of spending are made centrally. In effect, the health fund is a governmental budgetary institution largely financed by general taxation. Between 1998 and 2002 only about 20% of the fund's financial resources were derived from pay roll taxes and self-employed contributions.

Estonia

Estonia established 22 independent regional health insurance funds in 1992. A revenue sharing arrangement between them was planned, but this did not work in practice. As a result, a central health insurance fund was established in 1994 with the purpose of controlling and coordinating the individual funds. By 1995 the number of regional funds had fallen to 17, as mergers took place between the smaller funds, frequently due to management difficulties. In 1999–2000 the health insurance system was granted more autonomy through the establishment of the Estonia Health Insurance Fund (EHIF) (based on the previous Central Fund and the 17 separate regional funds) as a public independent organization. At the same time as the EHIF became more independent, there was a degree of centralization at regional level and the previous 17 regional funds, were first merged into 7 regional funds in 2001, and later into 4 regional departments in 2003. At present the national level is responsible for regulation, developing the purchasing strategy and establishing the benefit package, while the regional level is responsible for contracting decisions and reimbursement.

Box 2.2 Regional meso-level purchasing

Italy

Within the Italian National Health Service, reforms of 1992 granted regions the major responsibilities for the organization and management of their health care systems. There are now 19 regions and 2 autonomous provinces carrying out these functions. The regions receive the bulk of their budgets from central government on the basis of a weighted capitation formula and can choose how to allocate these resources among different programmes. The actual provision of services is devolved down to the micro or local level via local health units (LHUs) and to independent hospital trusts. In 2000, there were 197 LHUs covering average populations of 82 000 to 601 000 people.

Spain

A similar regionally based meso system operates in Spain. Until 2002, seven special regions (covering 62% of the population) had responsibility for purchasing health care whereas the remaining ten ordinary regions had health care purchased on their behalf by the central government. From 1 January 2002, however, the ten ordinary regions have also been allocated purchasing responsibilities. Thus all regions now have purchasing functions, with the central government retaining only broad regulatory functions.

A second category of meso purchaser includes the social health insurance based countries of Western Europe such as Austria, Belgium, France, Germany and the Netherlands (Box 2.3).

The third category of meso purchaser comprises those CEE/CIS countries that have made the transition from centrally planned, command-and-control systems to more devolved social health insurance schemes during the 1990s. These countries include the Russian Federation, the Czech Republic, Latvia and Slovakia. Although these countries have adopted Western European-style social health insurance schemes, their history and transitional status mean that they operate these schemes within a different economic, social and political climate and this inevitably affects their performance. For these reasons, there is a case for identifying them as a third and separate category (Box 2.4).

Micro-level purchasing

We use the term 'micro-level purchasing' to refer to situations where there is a high degree of local decision making. Purchasing budgets are devolved to local organizations (or may be raised locally, at least in part) and these organizations have varying degrees of freedom over the allocation of funding to providers. The Nordic countries – where there is a high level of local government

Box 2.3 Social-insurance-based meso-level purchasing in Western Europe

Germany

Statutory health funds and private health insurance companies act as purchasers of health care. The health funds are corporatist, non-governmental organizations, operating on a not-for-profit basis. In January 2003 there were 319 statutory health funds catering for about 70.9 million insured (about 50.3 million members plus their dependents). There are several varieties of health fund. In 2003, the largest category (257 funds) comprised company-based funds (BKK). Others include regional health funds (AOK), substitute funds (*Ersatzkassen*) and guild funds. Throughout the 1990s there have been a series of mergers between health funds, with the result that the number has fallen from 1146 in 1994 to 290 in 2004. The main reason were efforts by the sickness funds to increase economies of scale in pooling and distributing funds. In 2003, the private insurance industry comprised 52 private health insurance companies and provided cover for 7.1 million people who were outside the social insurance scheme. These people included those whose incomes were above the level for which social health insurance is mandatory; self-employed people who were excluded from social health insurance unless they were previously members of a scheme; and public employees who were excluded from social insurance and were reimbursed by the government for private health insurance expenditures.

The Netherlands

The Netherlands offers another example of meso purchasing based upon a mix of health funds and private insurers. Health funds are not-for-profit organizations that are responsible for purchasing health care for those people enrolled with them. Many of them have charitable origins and were originally regionally based. In the late 1980s there were over 40 regional health funds but these have been subject to considerable rationalization and amalgamation. In 2004, about 60% of the population was enrolled in 22 health funds operating nationwide. The remainder of the population whose income levels fall above the threshold for health fund eligibility under the Health Insurance Act, take out insurance with private insurers. Both health funds and private insurers have experienced a marked change in their roles as a result of the reforms that have taken place over the 1990s. Instead of fulfilling a primarily administrative function through the retrospective payment of claims, they have been expected to become cost-conscious purchasers of care. In addition recent reform proposals (currently planned for implementation in 2006) give a role to private insurers in the administration of basic health insurance.

France

France is a rather more complex, multi-level system with a strong meso-level component. The main health insurance scheme (*régime général*) has a network of 16 regional offices and 129 local fund offices. These health funds are responsible for purchasing health services: they make service agreements with providers on behalf of their insured and, at the national level, negotiate agreements with professional unions and set tariffs. The local fund offices are responsible for making payments to providers. All of these offices are not-for-profit organizations with their own boards and a degree of managerial autonomy, although they are subject to a supervisory function carried out by the national fund organization. A major change introduced in France in 1996 involved the establishment of regional hospital agencies as joint ventures between the state and regional associations of health funds. These agencies now have major responsibilities for purchasing through their ability to contract with hospitals, both public and private. In fact, their leverage over hospitals is a hybrid of purchasing (contracting), planning and funding.

Box 2.4 Social-insurance-based meso-level purchasing in the Russian Federation and the Czech Republic

Russian Federation

In the Russian Federation, the compulsory health insurance system introduced in 1993 created a purchaser–provider split through the establishment of a federal mandatory health insurance fund (MHIF) and territorial MHIFs at the regional level. The federal fund is responsible for supervising and regulating the 89 territorial funds, as well as implementing an equalization mechanism. The territorial funds collect and manage insurance revenues from a 3.6% payroll tax on employers on behalf of the working population, as well as regional government contributions on behalf of the non-working population (children, pensioners, unemployed, . . .) and distribute these funds to health insurance companies or territorial MHIF branches which purchase health services on behalf of their members.

Czech Republic

The Czech Republic currently has nine health insurance funds, which act as meso purchasers. The largest, the General Health Insurance Fund, is granted by the state and covers about 71% of the population (7.3 million people). The other funds each cover between 113 000 and 807 000 people. These funds are national (as in the case of the

General Fund), company-based or organized around professional groups. They are all public, not-for-profit organizations that receive delegated funds from the government, but have a degree of autonomy from the government.

responsibility – provide examples of micro-level purchasing (Box 2.5). Another, possibly stronger, example of micro-level purchasing that has emerged in recent years is primary-care-based purchasing. In this model, primary care organizations have control of budgets and are responsible for the purchase of secondary care services on behalf of their patients. England has the most highly developed version of this model, although Spain, Estonia and the Russian Federation have all experimented with some form of it.

Similar local-government-based decision-making powers are vested in county councils and municipalities in Norway, Sweden and Denmark, although the extent of purchasing varies. Sweden was one of the first countries in Europe to introduce purchasing and has gone through a succession of reforms with different models. These have included approaches based upon municipalities, counties and primary care. The city of Stockholm, in particular, has been associated with market-based reforms. At the moment, purchasing takes place in some of the 21 counties where the purchaser–provider split was introduced, but not in others. In Norway, 435 municipalities act as purchasers of primary care but not secondary care. Similarly, the 14 county councils purchase primary care and outpatient services in Denmark, but not inpatient hospital care.

Box 2.5 Micro-level, local government purchasing in Finland

In the Finnish system, purchasing responsibility rests with the 448 municipal councils, which cover populations of, on average, 11 000 people (in fact they range from less than 1000 to over 500 000). Each council is elected every four years by the inhabitants and appoints an executive board that is accountable to the council. The council also appoints members to various municipal committees, including health, education and social services. The municipal council, the municipal executive board and the committees are politically accountable to the electorate. Although the Finnish system has a long-standing reliance on local government (municipality) responsibility, it was the Government Subsidy Reform Act of 1993 that really turned municipalities into purchasers. This led to prospective, needs-based budgetary allocations to municipalities in the place of activity-related, retrospective reimbursement. Following the reforms, municipalities – by themselves or in association with other municipalities – were empowered to purchase secondary and tertiary care services from providers of their choice.

Turning to primary care-based purchasing, there have been a number of recent reforms in England that have led to the devolution of purchasing responsibility to locally based, primary-care-led organizations. Although the emphasis placed upon primary-care-led purchasing in England is certainly greater than in any other European country, there have been a number of pilot schemes experimenting with this form of purchasing elsewhere (See Box 2.6).

Box 2.6 Micro-level, primary-care-based purchasing in selected countries

England

The reform process began in 1991 with the introduction of purchaser–provider separation. As part of this process, selected primary care practices where allocated funding to purchase secondary care services for their patients. By 1998, there were 3500 of these GP fundholding practices covering 60% of the population. The new Labour government, which came into office in 1997, abolished fundholding and established a nationwide system of primary care trusts. Currently, all primary care doctors are assigned to a primary care trust, with each trust covering an average population of about 170 000 people. About 300 primary care trusts now have the major responsibilities for developing primary and community health services and for commissioning secondary care services. From April 2004, their purchasing budgets represent around 75% of the total National Health Service budget.

Estonia

Estonia has introduced purchaser–provider separation and, since 1998, family practitioners have undertaken a very limited form of fundholding. In 2002 they received a virtual budget representing slightly less than 20% of the total capitation fee with which they could provide and/or purchase selected services. However, the fact that 40% of the population live in sparsely populated rural areas and that over 80% of GPs are the only GP in their practice, places limits on the scope for budgetary devolution.

Spain

The Spanish region of Catalonia also piloted purchaser–provider separation under the Health Care Organization Law of 1990. Following these changes, a number of primary care developments catering for populations of 50 000 to 100 000 people were introduced and a form of GP fundholding emerged in the mid-1990s through the *Entitat de Base Asociativa* (EBA). Teams of EBA doctors and nurses receive budgets covering salaries, premises, diagnostic tests and specialist referrals for defined populations. Fifteen EBA teams were in operation by December 2002.

Russian Federation

Experimentation with primary-care-based purchasing also took place in the former Soviet Union between 1987 and 1991. In St Petersburg, Kemerovo and Samara, groups of GPs and primary-level polyclinics became fundholders receiving capitation-based budgets. They were able to purchase diagnostic tests, outpatient services and hospital care for their patients. Thus, in St Petersburg, groups of six doctors covering populations of 8000 patients were established, whereas in Kemerovo, polyclinics became purchasers. However, difficulties associated with a worsening economic situation meant that these schemes had only a limited life.

Sweden

There was some consideration of primary-care-based purchasing in Sweden, but it was never actually adopted. The situation arose because, in the 1990s, a number of Swedish county councils piloted different models of purchaser–provider separation. Within the Stockholm County Council pilot, a primary-care-led project was proposed in one district, Lidingo. But GPs' concerns over the personal financial risk that they would bear meant that they did not support the proposal and so it was not implemented. The only Swedish example of primary care doctors participating actively in purchasing occurred in Northern Dalecarlia, around Mora district hospital, where they provided expert support in the district commissioning process, but did not purchase directly themselves.

Horizontal organization

Horizontal organization refers to the nature of the market structure within which purchasers operate. Conventional economic analysis distinguishes between different forms of market structure based upon levels of concentration. These extend from monopoly (high concentration), through oligopoly and monopolistic markets (medium concentration), to perfect competition (low concentration). The level of competition or contestability is usually expected to increase as concentration decreases.

Chapter 5 analyses these purchaser markets in some detail, from both a theoretical and an empirical perspective, and assembles available evidence on the relative performance of different market configurations. In this section, we present an empirical overview of prevailing European purchaser market structures. The most striking message to emerge from this overview is how little competition seems to exist between purchaser organizations. Despite the rhetoric of market-based reform that has swept European health policy debates in recent years, the purchaser function is rarely carried out in a competitive environment. In the next section we provide some examples of non-competitive purchasing at the macro, meso and micro levels. The subsequent section presents information on meso purchasers in Germany, the Netherlands and the Russian Federation where some degree of purchaser competition appears to exist.

Non-competitive purchasers

Almost by definition, most macro purchasers are in a monopoly situation. Typically, a central government agency is responsible for purchasing or exerts strong control over lower-level organizations. As such, there is no scope for competition within the public system. In theory, private insurers could compete with the public monopoly purchaser but, in practice, private insurance is underdeveloped in such countries and there is not a sufficiently large sector to offer effective competition. Lithuania is an archetypal form of macro, non-competitive purchaser system. There is a single national health fund with ten regional branches. Consumers have no choice but to use the sole health fund and so there is no competition for the insured. Private insurers cover only negative list items not covered by the state health fund and so do not compete.

Those countries that allocate purchasing responsibilities to regional governments – such as Italy and Spain – can be described as meso purchasers operating in non-competitive environments. These governments typically have freedom to devise health systems that reflect regional preferences and there is therefore considerable variation in purchasing arrangements and patterns of service delivery between regions. In this sense, the national market is less concentrated and more heterogeneous than in a macro-purchaser, monopoly market. There may also be a degree of inter-regional rivalry that mimics competition, and some informal movement of patients who take out temporary addresses (with family or friends). However, for the most part, within a region there is no competition as residents are all served by the same purchaser. There is a spatial monopoly.

Some limited competition may exist within a region as the role of the private sector is more pronounced than in the macro-purchaser countries described above. In Spain, for example, around 10% of the population have some form of private health insurance, although this is mainly as a supplement to public coverage. In Italy, private insurance penetration is a good deal higher. In 1999 it was estimated that almost 30% of families were covered by private health insurance. This has resulted in significant resources being devoted to private facilities as an alternative to public supply.

The Czech Republic provides an interesting example of an attempt to introduce competition among meso-level purchasers (Box 2.7).

Box 2.7 Purchaser competition in the Czech Republic

Following the fall of communism, an employer-based social insurance scheme was introduced. There are nine health insurance funds in operation. Competition between funds was introduced in 1994, based on the offer of supplementary benefits. But the process of competition encountered difficulties. Many insurers experienced serious problems in funding the packages of care that they put on offer. As a result, reimbursement of extra services was limited in 1994 and completely abolished in 1997. Consumers are still formally free to choose among insurance funds – they may change funds on an annual basis – but because service coverage and contribution rates do not vary between funds there is little real competition.

Micro-level purchasing in Europe is not usually associated with demand-side competition, that is, competition between purchaser organizations for enrolees. The reason for this is that most micro purchasing is territorially based and therefore results in spatial monopoly. This state of affairs applies to both local government, micro purchasing in the Nordic countries and primary-care-based purchasing in England.

In the Nordic countries, county councils and municipalities generally cater for the needs of their resident populations. Markets are clearly delineated and as such there is no scope for any local government to compete with another for enrolees.

In England, there is some evidence that GP fundholders saw themselves in competition for patients over the period 1992–1998, and that this was one of the factors that led non-fundholders to become fundholders – as fundholders they were able to offer more and better services and therefore attract (or avoid losing) more patients. However, this was never more than a marginal consideration and, with the replacement of fundholding by larger primary care trust organizations, spatial monopoly has become far more pronounced.

Competitive purchasers

Despite the general absence of purchaser competition in European health care systems, there have been some cases where elements of competition have been introduced. Arguments for introducing market-type mechanisms into health care and the associated growth of new public management approaches to managing organizations have both been influential in Germany, the Netherlands and in the Russian Federation (Box 2.8).

Box 2.8 Competitive purchasers

Germany

In Germany, competition policy dates from 1993 when legislation laid the groundwork for increased competition among insurance funds and phased in free choice of funds for insurees. These measures were reinforced by further legislation in 1996 that sought to use competition to restrict the rate of premium growth among insurers and to encourage greater cost consciousness among patients by imposing additional copayments.

The growth of pro-competition policy has meant that the environment within which social health insurers operate now more closely resembles a private sector market environment than has traditionally been the case. Competition between funds takes place mainly in terms of price.

Information on contribution rates figures prominently in newspaper and magazine advertisements. Currently these rates vary between 11.5% and 14.9% of income, divided equally between the employer and the employee. However, the risk-adjustment redistribution formula between funds has led to some convergence of premiums and a reduction in competitive pressures. Moreover, there is little competition in terms of the range of services offered or quality because the catalogue of benefits is uniform and largely set by law. Nonetheless, the introduction of choice between funds has led to considerable movement of members between the funds. Over the three years from 1997 to 1999, membership in regional funds fell by nearly 1.2 million whereas membership in company funds increased by approximately 1.8 million. The data also indicates considerable shifting from sickness funds with higher (percentage of income) contributions to those with lower contributions.

The Netherlands

The Netherlands has also moved towards greater competition between purchaser organizations in recent years. Reform proposals set out in the Dekker Report (1987) envisaged a programme of both demand-side and supply-side competition within a managed or regulatory framework. Under these proposals, consumers were to have choice between insurers – both health funds and private insurers – with variations in premium levels expected to be one of the main sources of competition between insurers. Health funds were to lose their regional monopolies and were expected to compete with other insurers for enrolees. Similarly, private insurers were to be faced with pro-competition regulation such as open enrolment.

In fact, the actual pace of change was very slow. By the mid-1990s there had been a move away from a market-oriented approach back to one placing more emphasis on regulation and planning. But some change did occur. Since 1992, health funds have been able to extend their operations from a regional basis so that most of them are now able to operate nationwide.

Moreover, competition has been increased as private health insurers and large employers have obtained permission to establish new health funds and health fund members have been given more choice between the insurers with whom they register. From 1995 to 1999 one sickness fund gained a considerable number of members (approximately 100 000) while four others gained more than 20 000 members. There is also more price competition between health funds. In 2000, the lowest flat rate premium was about 30% less than the highest premium. Further pro-competition reforms were discussed in 2001 and 2003. These included the introduction of a mandatory social health insurance scheme for the whole population (in place of the current social plus private insurance system), with premiums payable to the central health fund. Both health funds and private insurers (for profit and not-for-profit) would be free to compete for insured and would receive payment from the central fund for those insured who register with them. The introduction of a common system of insurance (planned for 2006) is seen as offering a level playing field for competition between insurers.

Russian Federation

Yet another example of the introduction of competition between purchasers is provided by the Russian Federation. For the most part, spatial barriers prevent competition. The Mandatory Health Insurance Funds are regional, territorially based organizations and therefore also have spatial monopoly power. Moreover, the laws governing these funds practically rule out price competition. In some regions, however, the mandatory fund delegates purchasing functions to private health insurance organizations. To the extent to which competition takes place, it is through these health insurance organizations seeking to gain a larger share of the mandatory fund market, through formal and informal agreements with employers and local governments. A World Bank survey indicated that 54% of health insurance organizations reported competition. However, this sector currently accounts for less than one-third of the mandatory funds budgets, so competition is limited to a minority share of the market.

Summary

European health purchaser organizations display considerable complexity and diversity. In this section we have sought to identify some of their salient features. In doing so, we have suggested that a typology based upon macro, meso and micro levels of purchasing has some merit. These are not watertight categories and many countries have a mix of more than one level of purchasing. Like all analytical categories, they are a simplification of reality. But we believe that they provide some basis for distinguishing key features of vertical organization.

We have shown that highly centralized, macro purchasing is mainly associated with some countries of Eastern Europe but that even here it is being replaced by more decentralized models. Meso-level purchasing is a widespread model among both social health insurance (the Czech Republic, France, Germany, the Netherlands) and regional-government-based (Italy, Spain) purchasers. Micro-level purchasing through local governments (the Nordic countries) and primary-care-based purchasers (England) takes place to a lesser extent, but is a model that has attracted considerable interest from health policy makers.

On the horizontal dimension, we have shown that, despite considerable discussion of market-based reforms, competition between purchaser organizations is relatively rare. Only in Germany and the Netherlands does it appear to be developing to any extent. Elsewhere the presence of spatial monopoly constitutes a major barrier to demand-side competition at both the meso and micro levels.

Having identified the nature of purchaser organizations found in different European countries, we now move on to analyse their activities in terms of the three principal–agent relationships with citizens, providers and government.

Purchasers as the public's agent

The first agency relationship developed in Chapter 1 concerns the purchaser organization as the public's agent. To be specific: to what extent does purchaser decision making reflect the wants, needs and demands of the population on whose behalf it purchases health care services? Chapter 6 considers this question and shows that there are different ways in which patients and the public can influence purchasing decisions.

Drawing on Hirschman's analysis (Hirschman, 1970) it is possible to characterize the different mechanisms of the purchaser–consumer principal–agent relationship in terms of *voice* and *exit*.

Voice is primarily a political, administrative or legal means of influencing purchaser behaviour. It can take various forms, including public consultation, advocacy group activity, formal representation and, increasingly, through the establishment of patients' rights. Consumer choice and exit are, on the other hand, the classic market mechanisms for influencing organizational behaviour. Consumers choose to register with purchasers that meet their requirements and shun those that fail to do so. The quest for customers provides the incentive for the purchaser to act in the patients' interests.

To what extent do these mechanisms operate within European health care systems? In the remainder of this section, we consider some of these mechanisms in terms of each of the categories of voice and exit.

Patients' and public voice

The high level of government involvement in European health care systems – through finance, regulation and provision – means that political, administrative and legal mechanisms play an important role in offering patients and the public ways of influencing purchasers.

Informing and consulting the public

The provision of information to the public and consulting them about their views is the most basic means of public involvement. This usually operates at the collective rather than the individual level. However, the provision of information on purchasing to the public is by no means commonplace. The dissemination of routine information on what services are available from what providers is often very limited. This lack of information is particularly marked in Eastern European countries such as the Czech Republic, Hungary, Georgia and Latvia, but it is not unique to them.

On the other hand, there have been some imaginative innovations in the area of public involvement. In the Netherlands and in a number of Nordic countries, ambitious exercises have been undertaken in order to determine health care priorities in the face of limited public sector budgets. These have served as a mechanism for both consulting the public about their views and informing them about the hard choices that have to be made in allocating scarce resources. Public health considerations, especially population health needs assessment, as discussed in Chapters 7 and 8, have played a large part in these initiatives. However, health needs assessment as a distinct activity has been far less successfully integrated into direct purchasing activity.

One limited, but nonetheless interesting, approach to public consultation, took place in the United Kingdom through the use of citizens' juries (Box 2.9).

Box 2.9 Citizens' juries in the United Kingdom

A number of citizens' juries were established on a trial basis during the 1990s to assist with rationing or priority-setting decisions. A typical jury consisted of 12 to 16 members of the public selected in their capacity as ordinary citizens as broadly representative of their communities and with no special axes to grind. The jury was brought together for four days and fully briefed on the background to the questions it was considering through written information and evidence supplied by expert witnesses. The jurors were asked to scrutinize the information and cross-examine witnesses. At the end of the process the jury delivered its judgement in the form of a report that was submitted to the purchasing organization for its consideration. The recommendations had no legal or mandatory force but acted as a transparent input to democratic decision making, albeit on a limited scale (Coote & Lenaghan, 1997).

Advocacy groups

In many European countries there has been a marked growth in consumer and patient advocacy groups in recent years. Moreover, the style of advocacy has become more vociferous and forceful. In France, for example, patients' associations have played an important part in the development of public debates. The AIDS epidemic played a major role in transforming the approach of these groups. They are no longer satisfied simply to offer support for patients and engage in fundraising activities; rather, they seek to influence policy in their respective areas. Similarly, consumer organizations have influenced collective purchasing decisions by active political lobbying in the Netherlands. For example, their participation in public debate around the work of the Dunning Committee on setting priorities resulted in some dental services being returned to the basic health insurance package. In Italy, user groups have played a growing role in monitoring the quality of care in both the public and private sectors.

The growth in advocacy is not ubiquitous. Many countries have little advocacy, whereas in others they have little impact on purchasers because decisions about, *inter alia*, benefits packages are made through the legal system (for example, Germany, Hungary, Israel).

Formal representation

Formal representation of insured and user groups on purchaser boards and committees is found quite widely throughout Europe.

In Germany, for example, most health funds have boards elected by their insured and by employers, and an assembly of delegates responsible for deciding on bylaws and other regulations governing payments and the services to be offered. The Austrian governance structure of health funds corresponds quite closely with that of Germany. In the Netherlands, the majority of health funds have established a 'council of insured' (*ledenraad*) and some representatives of the insured sit on health fund supervisory boards. Similarly, in the Czech Republic, the law specifies that the insured should be represented on the supervisory board of the health insurance fund. The same type of arrangement applies in Estonia where the insured are represented on the supervisory council of the health insurance fund, and in Lithuania where non-governmental organizations, trade unions and municipalities are represented on health insurance boards.

Formal representation of the public has taken a rather different route in non-social-insurance-based systems. For example, the introduction of primary care trusts as purchaser organizations in England has been accompanied by the declared aim of making them more locally accountable. To this end, each trust is governed by a board with a lay (non-executive) chair and up to five lay members, as well as executive members. The non-executive members are required to live in the area covered by the trust and are supposed to be selected as champions of the local people. They are, however, appointed by the NHS Appointments Commissioner and not elected. This contrasts with those countries where purchasing is a local government responsibility – notably the Nordic countries – where elected members sit on health boards.

Despite the ubiquity of formal representation, a number of concerns arise about the representativeness of the members who sit on these boards and the scope of their influence. For example, in some countries (e.g. Lithuania) many of the elected members are doctors. This poses the problem of provider capture. In England, lay members are appointed, not elected. This has given rise to comments about a democratic deficit. This criticism does not apply in the Nordic countries, but to what extent are generally elected politicians appropriate for health care organizations? Furthermore, in some countries (for example, Spain) doubts have been raised about whether representation actually influences purchasing decisions. These issues are taken up in Chapter 6, and reviewed in Chapter 3, when questions of the effectiveness of formal representation arrangements are addressed.

Patients' rights

Throughout Europe there is a growing interest in both individual patients' rights, such as patient autonomy, and social or collective rights, such as the right to health care. Many countries have developed patients' rights legislation, whereas others have developed so-called patients' charters or ethical codes.

In France, for example, a law on patients' rights was enacted in 2003. The law – the first part of which is titled 'Democracy in the health care system' – contains numerous provisions for strengthening user influence. These include patient access to medical records; compensation for iatrogenic diseases; strengthening of user associations and the establishment of commissions with patient representatives in all hospitals.

The legal system has already been a channel for expression of patient dissatisfaction in several countries. In social-insurance-based systems, such as those in Germany and the Netherlands, officially lodged complaints have focused on disputes over entitlements, failure to update service baskets and the denial of free choice of provider. Since budget restrictions play a growing role in determining what care will be funded, patients are increasingly resorting to the courts to assert their rights in terms of the services that are available, their quantity and quality. Court rulings in the Netherlands have also been made – both positively and negatively – in relation to the denial of services based on clinical guidelines.

Similar cases have occurred in Italy, where several Constitutional Court rulings have centred on the citizen's constitutional right to health. The Court has taken the position that patients cannot be refused necessary care for reasons of cost. Clinical decisions relating to the need for drugs and other services should take precedence. However, the Court has also ruled that the right to health care is limited.

In the United Kingdom there has also been a strong movement towards strengthening patients' rights. A Patients' Charter was produced by the government in 1991 setting out the rights of patients and the standards of service that they could expect from the NHS. Since then there has been a raft of initiatives designed to improve the service's responsiveness to patients. In the case of complaints, individuals who feel that their case has not been dealt with adequately within the NHS are able to refer it to an ombudsman, the Health Service Commissioner. The Commissioner is independent of the NHS and able to investigate any aspect of care provided by it and for which it can be held accountable.

The European Court of Justice has also become increasingly involved with the subject of patients' rights. Recent judgments have clarified those situations when patients may travel abroad for treatment and have this reimbursed by their home-country purchaser organization. In general, these judgments have strengthened patients' rights of access to health care, particularly in relation to cross-border care when domestic waiting times are unreasonable.

Consumer choice and exit

Consumer choice and exit are the classic mechanisms for influencing an organization's behaviour in a market system. Consumers choose to purchase goods and services from those firms that meet their demands and decline to purchase from those firms that fail to meet their demands. Exit of consumers and the resulting fall in demand for its products is seen as the fate of failing firms, leading to the ultimate sanction of bankruptcy.

To what extent does this mechanism operate in relation to purchaser organizations in Europe? What opportunities are there for consumers to choose the organization that purchases on their behalf and to change organizations (that is, exit) if they are dissatisfied? We have already touched on the answers to these questions in our earlier discussion when we considered competition among purchasers. Also these are considered in more detail in Chapter 5. Freedom of consumer choice is a prerequisite for competition. But that review of the evidence indicated that consumer freedom of choice is not widespread.

There is little or no choice in countries as diverse as Estonia, Lithuania, the Russian Federation, France, Spain, Italy and the United Kingdom. Thus with regional-based purchasing in Estonia and Lithuania no choice is offered. In Russian Federation there is very restricted consumer choice. According to formal health insurance legislation, individuals can choose their health insurer but the standard rules do not specify how this right should be implemented. In fact, most choice is exercised by employers who contract with specific insurers on the part of their employees and regional/local governments who contract on the part of the non-working population. In this way, choice is exercised on behalf of individuals rather than by individuals themselves.

In France, consumers have free choice of providers, but they are not generally able to choose a purchaser. Affiliation to a health fund is based on employment status and place of residence. In Spain, people are formally entitled to be treated in any region in the case of emergencies, travel and so forth, and so there is some individual discretion around collective decisions. However, the absence of a financial compensation system for cross-boundary flows means that providers are often reluctant to treat patients from outside their region. In Italy and England, freedom to change purchasers is usually restricted to a change of residence and registering with a new territorial purchaser. There is, however, some freedom to change GP within the same purchaser organization.

On the other hand, as we have indicated before, choice of purchaser does exist in some countries. Germany, the Netherlands and the Czech Republic all offer some degree of choice. Box 2.8 describes how in Germany, individuals have been able to choose freely between health funds since 1996. As we pointed out earlier, insurees are now able to choose among funds on the basis of price, although there is little choice in terms of the range of services offered or quality because the catalogue of benefits is uniform and largely set by law. Nonetheless, expression of choice has led to considerable movement of insured between funds. Box 2.8 also shows how the Netherlands has placed a high priority on the extension of consumer choice. A round of reform proposals, put forward by the Ministry of Health in July 2000, asserted the importance of consumer choice. They aim to put in place a customer-oriented environment in which competing insurers seek to attract policy holders.

Choice is also offered to consumers in the Czech Republic, but in recent years the domain of choice has become rather limited. At the moment, consumers are free to choose between alternative health insurance funds. They may also change funds on an annual basis. In the early 1990s, different funds were able to offer different packages of care, and choice could be made on this basis. However, the inability of some funds to meet the costs of the packages of care that they were offering led to the abolition of competitive packages of care in 1994. Now all funds offer identical packages of care at the same contribution rates.

Summary

Our review of the evidence suggests that mechanisms for public involvement in purchasing decisions using patient and public voices are diverse and widespread. Mechanisms for formal representation, increasing advocacy group activity and growing emphasis on patient rights are found throughout Europe but questions remain about their overall effectiveness. Consumer exit and voice, on the other hand, have received rather more emphasis in the rhetoric of market-based health reform than in reality. With the exception of a few countries (for example, Germany and the Netherlands), choice of purchaser and exit are not found much in practice.

Purchasers and provider organizations

Our second agency relationship deals with that between purchasers and the providers of health care services. Here we are interested in the ways in which purchasers can influence the services that providers supply, particularly in relation to their mix, quality and cost. Several chapters in Part Two deal with aspects of this important relationship. Chapter 9 examines the contracting systems that are used between purchasers and providers in order to make explicit the services that are supplied and the terms on which they are supplied. Chapter 10 focuses on the way in which contracts and other tools are used by purchasers to make sure that providers adhere to certain quality standards of care. Chapter 11 looks at the ways in which doctors and hospitals are paid and how different systems affect performance. Chapter 12 examines different forms of provider organization on the grounds that these can influence the ways in which providers respond to purchasers.

In this section we highlight some of the main features of contracting, payment systems and provider organizations as they are found in different countries.

Contracting

Contracts are the most visible and practical part of purchasing. They are a key tool through which purchasers influence providers. They can be used to make clear what services are to be provided and the terms on which they are to be supplied. They also have an important function in specifying the risk-sharing arrangements that apply in the face of unplanned events on either the purchaser or the provider side. In short, contracts are a means of steering transactions and sharing risk.

The contracting process involves active negotiation and agreement between purchasers and providers. In the sense that we are using the term, it rarely takes place in health systems with macro-level purchasers. The existence of meso- or micro-level purchasers seems to be a necessary, but not sufficient, condition for contracting to play a role. Only in these systems do purchasers possess the levels of autonomy necessary to enter into contractual relationships with providers. In more centralized systems, line management replaces contractual relations. Even in some more decentralized systems, strong central negotiation and control replaces, or severely limits, contractual autonomy.

Current European experience suggests that active contracting is a fairly new activity in many countries, having only really developed during the 1990s. Nonetheless it is becoming an increasingly important feature of purchaser–provider relations in both Western Europe (for example, Denmark, Spain and the United Kingdom) and Eastern Europe (for example, Czech Republic, Estonia, Georgia, Kyrgyzstan, Latvia, Romania and the Russian Federation).

Of course, contracting can take many forms. In Chapter 9 distinctions are drawn between market entry contracts (covering licensing and accreditation), input contracts (covering fees and salaries), performance contracts (covering quality and cost) and service contracts (covering the types of services to be delivered). Payment systems can also vary between block and cost-per-case payments (for example, diagnostic-related groups, DRGs). Yet another important feature concerns the ability of purchasers to contract selectively, that is, to choose those providers with whom they wish to place contracts and to reject others. In Box 2.10 we elaborate on some of the major features of particular contractual arrangements, whereas in Box 2.11 we report on difficulties in implementing contracting systems.

Box 2.10   Contractual arrangements in selected countries

United Kingdom

A contracting system whereby purchasers (health authorities and GP fundholders) specified the services that they wished to purchase from providers and the terms on which they would be provided, was introduced as part of the internal market reforms in 1991. When a new Labour government was elected in 1997, contracts were replaced by service and financial framework agreements. Despite the change of name, these are forms of contracts that also set out the expectations of purchasers in relation to providers, although they tend to involve longer-term agreements (aimed at reducing transaction costs). In 2004, a new payment system based upon a variant of DRGs with national standard prices was introduced, with the aim of placing more emphasis on quality.

Spain

Hospital contracting systems have been developing in Spain since the early 1990s. These have tended to be pioneered in the Catalonia region and subsequently applied in other regions. The shift towards a contracts-based system reflects a desire to move towards agreed performance measures that permit comparisons between hospitals. In 1991, crude aggregate measures of activity were first developed as a basis for paying hospitals, and over time these have been refined. By 1998, new information systems based upon minimum basic data sets covered 90% of Spanish hospitals. Catalonia introduced a DRG-based payment system in 1998. It also pioneered contracts containing activity and quality targets. The contracting systems found in Spain set out the volumes of activity expected from hospitals and the payments to be made for these activity levels. To date, however, contracting has not been used on a selective basis in order to identify preferred providers.

Czech Republic

There are national-level negotiations between the insurance funds and providers on the types and levels of reimbursement. However, subject to compatibility with national agreements, contracts are negotiated between individual funds and providers. Individual funds are responsible for monitoring contract performance and for taking decisions about payment in the light of contract variances. This is a fairly common occurrence. There is also large-scale experimentation with a DRG system.

Estonia

A similar form of meso-level contracting within a macro-level framework exists in Estonia. Thus the Health Insurance Fund (HIF) signs yearly contracts with providers. The general terms of the contracts are negotiated between national bodies, that is, the Estonian Hospital Union, the Estonian Society of Family Practitioners and the Estonian HIF. However, the details of the contracts are the subject of negotiations between HIF regional departments and individual providers. The contracts are legally binding documents and specify the obligations of both parties in terms of, *inter alia*, levels of payment, service volumes by specialty and maximum waiting times. Contract performance is monitored by HIF regional departments, and financial penalties are applied in the case of contract variances. The HIF has made very effective use of contracts in the recent rationalization of hospital services in Estonia.

Box 2.11 Examples of difficulties in implementing contractual arrangements

Italy

In Italy, the 1992 reforms that were designed to introduce an internal market were never fully realized because of incomplete separation between purchasers and providers. In particular, local health units (LHUs) continue to carry out both purchaser and provider functions. Although the requirements for contracting have been set out, and many teaching hospitals have taken the status of independent trusts, few purchasers have yet signed contracts with preferred providers. The reliance of many LHUs on directly managed hospitals continues to hamper progress. So far, contracting experience has been mainly restricted to a few regions such as the Emilia-Romagna where LHUs have a history of signing agreements with hospital trusts operating in the region.

Lithuania

Territorial health funds contract with provider organizations in Lithuania. Contracts are negotiated on an annual basis and tend to rely upon historical data. As well as specifying the normal requirements in terms of price and volumes, contracts are starting to be used to achieve health reform objectives – for example, reductions in hospital beds and number of bed days. However, progress is slow because of weak incentive structures. There is currently limited use of contracts for provider selection because the health insurance law requires health funds to contract with all licensed providers.

Germany

In Germany, experience with autonomous contracting is limited. Relations between health funds and providers are based upon a strong corporatist system of high-level collective bargaining. This weakens the emphasis placed upon individual health fund–provider contractual relations. Associations of health funds and of different providers negotiate a uniform framework for all health funds for the payment of physicians. The absence of comparable corporatist institutions in the hospital sector means that individual hospitals contract with individual health funds. However, terms and conditions regarding services and remuneration are the same for all health funds and so do not vary within individual contracts. The framework for the introduction of the new DRG payment system and its prices are negotiated at the federal level.

In 2003 it was proposed that health insurance funds should be given new freedoms to contract selectively with providers and depart from collective contracts. The proposal anticipated the introduction of selective contracting in specialist ambulatory care. However, due to resistance from the associations of statutory health insurance physicians, these proposals did not come into effect. Some progress towards selective contracting was introduced in 2004. Subsequently, it has become possible for health insurance funds to conclude specific contracts for groups of providers and their patients who agree to sign up to disease management programmes. However, early experiences have suggested that modifying collective contracts is a difficult process.

Hungary

An even stronger reliance on a centralized purchasing system in Hungary compared to Germany, means that an active contracting system does not really exist. Higher-level laws and regulations are the basis for determining provider behaviour. The National Health Insurance Fund Administration monitors and controls hospitals through monthly activity reports. But it is not allowed to engage in selective purchasing. To the extent that contracts are used, they are often a formal exercise for establishing the basis for provider reimbursement.

Paying providers

The way that purchaser organizations pay providers can be expected to have a profound effect on provider performance. Chapter 11 looks at this subject in more detail. In doing so, it draws distinctions between payment systems used to pay physicians in primary and secondary care and payment systems used to pay hospitals. It also highlights differences between systems found in Western and Eastern Europe.

Paying doctors in Western Europe

Three main methods have traditionally been used for paying doctors, namely salary, capitation and fee-for-service. In primary and outpatient care, most doctors working in the public sector are paid on a salaried or capitation basis, and often a combination of the two. However, in some countries – such as Austria, France, Germany and Switzerland – extensive use is made of fee-for-service payments. This method of payment is the norm for primary and outpatient care delivered privately.

Within the public hospital sector, salary payments to doctors are widespread although, once again, fee-for-service was traditionally used in some countries with a recent trend of shifts towards a case-based payment system according to diagnosis related groups (for example, Austria and Germany). In other countries, marginal fee-for-service payments are sometimes used in the public sector as additional incentives related to specific policy objectives, such as achieving reductions in surgical waiting lists. Such systems have recently been used in Denmark, Portugal and the United Kingdom. Fee-for-service constitutes the mainstream method of paying doctors delivering inpatient care in the private sector in all countries.

Hospital payment systems in Western Europe

Methods of paying hospitals in Western Europe have gradually moved from systems of retrospective reimbursement to global budgeting and, increasingly, to elements of case payments based on diagnostic-related groups. Combinations of global budgeting with DRG/case-mix adjusters are found in Austria, Belgium, and the Nordic countries, France, Germany, Italy, Ireland, Portugal and Spain.

The Nordic countries provide a good example of the move towards activity-based reimbursement in place of capped global budgets. Activity-based financing was introduced in Norwegian hospitals in 1997 with the aim of increasing hospital productivity. Within this system, a proportion of the block grant from central government payable to the county councils was replaced by a matching grant determined on a DRG basis. This activity-based component has increased year on year. In Finland, hospitals are increasingly billing municipalities on a DRG basis. Similar billing systems are found in Sweden.

Spain provides another example of the move towards activity-based reimbursement. Following the introduction of purchasing, some method was needed to specify and cost hospital activity. Over time, the DRG system has been adopted for this purpose. In the Catalonia region, hospital activity is funded by prospective global budgets adjusted by case mix. Approximately 30% of hospital budgets are currently DRG based under this system.

Elsewhere, a DRG case-mix adjustment has been applied to hospital global budgets in Portugal since the early 1990s. In Ireland, around 20% of hospital budgets are DRG based, and in England a variant of DRGs is currently being used to specify national reference prices that will be used to reimburse hospitals.

Payment systems in Eastern Europe

As Chapter 11 points out, until the breakup of the Eastern bloc, health care budgets were dominated by the hospital. Activity was supply driven, with the hospital at the centre. Primary care and outpatient providers suffered from poor training and low status. As a result of this hospital provider dominance, hospital referral rates and admissions were excessively high and lengths of stay excessively long. A related problem was that physicians and nurses were underpaid, often relying on informal payments, and this led to low morale and poor productivity. Reform of payment systems was designed to address these problems.

In primary care, new payment systems based on capitation have been developed in many countries. These include the Baltic states, Bulgaria, Croatia, the Czech Republic, Hungary, Poland, Romania, Slovakia and Slovenia. In total, capitation payments now account for just over a half of primary care payments in CEE and CIS countries. In addition, some particular services, for example immunizations and minor surgery, are paid on a fee-for-service basis in some countries (the Czech Republic, Estonia, Romania and Slovenia).

Traditionally, payment of inpatient services in many CEE and CIS countries was based on inputs such as beds or doctors. During the reforms of the 1990s with the adoption of new social health insurance systems many countries introduced systems based on fee-for-service. However, these have tended to drive up activity levels and put financial pressures on purchasing organizations. Attempts to move away from these perverse incentives have led to greater emphasis being placed upon global budgets. These are seen as the next 'generation' of payment system and are developing in a number of countries, including Bosnia and Herzegovina, Bulgaria, Croatia, Slovakia and Ukraine.

As Chapter 11 points out, however, the reform of payment systems in Eastern Europe is very much an unfinished agenda, with problems continuing to revolve around fragmented public sector pooling and purchasing, poor coordination of payment systems, weak institutional structures and the persistence of informal payments.

Provider organizations

Purchasers do not supply health services to patients themselves. They have to secure these services through providers. Earlier sections looked at the ways in which contracts are being used by purchasers to make explicit the services that should be provided and the terms on which they are provided, and at the way that payment mechanisms can be used to influence provider behaviour. The success of contracting depends on how well these tasks are performed. But contracts and payment systems are just two elements among the mix of factors that will determine the extent to which providers respond to purchasers' objectives. Another important factor will be the nature of the provider organizations themselves. Their form of ownership, their degree of autonomy and scope for decision making and the type of market structure within which they operate will all influence the way in which they act as the purchaser's agent.

Chapter 12 examines provider organizations. It presents a typology of hospitals developed by Preker & Harding (2003) which distinguishes four main types of provider organization: budgetary, autonomous, corporate and private.

- *Budgetary* refers to old-style organizations where the budget is set by government and any surpluses or deficits are returned to or covered by the government. Managers are usually linked to a civil service hierarchy within a command-and-control system.
- *Autonomous* organizations are those in which funding is based upon global budgets and there are often performance-related payments. Managers are responsible for day-to-day decision making but are accountable to government for their actions.
- *Corporate* organizations have had their ownership transferred from the state sector to publicly owned but independent organizations. They are similar to private sector organizations with boards of directors and hard budgets. Surpluses remain with the organizations. There is usually dual accountability – managers are accountable to the board and the board is accountable to government.
- *Private* organizations can be either for-profit or not-for-profit. They operate in ways similar to private sector organizations elsewhere in the economy although they tend to be regulated more heavily in the health care sector than elsewhere.

From a behavioural point of view, a crucial feature distinguishing these different forms of organization is the degree of autonomy over decision making that they possess, including decisions regarding finance, service content, staffing and other areas. In budgetary organizations, line management through command-and-control prevails. On the other hand, in both autonomous and corporate organizations, managers accountable to a board have more freedom of action. As such, the responsiveness to purchasers lies far more within the managerial sphere of control. The categories are not tight – for example, a provider organization can have financial autonomy but little service content autonomy, or can be free to alter price but not volume or allocative priorities, and not overall coverage and so forth.

A review of European hospital systems indicates that autonomous or corporate organizations (in practice it is often difficult to distinguish between these two categories) are the dominant or emerging mode of organization. However, there are still some elements of a budgetary system of organization in a number of countries. There are also several recent developments associated with a larger role for private or privatized organizations. Some examples of these trends are reviewed in Box 2.12.

Box 2.12 Provider organizational trends

Italy

The majority of public hospitals are still managed within the budgetary mode but an increasing number of autonomous/corporate organizations were created during the 1990s. The new form of organization has been developed in the case of public hospital trusts. These provide specialized tertiary hospital care and have been granted the status of quasi-independent public agencies. In 1995 there were 82 hospital trusts; by 2000 their number had grown to 98. The Lombardy region was particularly active promoting hospital trusts over this period – the numbers grew from 16 to 27. Conditions for obtaining trust status relate to clinical complexity and managerial capability. They include: a divisional organizational structure, at least three highly specialized clinical units, a complete accident and emergency unit with an intensive care unit, and a complex case mix of patients. The trusts have regional and sometimes national catchment areas, and have been given financial and technical autonomy since 1993. Furthermore, recent national legislation in Italy has provided trust general managers with additional autonomy through the freedom to develop and implement three-year strategic plans, subject to compatibility with regional plans. However, although patients have freedom to travel for treatment at hospitals of their choice, providers do not really see themselves as competing for contracts from purchasers (LHUs).

Spain

The Spanish hospital system is also characterized by a traditional budgetary system. Most public hospitals are owned by the region. Managers within these hospitals are appointed by regional governments and are directly accountable to regional authorities and so there is limited autonomy. This lack of autonomy is further compounded because in some instances managers are chosen on the basis of political allegiances rather than professional or technical criteria. But the situation is changing rapidly with the development of a professional cadre of managers. Moreover some regions have been experimenting with privatization. Since the early 1990s there have been a number of pilots involving private-sector-style organization and management of hospitals, particularly in Catalonia and Andalusia. The 1999 Budgetary Law opened up the hospital sector for more flexible organizational forms on a national basis termed public foundations, although there was strong opposition from trade unions and popular opinion. Still, in some regions many hospitals have adopted this self-governing form of organization.

United Kingdom

The NHS reforms introduced in the United Kingdom in 1991 also transformed budgetary institutions into autonomous/corporate organizations. These reforms created NHS trusts as independent, non-governmental organizations. Although still within the NHS – and ultimately accountable to the Secretary of State for Health – these organizations were overseen by a board of directors and enjoyed greater autonomy and freedom of action than their predecessor directly managed units. This applied particularly in relation to employment policies and capital spending. Although NHS trusts were expected to compete for service contracts from purchasers – and limited competition did take place – it soon became clear that regulation of the newly emerging market severely limited their freedoms. Recently, the government has announced a new policy emphasizing local provider autonomy. This is to be achieved through the proposed creation of NHS foundation trusts. This policy will allow NHS trusts that are performing to a high standard to apply for foundation trust status that will bring them additional freedoms from central regulation and control.

The Netherlands

The Netherlands has a long-established system of autonomous/corporate hospital providers. Most hospitals are private institutions owned and operated on a not-for-profit basis by locally controlled independent boards. In fact, private for-profit hospitals are prohibited by law, although not-for-profit hospitals are permitted to make and retain surpluses. Since the late 1990s, many hospitals have started to operate on an increasingly commercial basis within a competitive environment. There have also been a number of developments in relation to for-profit provision. For instance, there has been growth in for-profit private clinics as an independent service offering diagnosis and short-term treatments. The private, for-profit sector has also responded to employers' demands by offering a range of workforce-focused services such as physiotherapy, counselling and health promotion. This process has been described as one of creeping privatization.

Summary

Our review of the relationship between purchasers and providers reveals a number of common trends and a common direction of policy development across Europe. Contracting is a clear mechanism through which purchasers can influence providers. It is a fairly new activity, having started to develop only during the 1990s. Furthermore, its development is uneven, with substantial development in some countries (the Czech Republic, Denmark, Spain, United Kingdom) but far more limited application of contracting in others (Italy, Germany,

Lithuania). Methods of paying providers have traditionally embodied many perverse incentives in both Western and Eastern Europe. Reforms aimed at addressing these problems have emphasized capitation payments in primary care and global budgets with activity-based elements (often based on DRGs) in the secondary care sector. Finally, our review of provider organizations suggests that autonomous or corporate organizations are the dominant emerging form.

Purchasers and government

In its *World Health Report 2000*, WHO maintains that the ultimate responsibility for the performance of a country's health system must always lie with its government. Governments discharge this responsibility through the exercise of their stewardship role. This function involves collective rather than individual responsibility and sets out to promote the welfare of populations through, *inter alia*, protection of the public, securing improvements in population health, ensuring responsiveness to public expectations and pursuing equity objectives. In short, stewardship has been described as the process through which government steers or guides the health care system.

In this book, we are concerned with the way in which this stewardship role is carried out in relation to purchaser organizations. We view purchasers as the government's agent – an agent that is expected to fulfil the principal's (that is, the government's) objectives in terms of its purchasing activities. Chapter 8 examines how stewardship is exercised to achieve this aim. In doing so, it identifies three core tasks of stewardship as previously set out by WHO (WHO, 2000) and these are:

- formulating health policy, in particular defining vision and direction;
- regulating the health sector; and
- collecting and using information.

Formulating the overall direction of health policy is a fundamental component of the stewardship function as seen by most national governments. To this end, health care legislation, health plans, guidance and other policy directives proliferate. However, very few of these activities focus specifically on the role of government in relation to purchasing. One area where this might have been expected to happen is in relation to government's role in improving public or population health. However, a number of countries demonstrate severe policy limitations or failures in this area, owing, among other things, to undeveloped health needs assessment and its use in purchasing.

There are some countries where the stewardship function in relation to health policy formulation is barely discernible. In some social health insurance countries, for instance, the Ministry of Health sets strategic health policy goals that need to be taken into account by the insurance funds in their purchasing plans, but there is no direct accountability of the insurance funds to local or national government and these goals often fail to be implemented.

Regulation is a key component of stewardship. It is the process through which governments ensure that purchasing and providing organizations comply with stated policy objectives and operate within a defined framework of action.

As many European countries have moved from integrated systems to contract models of health finance in the late 1980s and early 1990s, so the regulation function has increased in importance. Chapter 8 identifies the multiple forms that purchaser regulation can take, including setting benefits packages, strategic planning, regulation of price and regulation of purchaser budgets.

Setting the package of benefits that purchasers must provide for their populations is an almost universal aspect of regulation. Typically, these will specify the range of services for which people are eligible, and often their quality and cost. National benefit packages are found in countries as diverse as Armenia, the Czech Republic, Germany, the Russian Federation, Spain and Switzerland. In some other countries, negative lists – specifying what is excluded from the national package – are used. These are found in, for example, Germany, Finland, Latvia and Italy.

Regulation of purchasers' budgets is another widespread feature of European health care systems. This may take place in a number of different ways. In those countries where revenue is raised nationally, allocations are usually made to purchasers on the basis of (possibly weighted) capitation formula. This occurs in, for example, Armenia, Belgium, the Czech Republic, Estonia, Spain and the United Kingdom. In some other countries, such as Germany, contributions are collected by individual funds, but the contribution rates are regulated centrally. In those countries where sizeable amounts of revenue are raised locally through taxation (for example, Finland, Norway and Sweden), budgets are allocated (and regulated) locally.

Regulation through strategic planning has a number of different components. Hospital planning is, of course, a long-standing feature of government health planning. In fact, this is a particular aspect of the more general regulation of capacity. This form of regulation is traditionally seen as necessary to avoid supplier-induced oversupply. As such, it is mainly focused on providers rather than purchasers. Typically, it requires them to receive authorization before investing in new capacity. Social health insurance countries such as France and the Netherlands have extensive experience of legislation designed to restrict both public and private sector expansion in cases where it is dependent on public funding. But this does not work primarily through purchasers. There is, however, one area where regulation is being increasingly used to inform and assist purchasers. This concerns health technology assessment and the health technology assessment agencies as found in, for example, France, Sweden, the Netherlands and the United Kingdom. These agencies seek to influence the take-up of new technologies by informing purchasers about their clinical and cost-effectiveness. In some cases, favourable judgments by the agencies are a necessary condition of public reimbursement.

Price regulation often operates through the specification of national tariffs. These apply to providers but are important for purchasers because they relieve them from the need for price negotiation. Recent developments in this area centre on the adoption of centrally determined prices based upon DRGs. This system was first introduced in the United States during the 1980s as part of a Medicare prospective payment system designed to control costs. Since then a number of countries have adopted this general approach, with the Australian system about to be adopted in Germany. Both Italy and Spain also have initiatives in this area, as does the United Kingdom, where a move is under way to impose nationally specified prices based on health related groups (that is, a variant of DRGs).

Regulation also includes the question of monitoring the performance of purchasers. Countries such as the United Kingdom are putting a great effort into the purchaser reporting processes and performance monitoring.

One final aspect of regulation – as it is being developed in devolved systems – concerns the tension between central control and local autonomy. The United Kingdom (or, more specifically, England) provides a vivid example of this tension. Purchasing responsibility in England is being devolved to micro-level, primary-care-based purchasers, but this has been accompanied by increased central regulation to ensure national standards. New regulatory bodies, such as the recently created Healthcare Commission, have been set up to monitor standards and take action when these fall below acceptable levels.

Reconciliation of the tension between central regulation and local freedom of action is currently being pursued in England through the notion of 'earned autonomy'. This involves those organizations that demonstrate their ability to work in an effective and efficient manner being rewarded with greater freedom from central control.

France provides another example of a country where a tension between devolution of responsibility and central regulation exists. In 1996, a major shift of responsibility from the national to the regional level occurred when regional hospital agencies were given both planning and financial allocation responsibilities for the hospital sector, both public and private. Regional strategic health plans now set out the goals for hospital care over five-year periods. However, the central Ministry of Health retains a strong regulatory role. This regulation covers safety standards, quality and priorities in terms of service areas. These regulations and priorities have to be taken into account by the regional agencies when formulating their strategic plans and constitute a strong influence on their activities.

Both England and France provide examples of strong central regulation. Elsewhere the regulatory role of central government is much less pronounced. In the Russian Federation, for example, the federal government sets the general regulations governing purchasers but its powers of enforcement are weak. The federal Ministry of Health seeks to manage the system through the issue of 'orders' to regional and local health bodies but they are usually viewed as recommendations and are not always followed. In practice, most regulation is carried out by regional governments. Indeed, their stewardship role in relation to territorial MHIs and health insurance organizations is quite strong. Sometimes this is exerted through informal pressures as well as formal procedures.

Finally, the collection and dissemination of statistical and survey health information is the third main task of stewardship as identified by WHO. The extent to which European governments actually carry out this role varies. One area where there is consensus about the desirability of such activity, but where progress is patchy, is in relation to evidence-based medicine. Countries such as the United Kingdom and the Netherlands have invested heavily in evidence-based medicine information systems. In both the Russian Federation and

Estonia, clinical guidelines and protocols have been developed. Set against this, progress in countries such as Germany has been slow.

Conclusions

Our review of purchasing organizations has identified considerable variation between countries in terms of both vertical and horizontal organization, and the ways in which principal–agent relationships operate in three key areas, namely population–purchaser, purchaser–provider and government–purchaser relationships. This is hardly surprising. In seeking to understand the evolution of health policy, the theory of path dependency has much to recommend it (Wilsford, 1994). This argues that policies will follow paths constrained by structures that are themselves the culmination of past decisions and events. Policy will proceed along a predetermined trajectory until some major event disturbs the equilibrium. As such, the variations we observe in purchasing arrangements between countries are a consequence of past economic, social, political and legal influences. This explains why, despite the injection of common policy ideas in the 1990s and thereafter (for example, devolution, purchaser–provider separation, market-based approaches, and so forth), after having been filtered through particular national systems, considerable diversity remains. Significantly, it is in the countries of Eastern Europe where, following the demise of communist systems, convergence towards Western European models of health care has occurred. But even here strong elements of path dependency are evident in the ways that these systems are applied. While this variation between countries can be troublesome from an analytical point of view, it does provide a natural experiment for assessing the performance of different forms of purchaser system. This is the task we turn to in the next chapter.

References

Coote, A. and Lenaghan, J. (1997) *Citizens' juries: theory into practice*. London, Institute for Public Policy Research.

Figueras, J., Robinson, R. and Jakubowski, E., eds. (forthcoming) *Purchasing to improve health systems performance: Case studies in European countries*. Copenhagen, European Observatory on Health Systems and Policies, World Health Organization.

Hirschman, A. (1970) *Exit, voice and loyalty*. Boston, Harvard University Press.

Preker, A. and Harding, A., eds. (2003) *Innovations in health service delivery. The corporatisation of public hospitals*. Washington, D.C., World Bank.

WHO (2000) *The world health report, 2000. Health systems: improving performance*. Geneva, WHO.

Wilsford, D. (1994) Path dependency, or why history makes it difficult but not impossible to reform health systems in a big way. *Journal of public policy*, **14**(3): 251–263.

chapter three

Purchasing to improve health systems performance: drawing the lessons

Josep Figueras, Ray Robinson and Elke Jakubowski

Introduction

A central aim of this volume is to provide evidence to help policy makers improve purchasing performance in their respective health systems. As noted earlier, this work is grounded on two fundamental premises. First, all health systems exercise some form of purchasing, which in its most basic form constitutes the allocation of funds to provider organizations. Second, this function has the potential to play a key role in determining the overall performance of the health system. Moreover, we start from the hypothesis that performance improvements will result from the introduction of more strategic forms of purchasing. This is when purchasing goes beyond simple reimbursement for products and services and it is aligned to societal health needs and wishes, and results in the most cost-effective provision of services.

The chapters in this volume show a trend towards strategic purchasing in many countries of the European Region and elsewhere. This is not to say, however, that countries converge towards a single purchasing model, but rather that the rationale and some of the principles for strategic purchasing are being incorporated into different health systems. Some elements of strategic purchasing – such as linking of health needs, plans and priorities to the allocation of resources or decentralizing provider management and introducing competition among providers – appeal, albeit for different reasons, to both national health service (NHS) systems in Northern and Southern Europe and social health insurance (SHI) systems in Western and Eastern Europe.

Indeed, there is not one single organizational model of purchasing that can, or should, be applied to all health systems. As illustrated in Chapter 2, purchasing arrangements are chiefly determined by the main form of funding and provision in each country. Generally those organizations responsible for the collection and pooling of funds will also play a key role in purchasing. In the same way, the public–private mix and/or the degree of decentralization will shape the organizational relationship between purchasers and providers. Even if one could incontrovertibly demonstrate the superior benefits of a particular form of purchasing, the room for reform would still be constrained by each specific health system context. In other words as we argued in Chapter 2, purchasing systems are very much path dependent – that is, today's choices are limited by what has gone before (Putnam *et al.*, 1993).

The approach in this volume, therefore, is far from prescriptive. It does not put forward a normative model of purchasing that will work across health systems, nor does it respond to the question of what is the best form of purchasing. Rather the aim is to identify the main components of the purchasing function within different health systems and to put forward strategies to improve them and thereby increase overall health system performance. To do so we have adopted a broad systems framework, based on a triple agency model, and have argued that purchasing goes well beyond the mere contracting of providers to which it is often equated. As noted in Chapter 1, this conceptual framework also includes the central role played by the citizens and the government as well as the provider organizational forms that will enable effective purchasing.

Indeed, a central lesson derived from the analysis in this volume is that if policy makers are to achieve the desired results they will need to take a broad systems approach to purchasing and act upon all the various components of this function. When purchasing is narrowly focused on individual elements such as contracts, payment systems or provider competition it will not reach its full potential. For instance, the introduction of a new case-mix-based payment system to improve efficiency will only succeed if providers can count on the managerial and organizational ability to respond to these new financial incentives, and if the health interventions financed through the new payment system are informed by the evidence on cost and effectiveness and respond to the health needs and priorities of a particular population.

A definition of strategic purchasing, therefore, should reflect this systemic approach. Strategic purchasing aims to increase health systems' performance through effective allocation of financial resources to providers, which involves three sets of explicit decisions: *which* interventions should be purchased in response to population needs and wishes, taking into account national health priorities and evidence on cost-effectiveness; *how* they should be purchased, including contractual mechanisms and payment systems; and *from whom*, in light of relative levels of quality and efficiency of providers.[1]

Grounded in this approach, this chapter appraises existing evidence on purchasing and draws lessons for policy makers to improve the performance in their own systems. Thus, this chapter moves from Chapter 2's description of purchasing to an analysis of performance and suggested recommendations for policy makers. It is intended as a summary of the main lessons resulting from this volume and thus draws heavily from the chapters in Part Two as well as on the case studies specially commissioned for this analysis (Figueras *et al.*, forthcoming). It also takes into consideration the outcomes of other relevant research, including that resulting from the Health Systems in Transition profiles and from a number of Observatory volumes that have dealt with purchasing-related issues (www.observatory.dk). Explicit references to other materials and particularly to other chapters in this volume have been included in chapter endnotes to signpost relevant material for a more detailed analysis and discussion than could not be provided in this chapter, given its broad scope.

The chapter begins with an outline of the main objectives of a health system, against which we should assess the impact of purchasing arrangements. Next, it summarizes the theoretical rationale for purchasing and the expected benefits. The subsequent sections combine a discussion of existing evidence with a series of lessons for policy makers around five central themes for improving purchasing and which form the basis for the structure of this chapter:

- empowering the citizen;
- strengthening government stewardship;
- ensuring cost-effective contracting;
- developing appropriate purchasing organizations;
- improving provider performance.

The chapter concludes with a section reflecting on the existing evidence and the way forward.

Assessing purchasing

In attempting to assess purchasing we need first to define the main objectives of the health system. There is an ongoing debate about what constitute these objectives and about how to formulate and measure them. A wide range of objectives are often put forward in various mixes in different policy documents, including health gain, cost containment, solidarity, health outcomes, allocative and technical efficiency, consumer satisfaction, equity, access, choice, quality, transparency, accountability, citizen participation and provider satisfaction. These objectives may all be important but they exist on different levels – from the philosophical to the technical and operational – overlap with each other and are often difficult to define and measure.

One key contribution of the WHO's *World Health Report 2000* in this field is its proposal of a definition of health system boundaries and a set of what are termed primary or intrinsic goals, namely improving health, enhancing responsiveness to the legitimate expectations of the population and assuring fairness of financial contribution (WHO, 2000). The report argues that all other objectives will ultimately affect these three main goals. The health system's achievements against these goals are labelled *attainment* whereas *performance* is defined as attainment in light of what systems should be able to accomplish with given resources. Here we suggest a slight adaptation of this approach and propose the following health system objectives: health, responsiveness, equity and efficiency.[2]

- *Health* improvement is the *raison d'être* of the health system and it constitutes its primary or defining objective.
- *Responsiveness*, meeting the legitimate expectations of the population – and the satisfaction drawn from a responsive health service – is an important objective in itself, which goes beyond the health improvement resulting from an intervention. Responsiveness includes a wide range of dimensions such as choice, waiting time and quality of amenities (Valentine *et al.*, 2003).
- *Equity* refers to the distribution of health and responsiveness among the population and includes financial contribution, access, utilization and treatment according to need. Conceptually, equity of financial contribution is not linked to purchasing; hence, in this volume we are more concerned with equity of access for equal need.
- *Efficiency* comprises both technical efficiency or 'value for money' (minimizing costs or maximizing outcomes from interventions); and allocative efficiency (allocating resources among different sectors, for example between acute care and preventive services and interventions so as to maximize overall health levels from existing resources).

The formulation of the above objectives raises a number of questions about the appropriateness of the *World Health Report 2000*'s definitions as well as about the reliability and validity of the measures and indicators employed. These issues – including the rich methodological and political debate that followed the report's publication (Murray & Evans, 2003) – are important, but they go beyond the scope of this chapter and will not be addressed here.

An equally significant methodological challenge, and particularly relevant for this volume, is how to assess the impact of a health system function, such as purchasing, against those objectives. It proves very difficult, if not impossible, to disentangle the effects of the various health system functions on, for instance, health status and responsiveness and to demonstrate causality. This problem of attribution is compounded by the fact that purchasing itself has many different components, such as contracting or stewardship. These have different effects on health system objectives and need to be addressed separately. Moreover, there is very little evaluation available of the impact of various purchasing strategies on health system objectives.

These methodological complexities and the lack of evidence will render any evaluation of purchasing very difficult. Nevertheless this chapter will consider the framework of objectives outlined above when discussing evidence and drawing lessons from the analysis of the various purchasing components. The approach taken here is that of policy analysis, that is, considering not only the impact of particular policies but also the content of these policies and the processes to formulate and implement them (Walt & Gilson, 1994; Walt, 1998). In some instances, we adopt what has been termed an 'indirect research' approach, which considers whether the right conditions exist for a particular policy to succeed (Robinson & Le Grand, 1994).

One final point to consider is that the choice of health system objectives and the relative priority assigned to them will vary in different societies in light of their historical, cultural and political values. The scope of this exercise is to appraise purchasing against the framework of these objectives without making any judgments of their relative value.

Purchasing in theory

In theory, the introduction of purchasing is set out to meet a wide range of strategic challenges in different health system contexts. First, purchasing aims to link health needs, plans and priorities with the allocation of financial resources to different sectors and interventions within the health system. Hence, this should lead to a maximization of overall health gain from available resources, that is, increasing allocative efficiency. Purchasing addresses one of the main problems traditionally encountered by health planners – that of bridging the gap between plans and the budgetary allocation of resources. For instance, in many NHS systems these functions were carried out by separate departments with national health plans having little influence over the historical and incremental budgetary processes. Purchasing theory thus underlies the potential of this function when closely linked to the planning process.

Second, the introduction of purchasing addresses the bureaucratic rigidity resulting from command-and-control models and enables many of the strategies put forward by the managerial school, including management decentralization with the establishment of self-governing hospital structures, adoption of performance-related payment systems, introduction of quality and outcomes culture, and generally increased entrepreneurship in the public sector. These should all result in increases in technical efficiency. Finally, the proponents of health care markets also support the introduction of purchasing as an organizational mechanism that enables the introduction of market competition between the purchasers and the providers. So, in theory, purchasing should lead to an improvement in technical efficiency in those countries where there is some competition between providers and whenever services are contestable.

The appeal of purchasing theory to such different schools of thought could be termed the 'paradox of purchasing' and helps to explain its wide political acceptance. A review of the new institutional economics may provide a deeper insight into purchasing theory and its conceptual building blocks,[3] helping to further understand the paradox of purchasing. This literature makes clear that different forms of purchaser organization and systems of governance can be expected to generate different flows of costs and benefits. The concept of transaction costs is central to understanding these flows. In particular, it shows how different organizational forms based on markets, networks and hierarchies all vary in the costs and benefits they generate, depending upon the particular circumstances in which they operate.

Markets tend to have separately owned and controlled organizations responsible for purchasing and providing services. Contracts are a central mechanism for coordinating activities but these can have expensive transaction costs. Hierarchies are a means of economizing on transactions costs – but the incentive structures for efficiency may be weaker. Networks share some of the features of both markets and hierarchies. Ownership is dispersed, as in markets, but control is often exerted by a single organization, as in hierarchies. However, whereas hierarchies are characterized by authority and markets by arm's-length relationships, networks are characterized by cooperation and trust. These issues are discussed in more detail in Chapter 4.

As to the question of whether the separation of purchasing and providing will bring net gains, at least in terms of economic efficiency, organization theory highlights a number of factors. Markets appear to perform well when there is potential for a high level of competition, when investments do not tie providers to specific purchasers, when complexity and uncertainty are relatively low and when few economies of scale apply.

However, the absence of these conditions in health care has led attention to shift towards network models. These may involve partnership models, which retain purchaser–provider separation but encourage long-term relationships and integrated decision making. The relational contracts that are used in this model rely on trust to economize on transaction costs.

Partnership models resonate closely with political ideas of the 'third way', which has been described as an explicit rejection of both the old centralized command-and-control systems and of divisive market systems. It seeks to find a middle way that combines a commitment to social values with some of the benefits believed to flow from an entrepreneurial approach.

Following these short reflections on the theories underlying purchasing – and suggesting that 'in theory it ought to work' – the obvious question arising from this debate is whether the actual practice of purchasing meets these theoretical expectations. The following sections look at the evidence on the practice of purchasing around the five central themes introduced earlier in the chapter and suggest how policy makers can improve this function in their respective health systems.

Empowering the citizen

A central element in purchasing theory is that the purchaser agent represents effectively the wishes and needs of its citizenry. This section addresses the various strategies to ensure that citizens exercise effective leverage over purchasers and their decisions.[4] Strategies for citizen empowerment in purchasing are grouped here under four categories aimed at:

- assessing the health needs of citizens at aggregated population level and integrating this information into purchasing decisions;
- ascertaining the views, values and preferences of the citizenry with regard to purchasing priorities and transmitting them to purchasers;
- making purchasers directly accountable to the population in general and to individual consumers in particular;
- enabling individual choice of purchaser and/or provider.

It should be noted at the outset that these strategies primarily aim to increase health systems' responsiveness but also – to the extent that they reflect population health needs – improve health, equity and allocative efficiency. However, as noted in the discussions below, this will not always be the case and tradeoffs between these objectives will be necessary. One other preliminary consideration here is that, in addition to these mechanisms that strengthen downward accountability to the population, patient empowerment is also achieved through upward accountability of purchasers and providers to the stewards of the health systems – democratically elected governments. The stewardship role of the government is addressed later in this chapter.

Assessing population health needs

If purchasers are to make decisions that result in the health improvement of their populations, first and foremost they have to have a clear epidemiological picture of the health needs of those populations. This will serve them in allocating scarce financial resources and purchasing appropriate interventions across the whole spectrum of preventive, curative and rehabilitative sectors. At the same time this exercise will inform the development of a health strategy (see section below on building a health strategy into purchasing). Ostensibly the extent to which purchasers integrate health needs assessment into purchasing will be crucial in improving three key health system objectives: health status, equity and allocative efficiency.[5] Health needs assessment can be carried out by the purchasers themselves or by other public health organizations and its results incorporated in purchasing decision making.[6]

The review of the case studies (Figueras *et al.*, forthcoming) and the analysis of the literature reveal a disappointing picture. Despite its widely recognized importance, health needs assessment is not routinely carried out in many health systems and when it exists it is not always incorporated into purchasing decisions. This occurs for a variety of reasons, including the general deficiency of the public health function in many countries, the non-geographical delimited coverage of many purchasers – for example, sickness funds in many SHI countries – and the scarcity of public health skills in purchasing organizations, particularly those with small population coverage. Above all it reflects the lack of structural or functional integration of the public health function within purchasing.

The latter is particularly relevant in many SHI countries in Western Europe where public health has little influence on the work of the sickness funds with only a few exceptions, for instance France or the Netherlands where this function has gained in importance.[7] A worrying trend is that many of the new SHI systems in CEE and CIS seem to reproduce this problem and, with some exceptions, population health needs are not taken into account in purchasing decisions. This function seems to work better in NHS systems in which coordination or integration between public health and purchasing is easier. There are some illustrative examples in Norway, Sweden and the United Kingdom and in some regions in Spain and Italy. However, this can by no means be generalized to all NHS systems because in some of these countries there is a virtual absence of health needs assessment.

In sum, policy makers have a number of strategies available to incorporate evidence on population health needs into purchasing decisions. First, they should strengthen the public health function, including the epidemiological skills and information systems required to carry out health needs assessment.

Second, this should be carried out at all levels (national, regional, local) of the health system to inform the various levels of purchasing. It should also acknowledge that health needs differ between geographical areas. Third, health needs assessment should go beyond measuring the burden of disease and include health risks assessment (WHO, 2002), which will foster the prioritization of preventive interventions. Finally, policy makers should either integrate health needs assessment within purchaser structures or, alternatively, put in place organizational mechanisms that ensure a functional coordination between public health institutes and purchasers. Despite the inherent difficulties in SHI systems that, for instance, compartmentalize preventive and curative activities, the introduction of some innovative structures allowing for formal coordination between the actors have met with very positive results in a number of countries, for example France (Sandier *et al.*, 2004).

Issues concerning the integration of public health into purchasing are also relevant within other components of purchasing and are revisited in a number of sections below that address the establishment of a health strategy, the development of evidence-based contracts and the building of quality into the contracting process.

Ascertaining the views and values of citizens

A number of policy lessons arise from the analysis of the methods of assessing the public's views and values. To begin with, policy makers need to increase the use of consultation mechanisms in order to have a better understanding of patient views on purchasing priorities. Often, purchaser decisions do not reflect society's values. There are, however, a number of innovative experiences in Norway, Sweden, the Netherlands and the United Kingdom that we can draw upon to bring citizens' views into priority setting (Mossialos & Maynard, 1999). These are, however, not exempt of complexity. For instance, citizens' participation in determining the package of care has proven to be very problematic. Citizens are averse to reducing services and their views often lack consistency. Moreover, we should take into account the fact that the reflection of social values on purchasing priorities will not necessarily result in increases in equity and allocative efficiency, and tradeoffs will become necessary. The results of citizen consultations and debate on priorities in Sweden were reflected in a series of guidelines (McKee & Figueras, 1996). One important feature of these guidelines is that the elderly should not be discriminated against in view of their limited capacity to benefit from health interventions and, therefore, the principle of equity should prevail over that of efficiency. In strict utilitarian terms this implies that many interventions addressed to the elderly will have limited impact on the overall society's health status, as for instance on the total number of disability adjusted life years (DALYs) resulting from these interventions. On the other hand, one could argue that these interventions increase the overall equity as well as (from a broad societal perspective) the utility of the health system.

Another lesson arising from the review of the evidence is that consumer and patient advocacy groups can be very effective in shaping the purchasing agenda.[8] There has been a marked growth in the role of these advocacy groups in many countries of the region but much more needs to be achieved, particularly in parts of Southern Europe, the CEE and particularly in the CIS. Policy makers should thus endeavour to put in place the appropriate conditions to facilitate the establishment of these groups. Regardless of its actual impact on health system objectives, the active participation of advocacy groups in purchasing decision making is in itself an essential part of the democratic functioning of any civil society. And the efforts of international NGOs such as the Open Society Institute in CIS countries to support the creation of advocacy groups have met with significant success.

One qualification is in order here: the participation of advocacy groups will not always result in optimally increased health gain and responsiveness. For instance, consumer groups may be manipulated by particular interest groups such as the industry. Similarly, if patient groups advocate for interventions that are not very cost effective it can result in a reduction of health gain and allocative efficiency for society as a whole. This may also result in a reduction in equity by decreasing access by other disease groups with higher health needs amenable to more cost-effective interventions but with less lobbying power.

Finally, strategies of informing purchasing with patient views become truly effective when purchasers are held accountable through a mix of regulatory, legal and financial measures. This is the focus of the subsection below.

Enforcing purchasers' accountability

This section briefly outlines four sets of strategies to enforce purchasers' accountability to their populations[9] and summarizes the main lessons for policy makers: formal representation, statutory establishment of packages of care, patients' rights legislation and complaint mechanisms.

Formal representation of consumers in purchasing organizations is commonplace in many European countries. Clearly, providing consumers with statutory powers over purchasers and involving them in the day-to-day decision-making results in more responsive health systems. However, there are also some concerns, such as who is the best representative of consumers on those purchasing boards. For instance, to what extent do union representatives, elected politicians,[10] medical professionals or health academics – which occur in a number of countries – represent the views of the society as a whole? One lesson arising from the analysis is that there is a need to increase bottom-up, local and direct consumer representation. Still, as noted above, sometimes grassroot consumer groups are dominated by particular interest groups. Notwithstanding these complexities, policy makers should endeavour to increase consumer representation on purchasing boards and in doing so they can benefit from the wealth and breadth of experience in many European countries.

Another major strategy for enforcing purchasers' accountability is the statutory establishment of explicit packages of care with formal coverage guarantees. This is very much the practice in most SHI systems in Western Europe (Gibis *et al.*, 2004) but less so in the more recently developed SHI systems in Eastern Europe and in many of the national health service systems in Northern and Southern Europe.[11] In the latter group the package of care is often formulated in very broad terms and mostly left implicit. Establishing statutory guarantees of benefits is a key strategy for empowering citizens by allowing them to challenge purchasing decisions in light of these guarantees. There is an increasing number of examples of citizen groups effectively applying to the judiciary and even to the constitutional courts.

A key means of enhancing the role of consumers in purchasers' decision making and ensuring accountability is to stipulate their rights and the responsibilities of purchasers. In recent years, there has been a flurry of patients' rights conventions and declarations at national and international levels. Most countries have developed patients' rights legislation, whereas others have developed patients' charters or ethical codes. These charters stipulate what is expected from the purchasers in terms of treatment and access to services, and although they are not legally enforceable, they may have an impact on public awareness of provider and purchaser performance. However, there is still a danger that they might be merely rhetorical and symbolic commitments without any real impact on policy. Much more needs to be done in arming these charters with legal and financial sanctions such as, for instance, when public commitments on waiting times are backed by financial penalties against purchasers. For instance, in a number of NHS countries, if patients do not receive treatment in public facilities within stipulated target times, they are allowed to opt for private providers under the public purchasers' reimbursement. This is not to say, however, that these initiatives will always result in improving all health system objectives. For instance, the political imperative to reduce waiting lists may drive the allocation of limited resources to areas of lesser priority from a social health gain or allocative efficiency perspective.

In sum, the recognition of patients' rights by law and other means, although important, is only a first step to empowering consumers in health care. These rights need to be implemented and safeguarded in daily practice. It requires involving all stakeholders, educating professionals and patients of their rights and duties, and implementing a host of sanctions to enforce them.[12]

It is important to highlight here the role of patients' rights legislation at the European level, particularly in view of its likely impact on the role of purchasers. European Court of Justice rulings, based on economic principles of internal market and freedom of movement rights, are increasingly widening the range of circumstances in which consumers can seek treatment outside their national boundaries under reimbursement from their national purchasers (Busse *et al.*, 2002; McKee *et al.*, 2002). These rulings do undoubtedly empower patients, but their positive impact on social objectives is much less clear. While increasing access for some citizens, these may also have a negative impact on cost containment, priority setting and solidarity on the national level, thus juxtaposing individual rights to free choice against collective priorities.

One last mechanism to enforce purchasers' accountability and responsiveness to consumers is the use of complaint mechanisms. The use of voice, notably through formal complaint procedures, can be very effective in influencing individual purchaser decisions. This is particularly so in many SHI systems where, due to the contractual relationship, complaints are raised before the civil or administrative courts, or in quasi-judicial bodies. Most NHS systems have also put in place complaint systems, but the absence of legally enforceable entitlements in many of them reduces the scope for consumers to assert health claims. One related strategy that has shown important benefits across countries is the introduction of an ombudsperson not only to address consumer complaints but also to assist the enforcement of patients' rights.

In conclusion, the tension between individual rights and collective priorities has been summarized by den Exter in Chapter 6:

> [O]n an individual level, the patients' rights developments have resulted in effective tools for influencing purchaser decision making particularly when legally codified. Those developments may incur increased costs, threatening social solidarity and financial stability, but they are a consequence of a democratic evolutionary process in many health systems and cannot be ignored.

Increasing citizen choice

The strategies for citizen empowerment outlined above correspond, in Hirschman's terminology (Hirschman, 1970), to 'voice' mechanisms. Increasingly, health systems rely on exit mechanisms, notably choice of purchaser and/or provider, as the ultimate strategy to empower individual citizens. The issues related to the choice of purchaser are addressed in a separate section below on 'choosing between multiple purchasers'.

Consumers in most countries have the right to choose primary care providers. In SHI systems, consumers can also choose ambulatory specialists and hospitals (albeit in some countries – such as the Netherlands – through a gatekeeper). Choices are more restricted in NHS systems but this is rapidly changing in many countries; Swedish and Norwegian patients, for example, are allowed to choose any hospital outside their county of residence. In the same way, patients have seen hospital choice increased in the English NHS.

While increased consumer choice of providers clearly increases responsiveness, there is debate over its impact on other social objectives, notably equity, cost containment and allocative efficiency. There is evidence that choice tends to benefit the higher (and usually better informed) social classes and thus may lead to increasing health inequalities. The policy response, however, should not necessarily be to reduce choice in line with the 'equity in poverty' argument but rather to focus efforts to ensure wider access to information and to support choice among the underprivileged.

There are also tradeoffs between increased choice and efficiency, exemplified by the inappropriate use of specialist services in some SHI systems without gatekeeping. The introduction of cost-sharing schemes may reduce moral hazard and lead to a more appropriate utilization of services but these schemes have also had a negative impact on equity of access (Kutzin, 1998; Robinson, 2002). The higher costs in SHI systems in Western Europe may be explained by the higher level of provider choice, which in turn leads to increased provider responsiveness and population satisfaction (Figueras et al., 2004a), thus, according to some commentators, compensating for the higher costs.

A related tradeoff between choice-related responsiveness and efficiency occurs when the individual citizens' choices clash with those of their purchaser agent.

The 1990s introduction of purchaser–provider split schemes in NHS countries such as the United Kingdom was trumpeted by the principle that 'money will follow the patient', implying both activity-related financing and a more active role of the citizens in choosing providers. However, a guiding principle of purchasing is that purchasers will choose on behalf of their citizens. This is a central dilemma in SHI systems, such as Germany or the Netherlands, aiming to allow health funds to contract selectively among providers in light of quality and efficiency criteria. As this will severely curtail the current free choice of provider, it is bound to meet with major opposition from consumers. Experience with American managed care organizations offers a vivid example of how individuals used to free choice react against attempts to purchase on their behalf. Moreover, selective contracting interferes not only with user choice but also with professionals' freedom to act as they see fit on behalf of their patients. Finally, there is also a wide debate about the benefits derived from choosing purchasers or insurers, thereby introducing market competition between them. These issues are further discussed in separate sections below on competition of purchasers and providers.

One final strategy to exercise choice over purchasing is to introduce a voucher system that enables consumers to choose among care arrangements and effectively become the purchasers. This is still limited, having been used particularly with the purchasing of home care, and has met with some success but needs to be further evaluated. However, these strategies may play in future a significant role in the purchase of certain services.

Strengthening government stewardship

There is broad consensus among analysts and policy makers about the central role of government stewardship in ensuring the effective running of the health system. While widely championed by the *World Health Report 2000*, the notion of stewardship is not new and builds upon prior trends such as that of strengthening public governance, the introduction of the 'third way' political philosophy and the subsequent reinforcement of the steering role of government. Notwithstanding the complexities of exactly defining stewardship, most analysts would agree on its main functions, namely: formulating strategic policy direction, generation of intelligence, exerting influence through regulation and ensuring accountability (Saltman & Ferroussier-Davis, 2000; Travis *et al.*, 2003).[13]

The central question for policy makers is no longer whether strengthening the stewardship of purchasing is necessary but how to put it in place. Many countries are falling short of realizing their full potential for good stewardship, especially of the purchasing function. This section highlights three sets of instrumental strategies to affect government stewardship over purchasing: translating health policy into purchasing decisions; putting in place an enabling regulatory framework and strengthening government's capacity and credibility.

A preliminary consideration concerns the governmental level at which purchasing stewardship should take place – the role of central government vis-à-vis regional or local level and the accountability mechanisms. On the whole, devolution to lower levels of government tends to increase responsiveness to local needs. It may, however, decrease equity of access – especially for some minority groups – and compromise efficiency due to lack of economies of scale and duplication of facilities. Ultimately, though, the locus of purchasing stewardship is dependent on the organizational form and degree of decentralization of the health system.[14]

Translating health policy into purchasing decisions

As noted earlier in this chapter, a central aim for introducing strategic purchasing is to translate health needs and policy objectives into the allocation of resources to health interventions by means of a series of contracts with providers. In doing so, a purchaser will require, in addition to an appraisal of its population's health needs and wishes, a formulation of a clear set of health policy objectives and priorities to guide its decisions. Formulation of health policy is thus a key function of government stewardship but one that is either absent or poorly carried out in many countries and, as a result, its influence over purchasing decisions has been minimal.[15]

Although most countries in the European Region have signed up to the WHO's 'Health for All' strategy, they have not always translated it into national health policy strategy let alone implemented it (Marinker, 2002; Wismar *et al.*, forthcoming). This has been particularly the case in some SHI systems in Western Europe and the CEE, where there has been an absence of government leadership in health policy (McKee *et al.*, 2004). But even when countries have formulated national health policies, these are sometimes expressed in broad inspirational terms rather than in concrete, practical managerial terms (Marinker, 2002).

This situation is progressively changing with the development and adoption of quantitative targets to back up national policies. Although countries have been more effective in the formulation than in the implementation of targets, there are some successful experiences of implementation such as in Sweden, the United Kingdom and France, on the national level, and Catalonia (Alvarez Dardet, 2002) and North-Rhine-Westphalia (Weihrauch, 2002) on the regional level.[16] However, as shown by the experience with the implementation of the 'Health of the Nation' and 'Our Healthier Nation' national policies in the United Kingdom, this is not a simple matter (Fulop *et al.*, 2000).

A number of policy lessons can be drawn from the analysis of the failures, as well as successes, in implementing health targets. First, to enable implementation, the targets themselves should be realistic and achievable but challenging – not the mere projection of trends – transparent, technically and politically plausible, evidence based, reflective of health needs and priorities, and selective. Second, it is important to build broad ownership and support among key stakeholders, particularly the professionals involved in implementation, who should be included in setting the targets. Third, targets need to be supported with evidence for effective implementation policies. Fourth, experience with the development of targets at various levels of the health system shows the limitations of 'top down' targets, which may have limited relevance at the local level and stifle creativity and innovation. Subnational development of targets in combination with national formulation will increase the likelihood of their implementation. Finally, building targets within performance management systems, including financial incentives and performance reviews, will also facilitate implementation.[17]

On the whole, despite their many problems, health targets have significant potential to translate health policy into purchasing decisions. Their introduction into contracts, combined with appropriate payment incentives, may be one of the most effective approaches to implementing health policy. These issues are further discussed below under the section on cost-effective contracting.

Establishing an integrated regulatory framework

Regulation takes centre stage in health systems' adoption of purchasing structures. These typically involve the substitution of hierarchical managerial relationships with contracts, management decentralization and a plurality of public and private providers, all of which require increased regulation. There is a wide array of regulatory mechanisms available to decision makers to ensure the effective functioning of purchasing. This section outlines three general lessons in setting a regulatory framework[18,19] for purchasing and identifies those regulatory strategies shown to be most effective.

The first lesson for policy makers is to achieve an appropriate balance between pro-entrepreneurial regulation and regulation that sets boundaries to individual entrepreneurial behaviour, to ensure the achievement of health system objectives. Health systems that move from command-and-control authority to management autonomy can face opposite scenarios. Sometimes the development of purchasing is stifled by a host of constraining regulations without having mechanisms in place to facilitate entrepreneurship (such as enabling independent purchasing organizations and self-governance of public providers or introducing performance-based payment systems). The opposite has also been true in countries where command-and-control mechanisms have quickly been dismantled without having in place an appropriate regulatory framework. This has caused opportunistic behaviour by both providers and purchasers to the detriment of social objectives. Thus, a second complementary policy lesson is that there should not be deregulation without simultaneous re-regulation.

Purchasing's intricate components require a multilevel effort to achieve all policy objectives. Perverse consequences result from narrow regulatory efforts focused on single purchasing components, such as payment systems or on economic concerns such as cost control. A third general lesson is, therefore, that one should be able to regulate in a complex way, setting out a broad framework of regulations that integrates and coordinates the various aspects of cost-effective purchasing and deals with multiple objectives. The main regulatory mechanisms that should be part of such a framework are grouped into four main categories, as follows.

First, there are regulations to ensure citizens' participation and purchasers' accountability by ensuring the provision of information by purchasers about access to health services, formal participation of citizen representatives on purchasing boards, patients' rights legislation stipulating what citizens can expect from purchasers and complaint mechanisms including the office of the ombudsperson.[20]

Second, there are regulatory mechanisms aimed at monitoring purchasers' performance. One set of regulations focuses on their insurance role, ensuring equitable and efficient behaviour, and includes mandatory insurance with open enrolment, community-rated premiums and transfer of funds between purchasers by applying redistribution formulae to compensate for differences in the risk structure (Rice & Smith, 2002).[21] Another set of regulations relates to their purchasing function and aims to ensure operation within a fixed budget – by fixing the level of premiums and calling for external budget approval or budget ceilings – a standardized package of benefits and the participation of government on purchasing boards.

The third type of regulation aims at the contractual relationship between the provider and the purchaser. This includes setting up a framework and rules for collective contracting, specifying the roles of the various partners, including purchasers, associations of providers, professional organizations and the government as well as details of the contracting process, including negotiation and litigation rules. Specific rules and procedures for contracting include requirements to have open information for both purchasers and providers, the right of purchasers to evaluate implementation of contractual provisions, quality standards, payment system requirements and price regulation (via national tariffs by unit of output such as a DRG or requiring specific costing and pricing procedures). The extent and type of regulation required will depend on the degree of provider competition and the public–private mix of providers. This introduces the need for a series of additional regulations to ensure the efficient working of the market and aimed at, for instance, avoiding monopsony or monopoly situations – facilitating consumer choice and ensuring access.

A fourth set of regulatory mechanisms, is mainly directed at the providers and includes measures affecting strategic planning, technology and procedures for licensing, certification and accreditation.[22]

In setting regulations, governments need to recognize the potential for tradeoffs between the various objectives. For example, regulating for purchasers to provide consumers with information should empower consumers but, as noted earlier, it may well compromise equity. There is also an opportunity cost of regulatory measures to empower consumers as this money might otherwise be spent on health services.

Policy makers should not underestimate the enormous demands put on government to regulate in a complex way and to put in place an integrated regulatory framework. The current debate sometimes assumes wrongly that governments can effortlessly strengthen the regulatory function of purchasing.

Strengthening government's capacity and credibility

Governments face a series of technical, economic, political and cultural barriers that impinge on their credibility and ability to carry out effective stewardship of purchasing.[23] First of all, the technical and administrative abilities required are lacking, particularly in some of the CEE and much of the CIS (Figueras *et al.*, 2004b). When regulatory departments exist they are often understaffed and have poor information about the behaviour of purchasers and providers. Moreover, there are substantial transaction costs involved in formulating health policy and particularly in setting a regulatory framework, collecting information and monitoring purchasers. Although these costs should be offset by the efficiency gains derived from a well functioning purchasing system, they still pose an economic obstacle for some governments.

A larger economic and political obstacle is posed by the gap between the public guarantees of health care delivery and the public funding available. For instance, the violation by governments of their own obligations to finance health care services weakens their control over the purchasers.[24] Political obstacles are further increased by the weakness of some governments to enforce statutes and by the divergence of policies among different government bodies.

Many countries also face cultural and organizational difficulties in realizing stewardship of purchasing, including the existence of closed social networks between government officials, purchasers and providers that may prevent the enforcement of legal agreements. Moreover, in some countries, the former dirigiste culture of officials used to command-and-control functions may prevent them from adapting to the stewardship function.

These problems call for policy makers to establish well-staffed regulatory departments with appropriate information systems as well as systems of accountability and transparency that help to build trust in the action of government as steward. Clearly, however, there are huge variations among the countries analysed in this study. At one end of the spectrum, many SHI countries in Western Europe have long experience and major regulatory capacity, while at the other end, some countries in the CIS, until recently under integrated command-and-control systems, have no tradition of regulation.

One final reflection on the feasibility of government stewardship is pertinent here. The current debate on the subject assumes the ability of governments to move from their direct provider role to their new stewardship role. This may not be the case in a number of countries in the European Region with inadequate governmental functions. Indeed, as shown in this volume, the ability of some governments to stand back and steer purchasing is uncertain at best. Moreover, arguably, if governments do not have the ability to provide services themselves it is unclear why they should be able to exercise stewardship. As a result, policy makers in less developed countries of the region should adopt a step-by-step process of change, which at the outset should limit purchasing to few selected areas and maintain direct provision in all others. This should put fewer demands on government stewardship and may increase the long-term success of purchasing.

Ensuring cost-effective contracting

The central role of a purchaser is to translate its population's health needs and desires into the provision of a series of health services, taking into consideration both national health policy priorities and evidence on the cost-effectiveness of alternative interventions. Contracts are the main vehicle for purchasers to do so, to the extent that contracting is often considered synonymous with purchasing. Decision makers aiming to put in place a cost-effective contracting mechanism will typically face a number of questions. How can one ensure that contracts take into account population health needs and priorities informed by the best evidence on the cost-effectiveness of interventions? What are the main types of contracts available and their relative advantages for different client groups and health system contexts? Which are the best payment mechanisms to reward performance? Or how can one build quality measures into contracts to ensure that contracts lead to improved health outcomes? These and other questions will be addressed in the following sections on the main dimensions of cost-effective contracting.

Linking contracting with planning

Good planning is the linchpin to a properly functioning contracting system, and many authors in this volume have shown the need to ensure that contracting is linked to planning. This involves assessing population health needs, formulating health policy and priorities, and specifying the models of care that should be provided in light of the resources available. These will form the core of the purchasing strategy.

The purchasing strategy constitutes the starting point of the contracting process. More emphasis should be paid to requiring purchasers to develop strategic (long-term) and operational (annual) purchasing plans. These will signal purchasers' intentions by setting out service requirements, budget constraints and performance targets to be achieved through the contracts. They will also enable providers to produce their own business plans.

The contracting cycle continues with purchasers identifying and selecting providers, followed by contract negotiation, reaching agreements, managing and monitoring them. Clearly, the way this process is conducted depends on the degree of competition (see competition subsection below). In this regard, emphasizing collaboration over competition by involving providers and purchasers in joint planning exercises has shown positive results.

One final lesson here is to ensure an appropriate balance between the government stewardship and the roles of purchasers and providers in negotiating the main parameters of contracts, such as the activity, payment methods and selection of providers. In some countries, government determines these parameters and as a result the contracting parties are left with a merely symbolic role, making contracting a bureaucratic process with little effect on system objectives, whose sole purpose is to rubber stamp government decisions.[25]

Ensuring evidence-based contracts

As noted, specifying health care models and interventions to be incorporated in a contract is an essential component of planning and contracting. It could be said that part of the rationale for introducing contracts is to implement evidence-based health care by incorporating best practice guidelines. However, in practice, this potential is far from realized and contracts in most countries often make little or no reference to evidence-based practice.

The first step in evidence-based contracting is to ensure that the actual evidence on interventions and methods of service delivery is available to purchasers. In recent years there has been a flurry of initiatives under the evidence-based medicine movement, such as the Cochrane network. At the same time governments have established mechanisms that can draw on evidence to decide which interventions are effective. Most Western European governments now have some form of health technology assessment (HTA) in the form of national agencies such as the National Institute of Clinical Excellence (NICE) in the United Kingdom or the SBU in Sweden, although this is less the case in the CEE and in the CIS, where HTA is less common (Borowitz et al., 2004). These initiatives have yielded many valuable insights, but they often focus on individual technologies and interventions rather than looking at the overall organizational framework of health care within which the interventions are delivered. Overall, there is still very little research that can provide the information needed by purchasers and, despite their availability and good quality, there are too few nationally funded organizational research programmes.[26]

The second step is to incorporate the evidence on interventions and methods of service delivery into workable contracts for specific disease and client groups. This involves the development of treatment guidelines taking into account existing practice, the potential for change and the resources required, as well as a broad view of health improvement including both prevention and treatment options. This is an area of major potential, but it is manifestly underdeveloped in most countries. One exception, cited by many authors in this volume, is that of the National Health Service Frameworks in the United Kingdom, which provide a comprehensive approach to building health strategy, priority interventions, treatment guidelines and performance targets into contracts.[27]

Finally, policy makers need to consider the role as well as the ability of purchasers vis-à-vis other agencies in generating evidence and guidelines for contracts – see the section below on implementing contracting.

Moving towards cost and volume contracts

The contract is the most practical and visible part of purchasing, defining the relationship between the purchasers and providers.[28] Decision makers are often faced with the question of what is the most appropriate type of contract. Primarily, the answer to this question is rather context specific and will depend on the health system characteristics as well as on the availability of information and management skills. Issues of capacity and feasibility will be paramount in deciding the most appropriate form of contract.

On the whole, however, there seems to be a common trend towards service-(cost-and-volume) and performance-based contracts. In Western Europe, SHI countries are increasingly adopting more complex forms of cost-and-volume contracts, particularly concerning the definition of the product and inclusion of performance indicators. In Northern and Southern Europe, at the start of the purchaser–provider split reforms, NHS systems adopted block contracts that have become progressively sophisticated with better definitions of volume and product. Many SHI countries in the CEE began with retrospective forms of cost-per-case contracts aimed at increasing activity, but, given upward cost pressures, they have also been increasingly moving towards cost-and-volume contracting.

'Hard' (fully binding) contracts with providers are uncommon, particularly in those NHS countries like the United Kingdom and Sweden that abandoned internal market strategies in the mid-1990s where there is a trend towards 'soft' service agreements relying more on cooperation and continuity of relations than on competition.

Cost-and-volume contracts seem to have the most potential in signalling the appropriate incentives to providers. These contracts allow for purchasers to decide the volume of care required, define the product and determine cost-effective forms of intervention. At present, however, most of these contracts are still relatively unsophisticated. At their finest they define volume in terms of DRGs but, more often, activity is specified in rather broad terms such as number of total (or at best by specialty) cases or bed days. Although still uncommon, there is clear progress in incorporating measures of performance in access, quality and efficiency.

Decision makers need to further work on defining the health product against which activity is set, linking to payment incentives and developing perform-ance measures, particularly of quality. These issues are further discussed in the following three sections on payment, quality and the scope of contracts.

Paying for performance

Clearly the system of payment with its inbuilt financial incentives is the main mechanism for contract implementation, to the extent that often there is little difference between the contract and the payment system. In other words, con-tracts do not often go further than laying out the form and amount of reimbursement. In the same way, the method of payment may hinder some more sophisticated forms of contracting.

An optimal payment system should induce providers to deliver high quality treatments, responsive to patients' needs and with a high degree of technical efficiency. While these objectives are all desirable, no single payment system seems to achieve all of them and tradeoffs become necessary.[29] Generally, there is broad consensus among experts about the impact of different payment sys-tems. Retrospective methods of reimbursing providers by fee-for-service and/or *per diems* increase service productivity as well as responsiveness but may have a negative impact on cost containment and efficiency. When providers are reimbursed for finished cases through some case-mix measure the incentive is to treat cases more efficiently but problems with allocative efficiency and cost con-tainment remain. Retrospective systems based mostly on bed days were employed by SHI systems in Western Europe until the 1980s, when they were phased out and global budgets with activity caps were adopted in most coun-tries. In the same way, newly reformed SHI systems in the CEE reimbursed providers through fee-for-service and cost-per-case, which due to their upward cost pressures are being quickly abandoned in favour of prospective global budgets.

This is not to say that the answer lies simply in introducing prospective global budgets. Both historical incremental budgets – widely employed in many NHS countries in Western Europe – and input-based budgets in the former Soviet Union countries were effective in containing costs, but did not offer any incentives for efficient or responsive provider behaviour. The challenge is, therefore, to build incentives for improved efficiency, quality and responsiveness while maintaining the prospective nature of payment in order to ensure financial sustainability.

This is an area where trends in European countries seem to be backed by the existing evidence. Many countries in Western Europe have adopted a form of global budget based on prospective levels of activity and adjusted for severity through some case-mix measure such as DRG or one of its variants. Most countries also have an additional payment component based on retrospective cost-per-case reimbursement, usually for particularly expensive treatments or for cases treated by providers without a contractual agreement with the purchasers. This takes place in Sweden and the United Kingdom when patients are treated outside the geographical area covered by purchasers. Cost-per-case reimbursement is also employed to increase productivity, for example, to reduce waiting lists for some conditions.

The CEE and CIS broadly follow the same common trend, although there are still many countries in which no payment reform has taken place and providers continue to be financed through input-based budgets. At the other end of the spectrum, in a number of CEE countries that have undergone recent reform, providers are being paid retrospectively by fee-for-service and/or cost-per-case resulting in obvious upward cost pressures.[30]

Within this broad convergence in payment models there is still much diversity in aspects such as the choice of case-mix measure to adjust for severity and in the use of financial incentives to reach target levels of efficiency and quality. There are also many methodological aspects still unresolved. An important main methodological debate revolves around the definition and measurement of the health care product, which has led to the development of a host of case-mix measures such as diagnostic-related groups (DRGs), patient management categories (PMCs) and disease staging. While DRGs, or one of their methodological variations, seem to be the most widely used in European countries (Germany has been the latest country to adopt them) there are still very large differences in the types, numbers and costs of the diagnosis/treatment categories employed. This may reflect individual country differences but also shows substantial methodological uncertainty and detracts from the validity of these instruments. A more complex methodological challenge is how to pay for the treatment of diseases that require various episodes of care at different levels. As noted below, some experiences using disease management categories seem to go in the right direction but much more work and innovation remain necessary.

Another area that requires further emphasis and methodological innovation is linking payment incentives to quality indicators set out in contracts – for instance, providers' adherence to standards of care or fulfilling a series of health outcome and responsiveness targets such as reduced levels of hospital co-morbidity and increased access to services. There are still too few initiatives designed to pay providers for outcome improvements. The new general practitioner's contract in the English NHS is one of them (see Box 10.4 in Chapter 10) although it is too soon to know what impact it will have. We turn to quality measures again within the section below on promoting quality through contracts.

Finally there is also some uncertainty about how best to pay for the use of capital and capital development. The best approach to the former is to include a capital depreciation component when paying for activity. The financing of new buildings and equipment is often done through separate budgets and linked to planning standards and certificates of need. However, there is a concurrent view that providers should be given a broader scope and be allowed to undertake capital developments by borrowing from the private sector (for example, the private finance initiative in the United Kingdom) and then recoup those costs through recurrent payment systems. The private finance initiative approach very much fits the notion of further provider decentralization but hitherto has met with varied results.

In sum, payment systems are a central element of contracting and play a key role in improving provider performance. There is broad convergence towards global budgets setting out activity levels adjusted by severity and including performance targets. As noted above, however, there are a number of unresolved methodological issues that will require further innovation and development. A note of caution about the limits of payment systems is also pertinent here. Incentives often act as a double-edged sword; they can be easily 'gamed' by providers who invariably have better information than purchasers (Rochaix, 1998). Excessive reliance on payment systems may also detract from investing efforts in other possibly effective strategies. Moreover, there are also important tradeoffs in terms of the transaction costs and management skills required to implement complex payment systems. Policy makers, therefore, in some instances may prefer to opt for more transparent and easy-to-implement systems rather than more sophisticated systems with greater potential but greater difficulty of implementation and monitoring. This is a particularly important consideration in those countries where implementation resources are scarce.

Promoting quality through contracts

Contracts are often put forward as an effective vehicle to increase the quality of health services – a central policy aim in most countries and also a very elusive one to reach. One key strategy in increasing quality, which has already been addressed above, is the inclusion of guidelines and protocols into contracts. This subsection draws on the analysis carried in this volume[31] to suggest a number of quality improvement strategies that can be implemented through contracts.

Quality strategies can be examined in relation to the stages in the contracting process, including *negotiating* – specifying appropriate quality requirements; *monitoring* – requiring and checking provider quality reports, or getting feedback from the public; and *reviewing* – agreeing changes to improve quality via the contract. Specifying quality requirements prior to and within the contract is central to achieving quality.

Prior to entering into the contract the purchaser can establish a series of quality requirements and preselect only those providers who fulfil them. At a minimum, the purchasers should only contract with facilities and personnel that are licensed (this is also defined as a market entry contract). In addition, purchasers might set higher standards and contract only with certified personnel and accredited providers.

Accreditation measures have mostly been developed in the United States and, although they have attracted interest in Europe, they have been implemented at a relatively small scale with limited impact. A number of countries have rejected accreditation models based on external inspection and instead require providers to demonstrate that they are engaged in internal quality assurance activities. In the CEE, requiring accreditation and certification of providers as a precondition for contracts has resulted in significant improvements in the quality of hospital infrastructure and care. On the whole, however, while accreditation can integrate some quality regulations it does not guarantee quality of outcomes. Many accreditation systems do not require a comprehensive quality system.

A more effective approach is to specify a series of quality requirements within the contract to be agreed in negotiation. These would include a range of process and outcome targets that may be enforced through regulations, sanctions and/ or payment incentives. Three main types of quality requirements are:

- Establishing *standards of care* such as mandating providers to use a particular set of clinical guidelines is particularly useful in those cases were evidence is sound and uncontroversial – for example, adherence to diabetes care guidelines. These have proved effective but there are also some pitfalls. Enforcement bodies depend on being seen as independent of both government and purchasers but they are required to reflect the priorities of both. Also, while explicit standards have the benefit of improving consistency, they may also stifle initiative, deflect efforts to meet measurable goals (rather than sometimes less visible but more important ones) and promote opportunistic behaviour.
- Comprehensive *quality assurance initiatives* may be put in the contract by purchasers. However, the evidence for this type of initiatives suggests that sometimes they can lead to increased costs without significant results.
- *Quality targets* (process and outcome) can also be put in the contract. Process targets may include levels of provision or waiting times for certain interventions. Outcome targets may use surrogate measures such as blood pressure levels or hard outcome targets such as mortality from certain conditions, e.g. myocardial infarction. While this is very much the way forward, there are a number of significant methodological issues that need to be considered, particularly when quality targets are linked to sanctions and/or financial incentives. For instance, it is extremely difficult to adjust for differences in severity of patients and attribute differences to quality of care. Potentially, these targets could unjustly penalize those providers who care for populations at higher risk and, sometimes, may lead to reduced access for these patients. There are also problems with data measurement; often the number of cases is so reduced that there may be some random effect. These measures may also

lead to unintended negative effects by providers focusing solely on those aspects of care being measured and rewarded and leaving others unattended.

In addition to specifying quality requirements in contracts, purchasers need to monitor results and review the contracts accordingly. Performance monitoring is thus central to achieving improved quality. There is a need for regionally or nationally coordinated schemes, particularly when there is competition between purchasers and providers and a provider is likely to contract with several purchasers at the same time.

Redefining the scope of contracts: chronic diseases and public health

Contracting mechanisms and accompanying payment systems are predominantly aimed at interventions that are both well defined (such as elective surgery) and directed at individuals rather than populations. This reveals two areas of major limitations in contracting, namely, the management of chronic diseases and the delivery of collective interventions.

The combination of ageing populations with increased chronic diseases and new technologies demands complex models of care, requiring coordinated interventions by professionals at different levels of the health care system. However, most contracting systems make it impossible to contract for packages of care that span different sectors and levels of care. Many contracting developments reflect an opposite trend, seeking to package health care into well defined products and homogeneous interventions that can be easily linked to payment systems and incentives. Contracting, therefore, should move in an opposite direction, focusing on disease management programmes – rather than on episodes of care – which span different levels of the health care system and allow integrated care pathways. Given the complexities of drafting these contracts, there are only a few examples in the European Region, such as the contracts for disease management in Germany, that have been in place since 2002 (Busse, 2004).

One of the key theoretical advantages of strategic purchasing is that it is oriented towards health needs rather than demands and it considers interventions across the whole preventive and curative spectrum. Yet most public health interventions are typically population based and are of a 'public good' nature. Both characteristics set them outside the typical scope of most contract arrangements. This is particularly so when purchasers do not have geographically well defined populations and compete with each other for clients, as in many SHI systems.

In an analysis of prevention and public health activities in SHI systems, McKee *et al.* (2004) conclude that simply requiring that sickness funds pay for collective interventions does not mean that it will be done. Moreover, public health services in these countries have been able to undertake immunization programmes where the interventions are relatively straightforward but they have been less able to develop interventions such as cancer screening that depend on strong links to mainstream health services. To achieve more effective public health interventions in these countries, new structures are needed, such as the French regional hospital agencies, which provide a mechanism for formal coordination among the concerned actors including the public health authorities, health insurance and the care providers (Sandier *et al.*, 2004). In NHS systems such as Finland, Norway, Sweden, Spain and the United Kingdom, purchasers have well defined geographical populations and there tends to be better coordination between public health and purchasing activities. Still, coordination needs also to be improved in these countries.

With or without provider competition?

Most countries that discussed or introduced new forms of purchaser–provider separation during the 1990s did so on the assumption that there would be supply-side competition. It was believed that providers competing for contracts from purchasers would face the necessary incentives to spur greater efficiency and responsiveness to purchasers' requirements. Competition was to be the market-based lever for improved performance. In practice, however, competition did not always materialize in the ways theorists and policy makers intended. In some ways this was totally predictable. For one thing, health care markets are characterized by strong elements of spatial monopoly (resulting from patients' inability or unwillingness to travel), making competition difficult to achieve. In addition, it became clear that the political consequences of market failure – resulting from supply-side competition – could be unacceptable. This was vividly illustrated by the experience of the major London teaching hospitals in the United Kingdom. The advent of the internal market in 1991 led to major falls in their incomes as a result of purchasers shifting contracts to less expensive providers. The political outcry associated with the possible bankruptcy of these major institutions led to political intervention to save them. Thus, market regulation tempered the impact of supply-side competition.

In the same way the more recent move towards selective contracting and competition in a number of SHI systems has faced a number of political and institutional constraints including poor regulatory capacity and opposition from both providers and consumers. Also for selective contracting to work it requires spare bed capacity which is uncommon in many Western European countries facing long waiting lists. By contrast, selective contracting has met with some success particularly in some CEE and CIS countries which had an overprovision of hospital beds and the political will to implement hospital rationalization.[32]

It has also become clear that supply-side competition is expensive in transaction costs, and ways of economizing on these have been sought. As a result, a number of countries have sought to encourage longer-term collaborative arrangements between purchasers and providers. This raises the question of whether contracting can operate effectively when purchasers do not have a choice of providers. There is no clear answer to this question. On the one hand, the contracting process in itself is a mechanism for purchasers and providers to be more explicit about mutual expectations than would otherwise be the case; but, on the other hand, if a purchaser cannot move to an alternative provider in the case of unsatisfactory service from an existing provider, the stimulus for provider efficiency is seriously compromised. One possible way out of this conundrum is to rely on proxy competition. Regulators may benchmark provider performance and require change in the case of persistent failure. The concept of contestability may also be drawn upon: that is, new entrants to a market (through franchising arrangements, for example) may pose a threat to existing providers even if actual competition does not exist.

Implementing contracting

The analysis of the various strategies for cost-effective contracting outlined above reveals a common set of political, financial, managerial and organizational obstacles that will hinder implementation. Here we will outline some of the main obstacles and draw a number of lessons for decision makers.

The first major obstacle is the considerable complexity of most mechanisms, including the designing of contracts, developing appropriate payment systems, specifying quality requirements and monitoring performance, all of which require a high level of managerial and technical skill together with wide-ranging information systems that are not available to some purchaser organizations in several Western European countries, let alone in less developed countries in Eastern Europe. Moreover, these mechanisms are very resource intensive, which may pose an economic barrier to their implementation. The establishment of a contracting system, therefore, needs to be preceded by an assessment of the capacity of purchasing organizations and, when required, by investing in appropriate training programmes and information systems. In taking these decisions, however, policy makers need to set the costs of investing in new systems and the operating administrative costs against the expected efficiency gains.

Issues of implementation capacity, together with the investment and transaction costs and occasional uncertainty about their impact, call for an incremental approach to contracting implementation. This would include the wide use of pilot schemes to test the impact and implementation difficulties of some of the more complex mechanisms such as a new payment system. Policy makers may also wish to begin by limiting contracting to one set of services and products and increase the scope as results become available and implementation capacity increases. This is also a useful approach when political consensus between key health service actors is lacking.

In some countries, the organizational design and roles of purchasers and providers may also pose major obstacles to implementation. These include fragmentation of purchasing, poor complementarity of design among strategies, inappropriate organizational definitions of purchaser and provider roles, and institutional (legal and administrative) impediments. There is sometimes a fragmentation of purchasing, with many distinct purchasers and funding pools but little coordination. This is particularly a problem in the CIS, where newly emerging SHI often co-exist with the old financing mechanism of direct allocation by different levels of government to providers. The integration of these pools into a single purchaser model is key to the future development of purchasing in these countries[33] and a number of them, such as Kyrgyzstan, have already done so.

There are also issues of complementarity of design between different strategies that provide incongruent incentives such as financial incentives that are inconsistent with the quality indicators specified in the contract. Sometimes these problems apply to specific strategies such as the adoption of payment mechanisms across settings that do not complement one another and, hence, undermine allocative efficiency.[34]

Inappropriate definition of purchasers' functions is also likely to hinder implementation. In particular, there is much uncertainty about the roles of purchasers in the implementation of strategies such as health needs assessment, health strategy development, accreditation of providers and development of specification guidelines for quality indicators in contracts. As shown in the case studies (Figueras *et al.*, forthcoming), there is a variety of purchasing organizational models and functions available, mostly determined by the health system context. The main lesson derived from the analysis is that it matters less whether purchasers take responsibility for these functions than that there are formal structures to coordinate the actions of the organizations involved (for example the public health services, HTA agencies or accreditation bodies) to ensure coherent action.

The issues of organizational coherence also apply to provider organizations involved in contracts. For instance, the low autonomy of hospital providers constitutes one of the main obstacles to contracting implementation. For contracting to work, providers must have management and financial flexibility to respond to the contract's demands and incentives (discussed in the section on providers below). Further organizational reform of purchasers and providers is often blocked by institutional – legal or administrative – impediments. Many new models of purchasing organizations (both for purchasers and providers) have no chance to take root unless they are preceded by a broader reform of the civil service and the public sector where they are to be based. There are also issues with political agendas and cultural resistance from the civil service, which may prevent change.

Following capacity and organizational design, political and cultural issues make up the third category of obstacles to implementation. For instance, ministries of health often have vested political interests in not delegating decision making to purchaser organizations, particularly in areas such as the selection and contracting of providers. Moreover, in many countries, large hospital providers bypass the purchasers and appeal directly to ministries of health for special contracting conditions – thus fundamentally undermining the role and leverage of purchasers and the foundations of contracting. Issues of political power and balance between providers, purchasers and government are dealt with in the section below on providers.

Developing appropriate purchasing organizations

The previous three sections of this chapter have dealt with three important features of the purchasing function, namely how to empower patients and the public, how to strengthen government stewardship, and how to promote cost-effective contracting. In this section we consider what type of purchasing organization is likely to be able to best carry out these functions.

Finding the right purchaser

In Chapter 2 we described the range of purchaser organizations found in different European countries. An important distinguishing feature is the nature of their vertical organization. We showed how this could involve macro, meso or micro levels of purchasing. Given this variety, the obvious question is, what level of purchasing is likely to be most effective? As in many other areas of this book, methodological difficulties in tracing causes and effects and the weakness of empirical evidence make it difficult to offer an unambiguous answer to this question. Moreover, the history of the health service organizations in a given country and their current institutional structure will act as powerful constraints on feasible purchasing models. This point is illustrated vividly by the case of the Czech Republic, where attempts to radically reform social health insurance systems failed because of an inadequate institutional structure and led subsequently to a degree of retrenchment. Radical reforms proposed for the Netherlands during the 1990s could not be implemented in the way their designers intended because of the need to obtain the support of a wide body of stakeholders within the prevailing corporatist tradition. These difficulties suggest that a 'one size fits all' recommendation is not possible.

Beyond this, however, it is possible to make some observations that policy makers should take into account, albeit with a clear eye to their own national situations. One observation is that devolution of decision making seems to be associated with a number of advantages. Macro-level purchasing rarely offers the managerial autonomy necessary to improve local decision making. The new public management seeks to give managers the opportunity to manage rather than to act as inflexible bureaucrats. This is far easier to achieve within lower-level organizations. Entrepreneurship and innovation can be expected to follow. Similarly, responsiveness to patients and the public is likely to be increased as purchasing decisions are taken closer to users. Contracting also becomes a more effective mechanism as negotiations take place between local decision makers. Nonetheless, it has to be recognized that some functions do require a strong national focus. Public health goals and the pursuit of equity targets fall into this category. Clearly the appropriate level of purchasing will also depend on other conditions such as the types of services – tertiary, secondary or primary care – to purchase, the incidence and prevalence of different conditions, the number of places where the necessary services can be provided efficiently and the appropriate size of the risk pool to handle risk.

In sum, there is not 'one right type of purchaser' that would meet the needs of all countries in the region. Rather the approach taken in this volume is that decision makers should appraise the purchaser model in their own countries in light of a series of strategies to improve purchasing performance, which have been outlined in this chapter. Ultimately, the decision on the right purchaser will depend on the extent to which it represents and empowers the citizens, is accountable to government and has capacity to implement cost-effective contracting.

Choosing among multiple purchasers?

One of the most powerful ideas to influence public policy during the 1980s and 1990s was the belief that markets and competition have the capacity to improve efficiency. This idea has, of course, been the basis for widespread economic and social change in practically all European countries. In this book we are interested in the relevance of these ideas for purchasing in health care – specifically, whether demand-side competition will improve purchaser performance.

Chapter 5 examines this question in depth, considering both the theory and empirical evidence relating to demand-side competition in health care. Much of the empirical evidence derives from the United States, where health insurer competition for patients has been an established part of the health system for many years. More recently, the growth of managed care organizations has transformed the United States market, but they still compete for insurees. The American experience shows that insurer competition can offer wide choice but that it has a number of disadvantages. It can lead to adverse risk selection and is very expensive to administer. In Europe, proposals for the extension of consumer choice of insurer/purchaser and for greater competition among purchaser organizations[35] have sought to avoid the excesses of the American system. In the Netherlands, for example, policies designed to increase competition between insurers and sickness funds have devoted considerable effort to the derivation of appropriate risk-adjustment formulae in order to avoid adverse risk selection. Similar risk-sharing transfers of funds have been introduced in Germany as pro-competition policies have been pursued.

Notwithstanding these developments in Germany, the Netherlands and also Switzerland, the most striking finding to emerge from our study is that – despite the considerable pro-competition rhetoric that has characterized health service debates in Europe in recent years – many purchasing organizations continue to operate in non-competitive environments. Sometimes this occurs because macro purchasers are, by definition, monopoly purchasers. In other cases, it is because purchasers are territorially based, making effective competition difficult. In yet other cases, the requirement for purchasers to make standard packages of care available reduces the dimensions over which competition can operate.

Does the absence of demand-side competition matter? To those who argue that choice and competition are powerful stimulants for improved provider responsiveness and increased efficiency, the absence of competition is a cause for concern. However, if there is no effective provider competition and selective contracting – as in many SHI countries with insurer competition, it is unlikely that competing purchasers will lead to improved efficiency. Instead of exercising cost-effective contracting the purchasers may seek competitive advantage by selecting risks which will undermine equity of access. In addition, if the institutional structure within a country is such that it does not lend itself to purchaser competition – or if the downside of competition (reduced equity and increased transaction costs, for example) is considered too great – alternative mechanisms may be used to achieve similar ends.

Our discussion of empowering the patient and the public offers a number of options for using voice rather than choice as a means of increasing responsiveness. Benchmark competition within a strong regulatory structure can also be used. The English reforms involving micro-level, primary-care-based purchasing organizations also have potential to increase purchaser responsiveness, as do systems of local government accountability in the Nordic countries. Looked at overall, there does not seem to be a strong case for relying on demand-side competition as a mechanism for improving purchaser performance.

Improving provider performance

Previous sections have addressed strategies focused on the purchasers and their relationships with consumers, government and providers. Ultimately, however, the impact of purchasing on health system performance will be determined by the way in which and the extent to which providers respond to purchasers and increase quality and produce more value for money.

From a provider's perspective, purchasing can be conceptualized as a change in its external environment, which may require adaptive strategies such as increased autonomy and different forms of accountability. Assessing provider responses to these new demands, however, poses some considerable methodological problems. The introduction of purchasing is not the only change occurring in the external environment of providers. This makes it difficult to disentangle its impact from that of many other contextual factors such as the overall economy, technology innovation, consumer preferences or the regulatory regime in place, which may also have a substantial effect on provider behaviour. Moreover, changing provider performance through purchasing is a time consuming process. Bearing in mind the timing of most purchasing reforms, it is too early to draw firm policy conclusions. Nonetheless, it is possible to draw some general lessons about the main factors and conditions that influence providers' response to purchasing.[36] Three main sets of lessons are addressed here: increasing provider autonomy, making providers more accountable and managing a new power balance.

Increasing provider autonomy

Institutional providers in European countries vary greatly in their degree of autonomy – see Table 12.1 in Chapter 12 with features of hospital provider organizations in selected countries. Limited autonomy and flexibility to respond to the new contracting incentives have been a major cause of purchasing failure in many countries. Hospital autonomy has been characterized along four categories: budgetary, autonomized, corporatized and privatized; according to five critical determinants of provider behaviour: decision rights, residual claims, market exposure, accountability and social functions (Harding & Preker, 2003).

To achieve greater hospital autonomy and hence more flexibility for providers to respond, policy makers may extend decision rights on key areas such as hiring and firing; determining the number of staff and its skill mix; financial management (for example the ability to take loans), determining the level and scope of activities, and decisions on capital development including the number of beds and the technology mix. Moreover, decision makers may increase market exposure by introducing some form of provider market competition combined with a regulation of residual claims in such a way that 'leftover' resources remain with the providers. These measures will foster autonomy and act as powerful incentives to increase efficiency. However, as noted earlier, the results from experience with provider markets are mixed.

In general, the evidence shows that greater provider autonomy, such as in corporatized hospitals, leads to an increased response to contracting. This is not to say that this necessarily results in improved provider efficiency. For instance, there may be tradeoffs in terms of increased transaction costs due to the necessary regulation and monitoring arrangements.

Making providers more accountable

The requirements of purchasing and increased autonomy place a strong emphasis upon the accountability of the provider. There are several mechanisms to ensure *managerial accountability* linked to the contracting process. As noted earlier, contracts can specify rules to report on delivered volumes of care and the quality standards. In the same way, purchasers can negotiate performance targets with the providers, monitor the extent to which these have been achieved and, if not, amend or terminate contractual agreements.

The provider must also communicate its performance with patients and the public at large – *public accountability*. Information such as numbers of patients treated, complication rates, waiting times, and information about procedures can be made accessible in different media such as consumer journals, Web sites, newspapers or, alternatively, published on the hospital premises. There is growing emphasis upon a systematic and independent measurement of provider performance. This is increasingly used in countries to benchmark performance across providers such as, for example, the use of *hospital league tables*. There are still substantial methodological problems which at present undermine the validity of these rankings. Yet, provider autonomy needs to be accompanied by increased transparency and, therefore, these efforts to measure and benchmark performance are likely to continue and to grow.

Managing a new power balance

The introduction of purchasing, and its subsequent increase in provider autonomy, results in a different balance of power and incentives between purchasers, providers and consumers. Policy makers need to be aware of the range of provider responses to these new balances.[37] These may be positive or negative depending on whether providers see the introduction of purchasing as an opportunity or a threat. They may respond in a structural or a tactical manner. An example of a structural response is merging with other providers to increase market power. Tactical responses refer to how a provider operates in a concrete contracting process with the purchaser. A third distinction is that between a purchaser- and a provider-driven response. In purchaser-driven response models providers will respond opportunistically, for example by increasing activities in order not to miss out on extra resources that have become available. Contracting out, the creation of integrated health care delivery networks and initiatives to reduce waiting times are examples of provider-driven responses whereby providers usually proactively deploy initiatives to influence the purchaser. The strength of provider-driven responses will depend on the provider's ambition, and a distinction can be made between pioneers, followers and conservatives.

A final distinction is made between political, judicial and managerial responses. The political response, in particular, has caused the failure of purchasing in many countries in the region. Providers often mobilize political resources to increase pressure upon the purchasing agency and bias the contracting process in their favour. There are well known examples across the region with plans of purchasers to close or downsize hospitals. These providers have been very effective in mobilizing communities against those decisions. In many instances, therefore, providers continue to hold the balance of power against weak purchasers and exercise what has been referred to as 'provider capture'.

Conclusion

This chapter has sought to summarize the evidence about the impact of a series of strategies to improve purchasing and to draw the main lessons for policy making. The first challenge encountered in doing so is how to define 'purchasing'. Purchasing, like many other 'modern' terms in health policy, does not have a clear-cut definition that commands broad consensus among experts, nor does it translate easily from English to other languages. Pragmatically, and to avoid an endless terminological debate, purchasing is understood as the allocation of financial resources to providers, differentiating passive forms of allocation from proactive or strategic allocation in light of health gain, responsiveness and efficiency goals. From this viewpoint, therefore, all health systems exercise some form of purchasing, the central issue being how to move towards strategic purchasing and what mechanisms are most effective.

We analyse purchasing from a broad health systems perspective that considers the role of the purchaser as well as its agency relationships with, and the roles of, the consumer, provider and government. By taking this wide-ranging approach to purchasing we may lose some of its specificity in practical managerial terms; on the other hand, the analysis in this volume clearly shows that the ability to understand and integrate the various components of purchasing is central to its effectiveness.

Another related challenge is how to measure the overall impact of purchasing on health systems performance. It is difficult to distinguish the effects of purchasing from those of other functions of the health system such as delivery, resource creation or stewardship. There are no performance indicators specific to purchasing. Some of these functions, such as stewardship, also have an effect on the performance of purchasing itself. Finally, even if one could measure the overall impact of purchasing, it would be difficult to disentangle the effects of its various components. Despite these methodological difficulties, the policy analysis approach taken here permits some useful lessons to be drawn.

Analysis shows, unsurprisingly, a diverse approach to purchasing in different countries (Figueras *et al.*, forthcoming) but with some common general trends. Authors in this volume agree that, despite prevalent rhetoric, strategic purchasing is not in place in many countries and, as a result, the impact has been limited. However, they also agree in highlighting its significant potential to improve systems performance.

At a theoretical level, purchasing very much fits with prevalent European views of governance and network models of organization that combine the benefits of increased entrepreneurship with commitment to social values. More importantly, the analysis of some country experiences, albeit sometimes partial or of limited scope, illustrate the positive impact of strategic purchasing.

There is a wide range of purchaser organizations, which operate at macro, meso and micro levels of purchasing. Clearly, the organizational form of purchasing is linked to the characteristics of a particular health system, including its form of funding and its degree of decentralization. Hence, there is not much room for manoeuvre in determining who the right purchaser is in a particular country context. Rather, reform efforts need to focus on strengthening purchasers' ability to respond to consumer needs and to contract providers more cost-effectively.

Assessing consumer health needs at aggregated population level and integrating this information into purchasing decisions are central to the effectiveness of purchasing. Still, many health systems do not perform any health needs assessment and policy makers should further strengthen this function. By contrast, there has been an increase in mechanisms and activity to assess public views and values to inform purchasers. However, these only become fully effective when they are enforced through a host of legal, regulatory and financial measures and purchasers are held accountable for their decisions. They include establishing statutory packages of care, formal representation of consumers in purchasing boards, setting complaint mechanisms and the implementation of patient rights legislation and patient charters when these are underscored with financial and legal sanctions.

'Voice' mechanisms alone may be insufficient to empower consumers, and health systems increasingly rely on 'exit' mechanisms by expanding the range of provider choice. Individual choice of provider, however, may clash with that of the purchaser agent. This is a key unresolved question concerning purchasing systems. In many countries there are also calls for increased consumer choice of purchaser, thereby introducing market competition between purchasers. Overall, it is unclear whether the likely increase in transaction costs and reduced equity are compensated for by the yet to be proven improvements in efficiency.

Contracts are the main vehicle for purchasers to translate population health needs and wishes into the provision of appropriate health services. There is now substantial evidence on how to increase the cost-effectiveness of contracting. Volume and outcome contracts combined with prospective activity-based payment systems employing case-mix measures have resulted in improvements in provider efficiency. Contracts have also a major potential to increase quality by specifying standards of care and quality (process and outcome) targets.

However, these still face substantial methodological difficulties and require sophisticated information systems not yet in place in many health systems. In addition to implementation complexities, activity-based contracts have inherent limitations with the provision of public health interventions whose population-based characteristics set them outside the typical scope of most contract arrangements.

To be cost-effective, contracting needs to be integrated within the planning process and to be informed by population health needs, health policy and priorities, evidence on interventions and models of delivery, and monitoring of providers. In spite of increased emphasis on evidence-based initiatives in many countries, contracts often make little or no reference to evidence-based practice. This can be improved by increasing the breadth and relevance of this evidence and by translating it into best practice guidelines that can be incorporated into workable contracts. There is also some uncertainty about the roles of purchasers on health needs assessment, health policy development, accreditation of providers or development of evidence and guidelines. This will vary between countries and will depend on the health system context. Nonetheless, the issue is less whether purchaser organizations take responsibility for those functions than whether there are structures in place to ensure effective coordination among the various organizations involved.

Ultimately, the impact of purchasing on health systems performance will be determined by the extent to which providers respond to contracts. There are a number of strategies to improve that response. Increased hospital autonomy in the form of corporatized providers with extended decision rights in key managerial areas has resulted in some positive outcomes. To work, however, it has to be accompanied by appropriate regulation and strengthened accountability mechanisms, which at the same time raises issues of technical capability and increased transaction costs. Increased market exposure by means of introducing provider competition is widely championed as a strategy to increase provider performance. In light of the negative consequences of possible market failure and the increased costs associated with provider competition, there is some consensus about encouraging more collaboration while maintaining the principle of contestability. There are also substantial difficulties with the implementation of selective contracting, as it is opposed by both providers and patients who see their choice restricted.

Without effective government stewardship, strategic purchasing is bound to fail. Government needs to provide clear leadership by formulating health policy and establishing a set of health targets that can guide purchasing decisions and serve to evaluate its overall impact. The high complexity of strategic purchasing also requires a comprehensive regulatory framework to be put into place that integrates and coordinates the various components of purchasing. This framework needs to achieve a fine balance between regulation that favours, and regulation that limits, entrepreneurial behaviour so as to ensure the attainment of health system objectives. This is more easily said than done. In many countries, strengthening government's political and technical capacity as well as its credibility should be at the forefront of the policy makers' agenda.

Overall, the political, technical and financial ability to implement strategic purchasing is the single most important factor in determining its success or otherwise. Most, if not all, strategies reviewed here are very complex and require a high level of technical and managerial skills together with wide ranging information systems that are lacking in many countries. Strategic purchasing leads to a different balance of power among key stakeholders and, hence, it may often pose major political obstacles to implementation. This calls for an incremental approach using pilot schemes to test the most complex strategies; limiting, at the outset, the scope of purchasing to some services; and building political consensus to ensure the long-term sustainability of purchasing.

Finally, we hope that this volume not only confirms the potential of strategic purchasing in improving health system performance but also throws new light upon its understanding and provides a clear indication of what strategies are effective in realizing its full potential. Undoubtedly there is still much uncertainty; however, what is known should suffice to encourage policy makers to strengthen strategic purchasing within their own health system contexts.

Notes

1 This definition builds on the one put forward by the WHO's *World Health Report 2000*, 'deciding which interventions should be purchased, how and from whom'.
2 This framework of objectives has been employed to compare NHS and Social Health Insurance systems in Western Europe in a sister volume of the Observatory series (Figueras *et al.*, 2004a).
3 See Chapter 4 for a detailed discussion of the application of new institutional economics to purchasing.
4 A number of chapters in this volume deal with this question from different but complementary perspectives. In particular, Chapter 2 provides a short overview of the main strategies for citizens to exercise voice and choice, which are analysed in more detail in Chapter 6 on the role of the citizen. In addition Chapter 7 provides a complementary perspective on population health needs and Chapter 8 shows the importance of government stewardship in ensuring citizen representation in purchasing.
5 Clearly the extent to which health needs assessment achieves these objectives will depend on whether there are cost-effective and appropriate interventions available. These issues are dealt with later on in the chapter.
6 McKee and Brand in Chapter 7 show the central role played by health needs assessment in the purchasing process; review common methodological approaches, i.e. comparative, corporate and epidemiological assessment; and suggest a combination of these methods as the best way forward.
7 These challenges are analysed in more detail by McKee, Delnoj and Brand in a paper on prevention and public health in social health insurance systems published in a sister volume in the Observatory series (McKee *et al.*, 2004).
8 See a more detailed discussion of the role of advocacy and consumer groups in Chapter 6.
9 These are analysed in more depth by den Exter in Chapter 6.
10 Note that the role of government, including elected politicians, in purchasing is channelled through its stewardship role.
11 See also Chapters 2, 6 and 8.
12 See a more detailed discussion on patient rights in Chapter 6.
13 See Chapter 8 for a more detailed review of these tasks.

14 A separate study by the Observatory is looking at the broader question of the appropriate balance between centralization and decentralization in health systems (Saltman *et al.*, 2005).

15 Both Chapter 7 on public health and Chapter 8 on stewardship analyse, from complementary viewpoints, the main obstacles (as well as the ways forward) to translate health policy objectives into purchasing decisions.

16 See Chapters 7 and 8 for a discussion of experience with the implementation of targets.

17 Much more remains to be learned about target implementation. A separate volume in the Observatory series is looking at the issues involved in target implementation (Wismar *et al.*, forthcoming).

18 Regulatory framework refers to the spectrum of rules, procedures, laws, decrees, codes of conduct, standards that exist to guide a health system.

19 These lessons are drawn from a separate Observatory publication on regulating entrepreneurship (Saltman *et al.*, 2002).

20 See Chapters 6 and 8 for a more detailed discussion of some of these regulations.

21 See Chapter 5 for a detailed discussion on the regulation of insurers.

22 See a more detailed discussion in Chapter 10 on purchasing for quality.

23 See Chapter 8 for a more detailed discussion on the main barriers to implementing stewardship.

24 See Chapter 8 for a discussion of the problems caused by the lack of funding in many CIS countries.

25 See a more detailed discussion in Chapter 9.

26 For a fuller discussion of the incorporation of evidence into contracts see Chapter 7.

27 See a more detailed discussion on the NHS frameworks in Chapter 7.

28 See Chapter 9 for an analysis of the different types of contracts and an overview of developments in the region.

29 Chapter 2 provides a brief comparative overview of payment systems in Europe, which are dealt with in more depth by Langenbrunner and colleagues in Chapter 11.

30 See also Chapter 11 for a detailed review of these developments. Another detailed review of payment systems in Eastern Europe is provided by Dixon *et al.* (2004) in a recent Observatory volume.

31 A number of chapters in this volume have looked at quality issues from different viewpoints. More specifically, Chapter 10 looks at the various strategies to enforce quality through contracts. Chapter 7 on public health also looks at quality in the context of monitoring the performance of contracts.

32 Chapter 9 provides a more detailed analysis of the issues relating to competition and selective contracting.

33 See also Chapters 9 and 11.

34 See also Chapter 11.

35 A sister volume in the Observatory series provides a detailed analysis of insurance competition arrangements in social health insurance countries in Western Europe (Saltman *et al.*, 2004).

36 See a detailed discussion of these factors in Chapter 12.

37 See a detailed discussion of the range of provider responses in Chapter 12.

References

Alvarez Dardet, C. (2002) Spain. *In*: Marinker, M., ed. *Health targets in Europe: polity, progress and promise*. London, BMJ Books.

Borowitz, M. *et al.* (2004) Improving the quality of health systems. *In*: Figueras, J., McKee,

M., Cain, J. and Lessof, S., eds. *Health systems in transition: learning from experience.* Copenhagen, WHO.

Busse, R. (2004) Disease management programs in Germany's statutory health insurance. *System health affairs,* **23**(3): 56–67.

Busse, R., Wismar, M. and Berman, P., eds. (2002) *The European Union and health services – the impact of the single European market on member states.* Amsterdam, IOS Press.

Dixon, A., Langennbrunner, J. and Mossialos, E. (2004) Facing the challenge of health care financing. *In*: Figueras, J., McKee, M., Cain, J. and Lessof, S., eds. *Health systems in transition: learning from experience.* Copenhagen, WHO.

Figueras, J. *et al.* (2004a) Patterns and performance in social health insurance systems, 4. *In*: Saltman, R.B., Busse, R. and Figueras, J., eds. *Social health insurance systems in Western Europe.* Maidenhead, Open University Press.

Figueras, J., McKee, M., Cain, J. and Lessof, S., eds. (2004b) *Health systems in transition: learning from experience.* Copenhagen, WHO.

Figueras, J., Robinson, R. and Jakubowski, E. (forthcoming) *Purchasing to improve health systems performance: country case studies.* Copenhagen, European Observatory on Health Systems and Policies, WHO.

Fulop, N. *et al.* (2000) Lessons for health strategies in Europe: the evaluation of a national health strategy in England. *European journal of public health,* **10**: 11–17.

Gibis, B. *et al.* (2004) Shifting criteria for benefit decisions in social health insurance systems, 8. *In*: Saltman, R.B., Busse, R. and Figueras, J., eds. *Social health insurance systems in Western Europe.* Maidenhead, Open University Press.

Harding, A. and Preker, A. eds. (2003) *Private participation in health services.* Washington, D.C., World Bank.

Hirschman, A. (1970) *Exit, voice and loyalty.* Boston, Harvard University Press.

Kutzin, J. (1998) The appropriate role for patient cost sharing, 3. *In*: Saltman, R.B., Figueras, J. and Sakellarides, C., eds. *Critical challenges for health care reform in Europe.* Buckingham, Open University Press.

Marinker, M. ed. (2002) *Health targets in Europe: polity, progress and promise.* London, BMJ Books.

McKee, M. and Figueras, J. (1996) *For debate. Setting priorities: can Britain learn from Sweden?* London, BJM Books.

McKee, M., Mossialos, E. and Baeten, R., eds. (2000) *The impact of EU law on health care systems.* Berne, Peter Lang.

McKee, M. *et al.* (2004) Prevention and public health in social health insurance systems, 12. *In*: Saltman, R.B., Busse, R. and Figueras, J., eds. *Social health insurance systems in Western Europe.* Maidenhead, Open University Press.

Mossialos, E. and Maynard, A. (1999) Setting health care priorities: to whom and on what basis? *Health policy,* **49**: 1.

Mossialos, E., Dixon, A., Figueras, J. and Kutzin, J., eds. (2002) *Funding health care: options for Europe.* Buckingham, Open University Press.

Murray, C.J.L. and Evans, D.B., eds. (2003) *Health systems performance assessment debates, methods and empiricism.* Geneva, WHO.

Putnam, R.D., Leonardi, R. and Nanetti, R. (1993) *Making democracy work: civic traditions in modern Italy.* Princeton, NJ, Princeton University Press.

Rice, N. and Smith, P. (2002) Strategic resource allocation and funding decisions, 11. *In*: Mossialos, E., Dixon, A., Figueras, J. and Kutzin, J., eds. *Funding health care: options for Europe.* Buckingham, Open University Press.

Robinson, R. and Le Grand, J., eds. (1994) *Evaluating the NHS reforms.* London, King's Fund Institute.

Robinson, R. (2002) *User charges for health care. In*: Mossialos, E., Dixon, A., Figueras, J. and

Kutzin, J., eds. *Funding health care: options for Europe*. European Observatory on Health Systems and Policies Series. Buckingham, Open University Press.

Rochaix, L. (1998) Performance-tied payment systems for physicians, 8. *In*: Saltman, R.B., Figueras, J. and Sakellarides, C., eds. *Critical challenges for health care reform in Europe*. Buckingham, Open University Press.

Saltman, R.B. and Ferroussier-Davis, O. (2000) The concept of stewardship in health policy. *WHO Bulletin*, **78**(6): 733–739.

Saltman, R.B., Busse, R. and Mossialos, E., eds. (2002) *Regulating entrepreneurial behaviour in European health care systems*. Buckingham, Open University Press.

Saltman, R.B., Busse, R. and Figueras, J., eds. (2004) *Social Health Insurance Systems in Western Europe*. Maidenhead, Open University Press.

Saltman, R.B., Bankauskaite, V. and Vrangbaek, K., eds. (2005) *Decentralization in health care*. Maidenhead, Open University Press.

Sandier, S. *et al.* (2004) *In*: Thompson, S. and Mossialos, E., eds. *Health care systems in transition: France*. Copenhagen, European Observatory on Health Systems and Policies.

Travis, P., Egger, D., Davies, P. and Mechbal, A. (2003) Towards better stewardship: concepts and critical issues 25. *In*: Murray, C.J.L. and Evans, D.B., eds. *Health Systems Performance Assessment Debates, Methods and Empiricism*. Geneva, WHO.

Valentine, N.B. *et al.* (2003) Health system responsiveness: concepts, domains and operationalization, 43. *In*: Murria, C.L.J. and Evans, D.B., eds. *Health systems performance assessment debates, methods and empiricism*. Geneva, WHO.

Walt, G. (1998) Implementing health care reform: a framework for discussion. *In*: Saltman R.B., Figueras, J. and Sakellarides, C., eds. *Critical challenges for health care reform in Europe*. Buckingham, Open University Press.

Walt, G. and Gilson, L. (1994) Reforming the health sector in developing countries: the central role of policy analysis. *Health Policy*, **9**(4): 353–370.

Weihrauch, B. (2002) North-Rhine-Westphalia, 8. *In*: Marinker, M., eds. *Health targets in Europe: polity, progress and promise*. London, BMJ Books.

WHO (2000) *World health report 2000. Health systems: improving performance*. Geneva, WHO.

WHO (2002) *World health report 2002. Reducing risks, promoting healthy life*. Geneva, WHO.

Wismar, M., McKee, M. and Busse, R. (forthcoming) *Implementing health targets in Europe*.

part **two**

four

Theories of purchasing

Julian Forder, Ray Robinson and Brian Hardy

Introduction

Recent reforms of European health care systems have led to numerous changes in organizational structures. The separation of responsibility for purchasing health care services from the responsibility for providing them, and the subsequent development of the purchaser function, constitute a vivid example of this trend. In this chapter we look at some of the theories that have informed and bolstered these changes. We show how economic ideas have played a central role in underpinning many reforms. In the world of practical policy making, however, the theory drawn upon has often been fairly superficial. Basic textbook models of demand, supply and the benefits of competition have frequently been the sole theoretical foundation for change. In contrast, the recent academic literature has been characterized by an outpouring of work that takes a considerably more in-depth and sophisticated view of the performance of alternative organizational structures. This literature is generally referred to as the new institutional economics (NIE) or economics of organization (EO).

New institutional economics is a wide and fast growing area of intellectual inquiry. It has the potential to make a major contribution to our understanding of why different organizational forms emerge and how they can be expected to perform. It also provides the basis for some prescriptive recommendations, that is, how activity should be organized in order to meet predetermined objectives. The purpose of this chapter is to draw on some of the main elements of this literature in order to provide some deeper insights into the purchasing function in health care.

The chapter is divided into three sections. The first section sets out some of the conceptual building blocks that have been developed within the economics of organization literature. The next section takes one important area of the theory – that relating to transactions – and considers the dimensions of this process in more detail. Finally, the third section offers some reflections on the relevance of these theoretical developments for the development of purchasing.

Economic organization – conceptual building blocks

Organization is the central concept in this chapter. At the outset, it is worth posing the question of why, in modern economies, not just in health care, we have economic organizations. Economic organizations are 'created entities within and through which people interact to reach individual and collective goals' (Milgrom & Roberts, 1992: 19). But why do they exist? A fundamental observation about the economic world is that people can produce more, and realize economic gains, if they *specialize* in activities to produce goods and services, transacting with one another to acquire inputs and also final products and services. Specialization leads to organizations. However, whereas these gains to specialization can be massive, they can only be realized if, first, people's actions and decisions are coordinated so that one person's contribution is compatible and consistent with another's, and second, people are motivated to make the appropriate contribution.

Coordination and motivation

Modern health care systems have a high degree of organizational specialization. The development of distinct purchaser organizations is one of these. This division of functions gives rise to problems of *coordination* and *motivation*. Effective coordination requires the organization to decide what tasks need to be undertaken, how they should be accomplished and who should do what. For example, what health care services should be provided; how should they be produced and delivered to users; and who should do the commissioning and providing? An effective system of motivation requires appropriate incentives to be put in place to ensure that individuals and organizations behave in an efficient manner. As other chapters in this book explain, incentives can take many forms. They can be built into contracts between purchasers and providers; they can be pursued through payment systems; and they can be operated through government carrying out its stewardship function. The design of an efficient set of incentives will lead to appropriate behaviours and effective coordination.

Transactions and contracts

Specialization leads to the need for transactions. These are the core of EO theory. Through transactions, individuals and organizations plan and implement activities, and agree the terms on which resources will be exchanged. Contracts are the mechanism through which agreements between individuals and organizations are coordinated. Contracts can be far broader than formal legal agreements in the corporate world. They can be informal, verbal, not enforceable or even verifiable by a third party. They do, however, specify each party's actions and rewards for a range of circumstances or contingencies. Contracting is a continual process, with new agreements being reached as new contingencies arise.

Bounded rationality

The economics of organization differs from neoclassical economics in recognizing that individuals are subject to *bounded rationality* (Simon, 1951, 1955, 1957, 1961). This means that individuals are limited in their scope to act fully rationally because of limitations relating to both information at their disposal and their computational skills. This makes the writing of *complete* contracts impossible – hypothetically such contracts perfectly solve the coordination and motivation problems.[1] Put another way, in the real world, contracts are *in*complete, being costly to create and implement, and imperfect in solving the coordination and motivation problems. These limitations mean that new contracts are being continually determined and old ones adapted.

The principal-agent framework

Another conceptual building block of organization economics is the classification of people or parties involved in transactions. Transactions can be characterized by an imbalance of information, so there is likely to be a dependency relationship between the parties involved. In particular, one party to the transaction often has either more information and/or better bargaining power than the other. On this basis the theory identifies two types of parties to a transaction. The *principal* is a party who wishes to secure provision of some good or service but does not have the necessary specialized knowledge, skills or assets. The principal employs an *agent* to undertake this task and in the process delegates some control to that party (Grossman & Hart, 1983).

The problem faced by the principal is to secure some service benefit from the agent while not knowing the true value of those benefits, or being forced to accept those benefits the agent wishes to supply. Either way the information imbalance can make it difficult for the principal to be sure that the agent is acting in the principal's true interests. Even when the course of action that the principal wishes the agent to undertake has been established to a satisfactory extent, a motivation problem remains. The principal needs to put in place an incentive structure that motivates the agent to act appropriately.

Principal–agent relationships abound in health care because of specialization and information imbalances. Indeed this book has chosen to analyse the purchaser function in terms of a triple principal–agent relationship. In the first relationship, purchasers are the agents for patients, securing health care services on their behalf. The second relationship has the health care provider in the agent role with the purchaser now as the principal. In this relationship, the purchaser carries out a procurement function. This task involves securing services from providers, which means negotiating with or directing providers as to the characteristics of services to be provided and the terms of the transaction. In the third agency relationship the purchaser acts as agent for the state when ensuring that purchasing decisions reflect national health priorities.

Governance structures

Governance structures have been defined as the matrix of rules, regulations, protocols and conventions that relate to the transaction (Williamson, 1979, 1994; North, 1990).

The idea of governance structure is relatively simple, but actually defining such a structure is much less so. The literature has attempted to draw out several relevant dimensions. These include: ownership, control and agency (brokerage and devolution) (Williamson, 1975, 1985; Jensen & Meckling, 1976; Grossman & Hart, 1983, 1986; Coleman, 1990); contract form and reimbursement incentives (MacNeil, 1985; Milgrom, 1990; Laffont & Tirole, 1993; Hart, 1995; Forder, 1997; Lyons & Mehta, 1997); regulation (Stigler, 1971; Vickers & Yarrow, 1988; Spulber, 1989); and social environment (Hannan & Freeman, 1984; Feenstra, 1995; Granovetter, 1995).

The first dimension concerns the degree of integration of purchasing and providing roles, and *ownership* of the associated infrastructure. In this connection, it is useful to distinguish between ownership and control (Coleman, 1994). What is the distribution of ownership of the apparatus and assets of the purchasing and providing function? Are both purchasing and providing apparatus owned by the same (set of) stakeholders – such as the state – or are they separately owned? Whatever the distribution of ownership, it does not necessarily dictate the distribution of control between stakeholders over various functions. An organization with unified ownership may, for example, internally separate purchasing and providing. Or the owner of one set of assets may voluntarily pass or cede control to the owner of another set. In fact, the locus of real control (that is, how much authority is really shifted away from that vested originally by ownership) is perhaps the key factor in explaining strategic performance.

Reimbursement incentives have a fundamental bearing on the operation of economic systems in general (Laffont & Tirole, 1993), and health care systems are no exception (Frank & Gaynor, 1991; Ma, 1994; Propper, 1995; Forder, 1997). Oliver Williamson distinguishes types of incentives as either high or low powered (Williamson, 1985). Incentives are high powered when individuals can keep all the profits resulting from their efforts. Low-powered incentives feature some dilution of the relationship between profits/surpluses and efforts. Salaries are examples of low-powered incentives. Individuals receive income that is only indirectly related to their efforts. As Williamson notes, the power of incentives depends on whether providers have control over their own actions and efforts and have the right to appropriate net income, either as a result of ownership or because this right was ceded contractually.

The problem of *regulation* is to configure the health care system so that individual actors making decisions in their own best interests actually operate in the wider social interest. This is a key aspect of the evolving stewardship role of government (see Chapter 8). Regulatory activities normally relate to three main areas, namely the regulation of capacity, prices and quality. In each of these areas, government (or one of its agencies) sets standards that individual organizations are required to meet.

The *social environment* within which it takes place can exert a strong influence on the behaviour of health system actors. For example, Granovetter and others describe how actions that arise in specific transactions are *embedded* in conventions that exist in an individual's social sphere (Hannan and Freeman, 1984; Granovetter, 1985; Hamilton & Feenstra, 1995). These conventions may work against narrow economic considerations. For example, parties to transactions in societies that value personal honour may be less likely to exploit their position – to cheat – than parties in societies with more 'pragmatic' values (Granovetter, 1985; Hodgson, 1988; Sako, 1992).

Even restricting our attention to the above dimensions creates a multitude of possible governance structures. However, in practice, choices along particular dimensions tend to be correlated and can be grouped to reduce the number of alternative governance structures to just three main types, as follows.

Markets have separately owned and controlled organizations (or individuals) responsible for purchasing and providing goods and services. Contracts are determined in voluntary (bilateral) exchanges and contract adaptations are negotiated and resolved by both parties. Payment incentives are often high powered because ownership usually confers the right to appropriate residuals (profits). It is, however, possible for lower or mixed reimbursement incentives to be used if parties cede some of the rights to income in the contract.

Hierarchies are characterized by a decision-making authority that is vested with one party to a contract (the hierarchical superior – for example, managers), with this authority being ceded to them by the other party (the subordinate – for example, employees) accept the instructions of managers. Hierarchical subordinates are usually paid on a salary or equivalent low-powered incentive basis. Hierarchies commonly feature unified ownership although that is not always the case. Employees can always leave if they wish.

Networks share some features of both markets and hierarchies. Ownership is dispersed – as in markets – but control is often voluntarily ceded by one party and predominantly held by the other party, as in hierarchies. However, whereas hierarchies are characterized by authority and markets by arm's-length relationships, networks are characterized by cooperation and trust.[2] Purchasers, for example, are willing to give providers freedom to operate a service because they trust providers to not exploit this situation. Grant payment is very common. This arrangement mixes incentives regarding individual transactions. Although providers receive a lump-sum award and can keep the residual, this is usually spread over many transactions so allowing cost cross-subsidization. Moreover, there are often circumstances that allow retrospective adjustments to the payment.

These three governance structures are summarized in Table 4.1.

Governance structures: new public management

One area in which the components of EO theory have come together is in relation to the new public management (NPM). This has developed as a categorization of the broad set of reforms of the public sector described by commentators across the OECD countries. Despite a number of important inter-country differences, some of the main features of NPM can be identified as follows (Pollitt, 2001):

- a shift in the focus of management effort from inputs and processes to outputs and outcomes;

Table 4.1 Governance purchasing options

Dimension	Hierarchical	Network	Market, bilateral
Ownership–control–agency			
Ownership	Integrated	Dispersed	Dispersed
Control	Unified	Separate, but relational	Separate/ decentralized
Brokerage	Purchasing agent	Agent	Individual
Devolution	Strategic (central)	Tactical	Tactical (local)
Contract type			
Incentive type	Low powered (salaried)	Mid powered (grant)	High powered (provider keeps profits)
Specification	Minimal, informal	Minimal, informal	Detailed, formal
Length (duration)	Short, frequent	Short, frequent	Long, infrequent
Timing	Retrospective	Retrospective	Prospective
Contingency (linkage between payment and cost)	High, costs and reimbursement linked	Intermediate	Low, fixed prices
Regulation			
Contract-specific	Low – informal arrangements	Low	High – monitoring for compliance with respect to specifications
Supply-side regulation	Low – self-regulation	Low	High – regular inspection
Social environment			
Alignment of motivations by social convention	High	High	Low

- a shift towards more measurement, leading to an emphasis on performance indicators and standards;
- a preference for more specialized, 'lean', 'flat' and autonomous organizational forms rather than large, multi-purpose, hierarchical bureaucracies;
- a widespread substitution of contract, or contract-like, relationships for hierarchical bureaucracies;
- use of market or market-like mechanisms for the delivery of public services, including privatization, contracting out, the development of internal markets, and so forth;
- a blurring of the line between the public and private sectors (growth of public–private partnerships and hybrid organizations) (Osborne & Gaebler, 1992);

- a shift away from universalism, equity, security and resilience towards efficiency and individualism;
- growing consumerism.

The rhetorical basis for NPM can be traced to neoliberal and New Right ideologies. For example, in the United Kingdom, Mrs Thatcher's radical economic individualism drove her determination in 1979 to 'roll back the state'. Similar aims can be detected in the Dekker proposals and subsequent developments in the Netherlands. Even more dramatically, moves towards market-based systems in the former communist countries of Central and Eastern Europe are based on an embodiment of these principles.

In this way, NPM represents a move away from a hierarchical to a market form of governance. This involves a separation of ownership and control, arm's-length contracting, performance measurement and compliance monitoring. EO theory provides some normative underpinnings for NPM, although EO theory is far more restrictive about the conditions in which marketization would work (indeed, NPM precedes current version of EO theory).

Dimensions of transactions

One of the key components of the new institutional economics or economics of organization is the subject of transactions. This is the process whereby actors within an economic system interact with each other. The choice of governance structure and its outcomes are crucially mediated by the features of transactions. In this section, we take a closer look at the features or dimensions of transactions. These cover: measurement, bargaining and monitoring costs; costs arising from rent seeking and shirking; contract completeness; frequency, duration and reputation in carrying out transactions; complexity and uncertainty; competition and contestability; the role of the social context.

Above we noted the importance of complexity, contestability and frequency/duration of transactions. Complexity covers information problems relating to both uncertainty about the characteristics relevant to the transaction, for example population health needs, and asymmetric distributions of information, for example doctors knowing more about health care than patients, or hospitals knowing more than insurance funds. Contestability likewise breaks down into barriers to entry/exit (that is, levels of competition) and asset specificity – for example, medical technology that has only one purpose, that is, cannot be adapted for other uses without significant cost. To this list we would add the social environmental context of the transaction. These are distinguished from elements of the governance structure in that they are either given – outside the control of stakeholders – or at least immutable in the short run.

Measurement, bargaining and monitoring costs

Transactions typically give rise to measurement, bargaining and monitoring costs. Measurement costs arise because, in order to determine appropriate courses of action, the parties to a transaction need information on relevant characteristics – for example, the service in question, its quality, people using it, cost and so forth. In some circumstances there is wasteful duplication of effort as *both* parties (principal and agent) need to gather intelligence to negotiate from an informed position (Milgrom & Roberts, 1990). With suitable safeguards it would be much less costly overall for only one party to collect this information, sharing it with the other party without misrepresentation.

Bargaining costs are incurred in negotiating the terms of the contract. When both parties to the transaction have a significant contribution in determining how the benefits of the transaction are distributed, this bargaining can be quite protracted and costly.

Monitoring costs are incurred both *ex ante* and *ex post*. They are incurred in determining relevant characteristics that are pre-existing and private to a trans-action, for example about other parties' preferences. Such *ex ante* information contrasts with information about characteristics relating to the process and out-come of the transaction, for example quality of service or efforts of providers. Contracts determined without *ex ante* information cannot generally induce parties to divulge such information voluntarily (Baron, 1989; Laffont & Tirole, 1993; Forder, 1997). Yet, this information is needed for the transaction to work smoothly and efficiently, making gathering at least some of it – thus incurring monitoring costs – worthwhile. It should also be noted that there is often an inverse relationship between *ex ante* and *ex post* costs, so that if, for example, a purchaser invests time and money in developing more complete contracts, the costs of monitoring are likely to be reduced.

A major advantage of hierarchies and networks over markets as a system of governance is the low level of measurement and bargaining costs they entail. Where control is ceded to a higher authority or network partner, duplication of measurement is avoided. In addition, because one party is given authority voluntarily, protracted bargaining is unlikely.

Rent seeking, poor incentives and coordination problems

Rent seeking occurs when stakeholders expend effort in an attempt to gain a greater share of the total surplus (profit) of a transaction and in doing so actually reduce the total surplus generated (Milgrom & Roberts, 1990). Such behaviour can take many forms. It may be characterized by providers exploiting low con-testability to restrict supply and push up prices (that is, monopoly markets). Another form involves principals renegotiating contracts with agents after those agents have made substantial investments. Principals thereby acquire some of the benefits of that investment without bearing a share of the costs. In response, in anticipation of this danger, agents may underinvest and so reduce total future income prospects for both parties. For example, a purchaser organ-ization may contract with a hospital to provide emergency medical services. Ideally, a dedicated, specifically built unit would be provided. However, in anticipation of the possible rent seeking by the purchaser, the hospital may build a less specialized unit that can be adapted for other purposes so as to limit the possibility of contract renegotiation.

Given the inherent complexity of health care, its provision is fraught with *risk*. If this risk is inappropriately distributed then principals and agents might alter their behaviour to protect themselves but in ways that usually involve a reduction in the overall benefits of the transaction.

Poor production incentives may result in coordination problems, specifically poor incentives to cut costs and also to be responsive to changes in demand – that is, slacking. For example, if agents are salaried, efforts to cut costs are not rewarded (at least not directly) and they may instead opt for less stressful, more leisurely activities. Likewise, altering supply in response to purchaser requests may generate few benefits for providers although they are likely to face additional costs. For example, a doctor as agent for the patient might not fully research all possible diagnosis and/or treatment options for the patient. Waste, or *x-inefficiency*, will result (Leibenstein, 1966, 1980).

Motivation failures: problems of shirking

Motivation failures arise because principals often have poor information about production processes and costs and may have a hard time assessing the contribution or effort of individual agents (Holmstrom, 1982). Agents might then *shirk*, that is, engage in behaviour disguised amid the usual fluctuations in output that result from external conditions. The problem is akin to the incentives coordination problem described above. The coordination problem hinged on the comprehensiveness of instructions to agents to improve productivity; the motivation problem rests with principals not being able to determine whether their instructions are being followed (or perhaps the inability of purchasers to specify their instructions in a way that is verifiable).

Shirking on quality is also a problem, with agents being able to undersupply service quality since principals have only imperfect quality indicators (or 'noisy signals' of quality). The quality of health care, particularly in terms of outcomes, is difficult to measure and therefore to write into contracts; purchasers may simply not know whether the services provided are of good quality, especially at the time of purchasing before the service is used. Similarly, the cost characteristics of services (affected by the types of user needs) are much more precisely known by providers. Where reimbursement is affected by cost characteristics, providers will have incentives to overplay these costs – so-called 'up coding' (Forder, 1997).

A related form of motivational failure is cream skimming, whereby providers try to avoid treating potentially high-cost patients and thereby reduce costs relative to a fixed income based on an average across all cost types (Matsaganis & Glennerster, 1994).

Contract completeness

In theory, all of these motivation and coordination problems could be overcome by using appropriately crafted contracts – that is, complete contracts – accompanied by monitoring for *ex ante* information (Milgrom & Roberts, 1990). For example, rent seeking could be addressed by having parties to the transaction share the initial investment cost. Shirking could be stopped by having the contract pay according to providers' efforts. Similarly, poor incentives could be overcome by having a contract that rewards specific behaviours and penalizes inappropriate ones. These contract clauses would just need to be determined. However, contracts are not complete because extending the circumstances covered by the contract is a costly business: contracting incurs transaction costs as described above. At some point, the benefits of overcoming motivation and coordination problems do not justify the extra transaction costs that would be incurred.

Frequency, duration and reputation

Frequency and duration are key features of transactions. Parties engaged in frequent interactions (of relatively short individual duration) – but part of a long, close relationship – have greater opportunities to grant or deny favours to each other. This ability has significant implications for the motivation problem outlined above, and usually means lower costs of transacting. It will also affect opportunities for reputation that have a bearing on behaviour. Reputation is a very powerful mechanism for economizing on transaction cost: in repeated transactions stakeholders have every incentive to maintain a good reputation because the outcome of future transactions depends on it (Kreps & Wilson, 1982; Milgrom & Roberts, 1982; Roth & Schoumaker, 1983; Fundenberg & Tirole, 1992).

This mechanism is central to the operation of hierarchies where subordinates (for example, employees) are willing to cede control (and thereby risk exploitation) because the employer has a reputation to protect (Kreps, 1990, 1996). Reputation is needed to ensure that employees can expect a reasonable share of the surplus generated by the relationship.[3] A similar argument applies to networks; minimum specification, adaptive ('relational') contracts are sufficient since concerns about reputation commit the stakeholders to act reasonably with reference to non-contracted contingencies.

Complexity and uncertainty

Transaction costs tend to increase as the complexity of a transaction increases and fall as a contract becomes more complete. Where complexity is high, there is a danger of a detrimental effect because of contract incompleteness. The form of this effect depends largely on the type of governance structure being used. In markets, where parties own assets, they are residual claimants and shirking will take the form of reducing production costs, for example by quality shirking, cream skimming and so forth. Where parties are not residual claimants, for example in hierarchies, and they face low-powered incentives – such as salary reimbursement – then shirking usually takes the form of slacking.

The negative effects on outcomes of these different behaviours are hard to judge *a priori*. Transaction costs might be lower in hierarchies, so it is less costly to adapt contracts for a resolution. For example, following a change in demand patterns or production technology, managers in hierarchies can simply change instructions to employees in the provider division. Or, the doctor – as hierarchical superior to the patient (see below) – can prescribe a different course of treatment for the patient. In markets, the new round of contract renegotiation will involve duplicated measurement, bargaining between parties and so forth.

Nonetheless, it is still the case that contract incompleteness will be problematic in hierarchies, especially because managers are the people determining the contract (with control ceded by subordinates) and they are the ones facing the relatively high contracting costs if transactions are complex. Hierarchical superiors (for example, managers) will adopt relatively simple contract forms, which commonly take the form of salary reimbursement (which may lead to slacking, as mentioned). Alternatively, they may issue only straightforward instructions that represent slack – for example by not fully responding to the patient's needs, or leaving scope for slacking by hierarchical subordinates.

The problem of slacking is particularly significant in *public* sector hierarchies where managers themselves are unlikely to benefit substantially from efforts to be creative in motivating employees. This problem is at the heart of criticisms of large public, bureaucratic hierarchies such as national health services where staff on the ground have few incentives other than their own professionalism or altruism to contribute to the effective functioning of the organization. Decision making is centralized and so can suffer inertia. It tends to be supply led and non-responsive to local needs (Savas *et al.*, 1998).

Generally speaking, the greater the complexity of a transaction, the greater is the associated *risk* as there are more variables in the equation. From a governance point of view, hierarchies may be slightly better placed to deal with risks. For one thing, they tend to be large and less fragmented (which enables risk spreading and pooling by internal transfer). Providers in markets and networks would be less able to share risks with purchasers without the use of sophisticated and costly 'contingent' contracts. Hierarchies also tend to use salary reimbursement, which is less subject to fluctuation and protects employees who are most sensitive to risk. By contrast, where parties are residual claimants by virtue of asset ownership, fluctuations are not absorbed.

Competition

The degree of competition has an important bearing on transaction costs. First, transaction costs relating to bargaining depend critically on the level of competition. If there is only one provider then negotiation can become protracted, but add one more provider and haggling and bargaining can be cut short by the threat of the purchaser playing suppliers off against one and other. Second, high levels of competition largely undermine rent-seeking behaviour because competition forces providers to act efficiently in order to survive (Tirole, 1988). Even in the absence of actual competition, potential competition or contestability may address problems of monopoly. Third, competition can help address some shirking (and slacking) problems by allowing benchmarking of competitors – that is, by allowing principals to compare agent/providers' observed behaviour. This process is called yardstick competition (Schleifer, 1985). Fourth, when competition is healthy, prices in markets are good mechanisms for transmitting information, which acts to reduce measurement costs (Milgrom & Roberts, 1992).

Specialization leads to the dependence on assets that are specific to a transaction in the sense that they have very limited use elsewhere (asset specificity). For example, a supplier may gear production to provide proprietary components that are used for a single final product. This may yield economies of scale and improved quality but also locks the provider into a transaction because to switch to an alternative buyer would require costly modification or even retooling of the production process. In this way, acute hospitals with specialized technologies, and catchment areas defined by patients' unwillingness to travel large distances, are often locked into a particular local purchaser. At the same time, new entrants to the market may find it difficult to challenge an established provider because of the incumbent firm's sunk costs in specific assets. These factors lead to low contestability.

In this way, asset specificity reduces potential competition and can cause underinvestment. It is, however, less of a problem in hierarchical governance structures where both production and purchasing (physical) assets are under unified ownership (Grossman & Hart, 1986). Networks would partially address these problems because control is often ceded to one party, even if ownership is still separate.

Social context and values

The social context within which they take place can exert a strong influence on transactions. Transactions tend to be embedded in conventions that exist in the social sphere (Hannan & Freeman, 1984; Granovetter, 1985; Hamilton & Feenstra, 1995). These will act as determinants of behaviour and may well act in the opposite direction to economic influences. Thus a strong attachment to personal honour will make it less likely that individuals will exploit their position – for example, cheat – compared with situations displaying more pragmatic values (Granovetter, 1985; Hodgson, 1988; Sako, 1992). Social capital or, more generally, inherent trust can produce very similar effects to reputation (Kreps, 1996). Where trust is high, transaction costs will be considerably reduced. In markets with high trust relations, many of the formal mechanisms of arm's-length contracting become redundant.

Implications for purchasers

Purchaser organization: markets, hierarchies or networks?

So what does economics of organization theory tell us? First, by focusing on transactions and identifying the governance structure that frames them, organizational theories have been used by analysts to understand why complex organizations exist, and in what circumstances different types of organization occur. The key theoretical proposition is that a relationship exists between choice of governance structure and outcomes, mediated by the features of the transaction and the principal–agent configurations involved.

The theoretical basis of this proposition varies between the different schools of thought. *Contract theory* argues the central role of asymmetric information (Milgrom & Roberts, 1990; Hart, 1995; Kreps, 1996). *New institutional economics* of the Williamson variety sees asset specificity (a type of contestability problem) at the core. *Social exchange theory* emphasizes the importance of trust and social capital to exchange relationships, which it sees as deriving inherently from fundamental social and cultural values and norms rather than being primarily calculative (Coleman, 1994). Notwithstanding these differences of perspective, in this section we have drawn on some of the key features of the economics of organization literature to comment briefly upon possible governance structures in the case of the three main principal–agent relationships used in this book.

Purchaser as the agent for the patient

Transactions between the purchaser (for example, gatekeeping doctor) and the patient are usually conducted in hierarchical or network governance structures: patients voluntarily cede a large element of control and authority over health care decisions to the purchaser (Evans, 1981). This arrangement relieves the patient of the huge measurement cost burden incurred in determining the extent and range of required health care services themselves. If the agency relationship performs well it avoids the wasteful duplication of effort incurred when both parties attempt to gather information to negotiate from an informed position (Milgrom & Roberts, 1990). The adoption of hierarchical arrangements is very much driven by the complexity of the service needed by the patient.

High frequency is also important because reputation is paramount in protecting the patient from motivation failures such as supplier-induced demand (Evans, 1974; Cromwell & Mitchell, 1986; Rice & Labelle, 1989; Grytten & Sørensen, 2001), or slacking (depending on how the doctor is paid). Kreps (1990) notes that it need not be the same patient in frequent contact with the doctor. A sequence of different patients seeing that doctor, who are able to feed back their experience to others, would be sufficient.

Trust and social capital in networks can also perform this protection role. If there are social sanctions that effectively prevent purchasers from exploiting their position then such governance structures can be very efficient. Transaction costs will be low since measurement is mainly undertaken by only one party and negotiation is at a minimum. Transactions benefits will be reasonably high because safeguards against motivation failure, in particular, are effective.

Market governance structures are not completely ruled out, however; for example, informed patients may employ the purchaser more in a broker role to arrange provision of the service whose nature is specified by the patient. But given the repeated nature and high measurement costs, and also the barriers to entry that restrict competition – such as memberships of professional associations – market transactions are not likely to be optimal.

Purchaser as the agent of the government

The choice of governance arrangements depends in part upon the weight that is given to alternative objectives. Government as steward of the health care system has the ultimate responsibility for ensuring that the health care needs of the population are met. Among other things, this entails making sure that organizations responsible for purchasing health care services operate in ways that are consistent with national objectives. In most public health care systems this objective is pursued within a hierarchical governance structure. In some cases, this is a tight command-and-control system. Increasingly, however, power over decision making is being devolved to regional or local organizations, but these local organizations are subject to national monitoring and regulation.

Greater local autonomy is consistent with the tenets of new public management. There are, however, usually widespread problems of coordination and motivation. Lack of accurate information on local purchaser performance can also restrict the principal's capacity to get local agents to act in ways that are totally consistent with its aims. For example, gaming is a widespread problem encountered by governments that try to micromanage through target setting.

Market governance arrangements between government and purchasers are far less common, although sometimes there is some form of contracting out of purchaser responsibilities. Medicare and Medicaid payments to health maintenance organizations in the United States are one form of this type of arrangement. The allocation of budgets to GP fundholders in the United Kingdom between 1991 and 1997 was another example (Glennerster & Matsaganis, 1993; Light, 1995).

A market arrangement is considered advantageous if responsiveness is an important goal. Conversely, economizing on transaction costs probably favours hierarchy.

Provider as agent of the purchaser

The purchaser assumes the role of principal in relationships with providers. Again, there is a range of possible governance structure options and indeed the NPM literature mostly concerns this relationship. Central to the choice of options is the nature of the service to be procured by purchasers. Mainstream, high-volume services have quite different transaction features from specialized low-use services. In the case of mainstream services, transactions are repeated frequently so reputation will be an important mechanism in dealing with motivation and coordination problems. Competition levels could potentially be quite high. In fact, different health services have rather different characteristics. Some are harder to measure or more difficult to define, with more specific assets, than others. In consequence, some services lend themselves more to market arrangements whereas hierarchies are more appropriate for others (Ashton, 1998).

The choice of markets over hierarchies will depend greatly on the amount of knowledge amassed by purchasers as a result of their dealings with the health ministry (as discussed above). If purchasers are not tightly constrained in this way, it will make sense to use hierarchical arrangements and so save significant transaction costs by ceding control to the provider division. The downside is slacking. In particular, high production costs and services that are supply led are characteristic of public providers (Department of Health, 1990; Bartlett *et al.*, 1998). Purchasers can develop means to motivate providers to slack less but lose some of the low transaction cost advantages in doing so. Also, with public hierarchies the problem may lie more with the incentives provided to managers rather than to subordinates. Managers may also find that they lack the authority to make changes without the powerful threat of exit provided by competition (Hirschman, 1970). Overall, if providers can be made to compete, markets make a great deal of sense from a governance perspective. But, given the barriers to entry and exit in, for example, hospital markets, attaining sufficient competitiveness in markets is far from certain (Dranove & White, 1994; Propper, 1996).

Conclusion

Given the complexities of health and social care systems resulting from the massive opportunities for specialization, policy makers are faced with a great many choices regarding appropriate arrangements for governance. These choices have ranged from strategic issues about ownership and control of the apparatus of purchasing and provision, through choices about contracts and incentive structures, to ways of monitoring and regulating to ensure standards. Good governance ensures that the right services are produced and delivered to the right people at the right time, and at the optimum cost. But governance activities also divert resources and so have a cost. New manageralism embraces these ideas, emphasizing the need for policy makers to consider their governance options, taking account of governance costs and benefits as they apply in given local situations.

This chapter has shown how concepts developed in the economics of organization (EO) theory are relevant to the choice of governance arrangements. Economics of organization, although a rather amorphous set of theories, has transactions as the unit of analysis with boundedly rational individuals. Economics of organization theory compares governance arrangements according to the net transaction costs of undertaking transactions. Its relevance to policy analysis is in drawing relationships between choice of governance structure and outcomes, mediated by the features of the transaction and the principal–agent configurations involved. This theoretical relationship allows, first, a given set of reforms to be assessed, and second, for normative interpretations of the theory to be used to underpin development of health care reform policy.

There are, of course, alternative theoretical perspectives. For example, system theories, which focus on groups rather than atomistic individuals, the idea being that organizations are greater than the sum of their (individual) parts (Hodgson, 1993). The underlying theory is therefore in an ongoing process of development and as a result its emphases may be subject to change.

As to the question of whether the separation of purchasing and providing will bring net gains, at least in economic efficiency terms, economic organization theory points to a number of conditional factors. Markets appear to perform well when there is potential for high competition, investments do not tie providers to specific purchasers, complexity and uncertainty are relatively low and/or when few scale economies apply. But these are not, arguably, characteristics of health care. As such, the theory does not point to the unambiguous superiority of market mechanisms. What empirical findings there are tend to support this view (Propper, 1993; Mills, 1998; Shirley & Xu, 1998).

These conclusions of EO theory are in many ways at odds with the theory that drove the NPM agenda and they have led to a reassessment of policies encouraging the widespread introduction of market forces in welfare services (Bartlett *et al.*, 1998). As a result, attention has shifted somewhat to looking at network forms of governance. These may involve, for example, partnership models, which retain purchaser–provider separation but encourage long-term relationships and integrated decision making (Rhodes, 1995; Osborne, 1997). The relational contracts that are used in this model rely on trust to economize on transaction costs but still promote reasonable productivity. Partnership models resonate closely with political ideas of the 'third way' (Blair, 1998; Giddens, 1998). This has been portrayed as an explicit rejection both of the 'old centralized command and control systems of the 1970s' and of the 'divisive internal markets systems of the 1990s' (Osborne, 1997).

Looked at overall, it appears that health care governance issues are being pushed higher up the policy agenda. The problem of assessing complex issues such as governance is inherently difficult – sometimes impenetrable – but the latest analyses suggest that substantial potential gains can follow from improving governance choices.

Notes

1   As to coordination, the contract would specify all contingencies for all possible circumstances. Moreover, with reference to the motivation problem, the contract could arrange the distribution of realized costs and benefits between stakeholders in each contingency so that each stakeholder individually finds it optimal to abide by the contract terms (Milgrom & Roberts, 1990, 1992).

2   This is not to say that markets and hierarchies do not feature trust and the effects of social conventions. Indeed, many commentators do not distinguish 'networks' as a separate category, instead emphasizing that markets and hierarchies are embedded in social networks (Granovetter, 1985).

3   This reasonable distribution can be quite modest; because employees are risk averse they are willing to trade short-term risks of exploitation against longer-term risks of starting up a business venture of their own.

References

Ashton, T. (1998) Contracting for health services in New Zealand: a transaction cost analysis. *Social science and medicine*, **46**(3): 357–367.

Baron, D. (1989) Design of regulatory mechanisms and institutions. *In*: Schmalensee, R. and Willig, R., eds. *Handbook of industrial organization*. Amsterdam, North-Holland Publishers.

Bartlett, W., Roberts, J. and Le Grand, J. (1998) The development of quasi-markets in the 1990s. *In*: Bartlett, W., Roberts, J. and Le Grand, J., eds. *A revolution in social policy: quasi-market reforms in the 1990s*. Bristol, Policy Press.

Beveridge, Sir W. (1942) *Report on social insurance and allied services*. Cmnd. 6404. London, HMSO.

Blair, T. (1998) *The third way: new politics for the new century*. Fabian Pamphlet 588. London, The Fabian Society.

Coleman, J. (1990) *Foundations of social theory*. Cambridge, MA, Harvard University Press.

Coleman, J. (1994) A rational choice perspective on economic sociology. *In*: Smeltzer, N.J. and Swedberg, R., eds. *The handbook of economic sociology*. Princeton, NJ, Princeton University Press.

Cromwell, J. and Mitchell, J. (1986) Physician-induced demand for surgery. *Journal of health economics*, **5**: 293–313.

Department of Health (1990) *Community care in the next decade and beyond: policy guidance*. London, HMSO.

Dranove, D. and White, W. (1994) Recent theory and evidence on competition in hospital markets. *Journal of economics and management strategy*, **3**: 169–209.

Evans, R.G. (1981) Incomplete vertical integration: the distinctive structure of the health care industry. Paper read at Health, Economics and Health Economics.

Forder, J. (1997) Contracts and purchaser–provider relationships in community care. *Journal of health economics*, **6**: 517–542.

Frank, R.G. and Gaynor, M. (1991) *Incentives, optimality and publicly provided goods: the case of mental health services*. Cambridge, MA, National Bureau of Economic Research.

Fudenberg, D., Holmstrom, B. and Milgrom, P. (1990) Short-term contracts and long-term agency relationships. *Journal of economic theory*, **51**: 1–31.

Fundenberg, D. and Tirole, J. (1992) *Game theory*. Cambridge, MA, MIT Press.

Giddens, A. (1998) *The third way: the renewal of social democracy*. Cambridge, Polity Press.

Glennerster, H. and Matsaganis, M. (1993) The UK health reforms: the fund-holding experiment, *Health policy*, **23**: 179–191.

Granovetter, M. (1985) Economic action and social structure: the problem of embeddedness, *American journal of sociology*, **91**(3): 481–510.

Granovetter, M. (1995) Coase revisited: business groups in the modern economy. *Industrial and corporate change*, **4**(1): 93–129.

Grossman, S. and Hart, O. (1983) An analysis of the principal–agent problem. *Econometrica*, **51**(1): 7–45.

Grossman, S. and Hart, O. (1986) The costs and benefits of ownership: a theory of vertical and lateral integration, *Journal of political economy*, **94**(4): 691–719.

Grytten, J. and Sørensen, R. (2001) Type of contract and supplier-induced demand for primary physicians in Norway. *Journal of health economics*, **20**: 379–393.

Hamilton, G. and Feenstra, R. (1995) Varieties of hierarchies and markets: an introduction. *Industrial and corporate change*, **4**(1): 51–91.

Hannan, M. and Freeman, J. (1984) Structural inertia and organizational change. *American sociological review*, **49**: 194–264.

Hart, O. (1995) *Firms, contracts and financial structure*. Clarendon Lectures in Economics. Oxford, Oxford University Press.

Hirschman, A. (1970) *Exit, voice and loyalty*. Cambridge, MA, Harvard University Press.

Hodgson, G. (1988) *Economics and institutions: a manifesto for a modern institutional economics*. Cambridge, Polity Press.

Hodgson, G. (1993) Transaction cost and the evolution of the firm. *In*: Pitelis, C., ed. *Transaction costs, markets and hierarchies*. Oxford, Blackwell Publishing.

Holmstrom, B. (1982) Moral hazard in teams. *Bell journal of economics*, **13**: 324–340.

Jensen, M. and Meckling, W. (1976) Theory of the firm: managerial behaviour, agency costs and ownership structure. *Journal of financial economics*, **3**: 305–360.

Kreps, D. (1990) Corporate culture and economic theory. *In*: Alt, J. and Shepsle, K., eds. *Perspectives on positive political economy*. Cambridge, Cambridge University Press.

Kreps, D. (1996) Markets and hierarchies and (mathematical) economic theory. *Industrial and corporate change*, **5**(2): 561–595.

Kreps, D. and Wilson, R. (1982) Reputation and imperfect information. *Journal of economic theory*, **27**: 253–279.

Laffont, J.-J. and Tirole, J. (1993) *A theory of incentives in procurement and regulation*. Cambridge, MA, MIT Press.

Leibenstein, H. (1966) Allocative efficiency vs. 'x-inefficiency'. *American economic review*, **56**: 392–415.

Leibenstein, H. (1980) *Beyond economic man*. Cambridge, MA, Harvard University Press.

Lyons, B. and Mehta, J. (1997) Contracts, opportunism and trust: self-interest and social orientation. *Cambridge journal of economics*, **21**: 239–257.

Ma, C.-T.A. (1994) Health care payment systems: cost and quality incentives. *Journal of economics and management strategy*, **3**(1): 93–112.

MacNeil, I. (1985) Relational contracts: what we do and do not know. *Wisconsin law review*, 483–525.

Matsaganis, M. and Glennerster, H. (1994) The threat of 'cream skimming' in the post-reform NHS. *Journal of health economics*, **13**(1): 31–60.

Milgrom, P. and Roberts, J. (1982) Predation, reputation, and entry deterence. *Journal of economic theory*, **27**: 280–312.

Milgrom, P. and Roberts, J. (1990) Bargaining costs, influence costs, and the organization of economic activity. *In*: Alt, J. and Shepsle, K., eds. *Perspectives on positive political economy*. Cambridge, Cambridge University Press.

Milgrom, P. and Roberts, J. (1992) *Economics, organization and management*. Englewood Cliffs, Prentice-Hall.

Mills, A. (1998) To contract or not to contract? Issues for low and middle income countries. *Health policy and planning*, **13**(1): 32–40.

North, D. (1990) *Institutions, institutional change and economic performance*. Cambridge, Cambridge University Press.

Osborne, S. (1997) Managing the coordination of social services in the mixed economy of welfare: competition, cooperation or common cause? *British journal of management*, **8**: 317–328.

Osborne, D. and Gaebler, T. (1992) *Reinventing government*. New York: Addison-Wesley.

Pollitt, C. (2001) Convergence: the useful myth? *Public administration*, **79**(4): 933–948.

Propper, C. (1993) Quasi-markets, contracts and quality in health and social care: the US experience. *In*: Le Grand, J. and Bartlett, W., eds. *Quasi-markets and social policy*. Basingstoke, Macmillan.

Rhodes, R.A.W. (1995) The new governance: governing without government. Paper read at The State of Britain Seminars.

Rice, T. and Labelle, R. (1969) Do physicians induce demand for medical services? *Journal of health politics, policy and law*, **14**: 587–600.

Roth, A. and Schoumaker, F. (1983) Expectations and reputation in bargaining: an experimental study. *American economic review*, **73**: 362–372.

Sako, M. (1992) *Prices, quality and trust: inter-firm relations in Britain and Japan.* Cambridge, Cambridge University Press.

Savas, S. *et al.* (1998) Contracting models and provider competition. *In*: Saltman, R., Figueras, J. and Sakellarides, C., eds. *Critical challenges for health care reform in Europe.* Buckingham, Open University Press.

Schleifer, A. (1985) A theory of yardstick competition, *Rand journal of economics*, **16**, 319–327.

Shirley, M. and Xu, L. (1998) Information, incentives, and commitment: an empirical analysis of contracts between government and state enterprises. *Journal of law, economics, and organization*, **4**(12): 358–378.

Simon, H. (1951) A formal model of the employment relationship. *Econometrica*, **19**: 293–305.

Simon, H. (1955) A behavioural model of rational choice. *Quarterly journal of economics*, **69**: 99–118.

Simon, H. (1957) *Models of man: social and rational.* New York, Wiley.

Simon, H. (1961) *Administrative behaviour.* New York, Macmillan.

Spulber, D. (1989) *Regulation and markets.* Cambridge, MA, MIT Press.

Stigler, G. (1971) The theory of economic regulation. *Bell journal of economics and management science*, **2**: 3–21.

Tirole, J. (1988) *The theory of industrial structure.* Cambridge, MA, MIT Press.

Vickers, J. and Yarrow, G. (1988) *Privatization: an economic analysis.* Cambridge, MA, MIT Press.

Williamson, O. (1975) *Markets and hierarchies.* New York, Free Press.

Williamson, O. (1979) Transaction cost economics: the governance of contractual relations. *Journal of law and economics*, **22**(2): 233–261.

Williamson, O. (1985) *The economic institutions of capitalism.* New York, Free Press.

Williamson, O. (1994) Transaction cost economics and organization theory. *In*: Smeltzer, N. and Swedberg, R., eds. *The handbook of economic sociology.* Princeton, NJ, Princeton University Press.

chapter five

Role of markets and competition

Peter C. Smith, Alexander S. Preker, Donald W. Light and Sabine Richard

Introduction

As described in Chapter 2, health care purchasers can take numerous forms, such as competitive insurers, social funds or local governments. They operate in two broad types of market: the market for members (or potential patients) and the market for clinical goods and services (hospitals, clinics, diagnostic services). In the first they operate as sellers of services to the general public and in the second as buyers of services from a range of clinical and other providers. Other chapters in this book examine various aspects of the buying role of purchasing organizations. Although we make some reference to the role of purchasers as buyers, the main focus of this chapter is on the market (if any) *between* purchasers, however defined, and the extent to which competition between purchasers affects their actions and the outcomes for patients. Although this concern may appear superficially to relate only to health care systems with competitive insurance markets, the potential for competition in purchasing is relevant to almost all types of health care systems.

We address the instances where a purchasing organization has been established and do not consider the extreme case in which the only purchasers of clinical services are individuals or households. Collective purchasers can be thought of as insurers or budget holders, each of which may offer a single package or a menu of different health care plans to potential members. The characteristics of the purchaser market can then be considered along a number of dimensions:

- the number and size of purchasers; there are enormous variations within Europe;
- the degree of patients' choice of purchaser to represent them (see also Chapter 6);

- the degree of patients' direct say in purchasers' policies (see also Chapter 6);
- the degree of purchasers' choice of which patients to accept;
- the degree of purchasers' control of the clinical services used by patients;
- the extent of variation in purchasers' packages of care;
- the extent of variation in premiums and charges levied by purchasers; and
- the extent to which purchasers compete for contracts with providers.

At one extreme one can envisage a largely unregulated purchaser market in which a large number of purchasers offer a broad spectrum of packages of care and payment mechanisms to the general public. At the other extreme, a health care system might offer no choice of purchaser, or seek to regulate virtually all aspects of health care, rendering meaningless any nominal choice. Across this continuum, effective purchasing of any sort relies on the existence of an orderly and effective state that can ensure that contracts are enforceable, transactions are honest, and crimes or corruption are prosecuted. No system of collective health care purchasing can function in the absence of these fundamental stewardship functions (see Chapter 8).

There are numerous examples of purchaser markets in health care. The prime case is the United States, which exhibits a unique plurality of purchasers and providers, reflecting a policy preoccupation with employer and individual choice (Reinhardt, 1996). In principle, citizens can choose insurance arrangements from a diverse spectrum of health care plans offering different payment mechanisms, coverage and quality. In practice, the choices of most citizens are seriously circumscribed, either because they are locked into particular plans through their employment, or because they lack the means to insure, or because insurers are able to decline those they perceive to be bad risks. The United States insurance market is characterized by a high degree of market segmentation and niche formation (Grembowski et al., 2000).

In Europe, many of the systems of social insurance (the Netherlands, Germany, Israel, Switzerland and Belgium) have reformed in order to offer citizens a choice of insurers (Normand & Busse, 2002; Saltman et al., 2004). In contrast to the American case, the principle of social solidarity has led to a requirement that coverage should be universal and offer similar packages of care. Furthermore, an insurer in such systems should set the same rate of premium for all members, unrelated to risk, and cannot turn away any application for membership. Thus they are in principle expected to compete on efficiency and quality of services, and not on the basis of selection of membership. Some attempt is usually made to compensate insurers for variations in the risk profile of their memberships using risk adjustment methods and, in general, packages of care and copayment rules have been highly regulated. Hitherto there has in practice been little realistic choice for consumers, although there is evidence that some differentiation is beginning to emerge in countries such as the Netherlands.

Even unitary systems of health care have sought to offer citizens some choice of purchaser. For example, the United Kingdom experimented for seven years with a system of general practitioner fundholders, which could in principle offer patients a choice of purchaser, albeit within fairly circumscribed rules as to the range of services available (Audit Commission, 1996). In practice there was little evidence of patients switching GP, although fundholders did appear to secure some efficiency and quality improvements (in the form of lower expenditure and lower waiting times than their non-fundholding counterparts). It is also important to note that many systems with no nominal choice of mainstream health care insurer exhibit flourishing markets in private supplementary insurance.

The purpose of this chapter is to examine the role of markets in health care purchasers, and to discuss the circumstances in which some sort of market organization among purchasers may lead to better outcomes than other forms of purchasing. We first sketch some rudimentary economic and sociological theory concerning the nature of markets and competition in general. We then examine some of the incentives associated with a competitive market and note that any market in health care purchasers must be carefully regulated. We briefly discuss the implications of the different types of provider markets for the purchasing function. The chapter then summarizes experience with purchaser markets in health care, and concludes with some policy advice on issues to be considered when moving towards purchaser markets.

Markets and competition

It is first worth recalling the rudimentary components of a market, as construed by neoclassical economists (Roberts, 1987). Among the most important are:

- There must be many buyers and sellers so that no one's actions are large enough to affect the market overall. In particular there is no monopoly of supply or demand.
- Buyers and sellers have no relations with each other that might affect their economic behaviour.
- There are no barriers of entry or exit of sellers. Failing sellers drop out of the market and sellers with better products or prices can enter the market easily.
- There is freely available information about services, products, prices and quality.
- Buyers choose to maximize their individual utilities.
- Providers seek to maximize some notion of profit or surplus.
- Market signals are instantaneous and the market quickly clears differences between supply and demand through price fluctuations.
- Price conveys all that buyers need to know in order to identify their opportunity costs.
- There are no externalities to these transactions so that only the buyers experience the benefits and liabilities of their purchases.
- There are no transaction costs to inhibit trade.
- Any contract made in the market is complete and enforceable.

The extent to which these conditions are met has a profound influence on the outcomes for society and the associated policy prescriptions. No pure market in the sense envisaged by neoclassical economists has ever existed. A great deal of contemporary microeconomic theory therefore focuses on certain departures from the pure neoclassical assumptions, such as information asymmetries, incomplete contracts, transaction costs, externalities, public goods and various other aspects of market imperfections. Numerous policy prescriptions flow from these adapted neoclassical analyses, such as various forms of regulation, information provision and motivational instruments. Many of these have been highly influential with policy makers. In particular, economists have extended analysis of markets to situations of imperfect competition, many of which are likely to apply in health care systems (Eatwell *et al.*, 1989). For example, they have examined the implications of:

- monopoly supply, under which an unregulated monopolist produces lower quantities at higher prices (or lower levels of efficiency) than under competition;
- oligopoly supply (a small number of providers), which leads to a solution intermediate between perfect competition and monopoly if providers do not collude, but reverts to the monopolistic outcome if collusion is possible;
- monopolistic competition, another situation intermediate between monopoly and perfect competition, under which a large number of suppliers compete with products that are qualitatively different, and therefore imperfect substitutes;
- monopoly purchasing (or monopsony), under which the purchaser can secure higher quantities at lower prices than under competition.

Furthermore, there are circumstances in which there may be a small number of buyers or sellers, but the market is effectively competitive, or contestable, in the sense that new entrants could enter readily if the existing players failed to behave competitively.

A particularly important principle underlying welfare economics is known as the theory of second best. This states that if a market imperfection exists in the economy that cannot be directly remedied, the optimal policy response may require the introduction of a second 'imperfection' to counteract the first. For example, there may be circumstances in which, rather than break up a monopoly supplier, it might be preferable to introduce a monopoly *purchaser* to counteract its power.

One particular feature of the economist's notion of a market is that it is preoccupied mainly with efficiency. The only considerations it gives to equity are the assumptions that legitimate property rights should be respected and that all actors should be treated procedurally fairly – for example:

- no actor is to be given preferential access to the market;
- all services are to be provided with clear terms and conditions;
- comparable information on price and quality is to be available to all;
- no cost shifting onto third parties is permitted;
- payment should be prompt.

Unequal outcomes are considered immaterial in the conventional analysis of markets. Where economists have considered equity issues (for example, in the optimal taxation literature), the general presumption has been that this is a redistributive function of government and not a concern of the market (Myles, 1995).

In contrast, the sociological viewpoint is that all economic action is socially situated, and is embedded in networks of social relations. Individual actors are rarely, if ever, autonomous. All markets are therefore constructed realities in which societies (or those engaged in transactions) decide what can be competed over, who can buy and sell, and how transactions will take place (Light, 1994, 2001; Rice, 2002). From this perspective, there arises a need to analyse the rules and boundaries of purchasing in order to understand the roles and functions of purchasers that society wants to develop. In particular, one would attend to relations between powerful buyers and sellers (or their agents) in order to assess how their relations affect their economic behaviour. From this perspective, health care purchasing is shaped by institutions, power relations, networks and common practices (Smelser & Swedberg, 1998).

Markets, competition and health care insurance

Causes of market failures

The question addressed by this chapter is not whether markets work perfectly in health care. In this context, it is worth noting the serious government failures that can arise when organizing health care purchasing on non-market principles (Wallis & Dollery, 1999). Rather, our purpose is to address whether some sort of market organization among purchasers leads to better outcomes than other forms of purchaser organization, and what the best form of market organization might be. This section therefore first examines the hypothetical operation of an unfettered insurance market. It then discusses some of the market imperfections that arise in health insurance, and concludes with a discussion of the regulatory issues that this gives rise to.

The argument that a market in health care purchasers could lead to beneficial outcomes goes as follows. Let us assume a system in which citizens are free to insure with a purchaser of their choice (or none at all) at a premium reflecting expected personal costs of care. The mobility of patients requires that purchaser surplus depends on winning and retaining profitable membership. Purchasers are expected to maximize some concept of long-run financial surplus, and might therefore seek out competitive advantage by:

- offering higher quality of care than competitors;
- designing packages of care that attract particular client groups (specialization or 'niche marketing');
- seeking out and offering new (often costly) procedures that attract popular support;
- securing cost efficiencies that enable them to offer lower premiums than competitors.

In principle, these actions should promote, respectively: quality, choice, innovation and efficiency. The proponents of a market in purchasers argue that the joint attention to demand side preferences and supply-side cost-effectiveness will advance the objectives society wishes to attach to its health care system (Cutler & Zeckhauser, 2000).

In practice it is difficult to envisage any sector of the economy that departs further from the neoclassical ideal of a competitive market than health care

Table 5.1 Market imperfections in purchasing health services

Functional markets	Insurance provider market	Patient provider market
Perfect information	Medium asymmetry	High asymmetry
Many sellers (no barriers to entry and exit)	Monopoly or small numbers of sellers (high barriers)	Monopoly or small number of sellers (high barriers)
Many buyers (no barriers to entry and exit)	Monopsony or small numbers of buyers (high barriers)	Many buyers but catastrophic care unaffordable (high barrier)

insurance (Evans, 1997). Table 5.1 summarizes some of the key market imperfections that often prevail in the purchasing of health services. In the following paragraphs we focus on four key market imperfections related to: information asymmetry, barriers to entry, principal–agent problems and transaction costs.

Information failures

Purchasing is a transaction that involves serious information and measurability failures due to the nature of health services (see Box 5.1). Although collective purchasers are in a better position to address information and measurability failures than individual consumers, this information asymmetry easily impedes efficient functioning of markets. Similarly, consumers usually lack adequate information with which to compare competing insurers.

Barriers to entry and exit

Significant natural and constructed barriers to entry limit the role competitive forces can play. In practice, even health systems with apparently competitive purchaser markets severely constrain the extent to which purchasers are allowed to fail, or new players can enter the market. Non-competitive systems can secure change only through mechanisms such as merger or other modes of managerial change, such as franchising or electoral accountability.

Principal–agent problems

Both purchasers and providers behave as imperfect agents for the patients that they are supposed to represent, frequently demonstrating conflicting interests. These problems can be addressed through incentive alignment, monitoring, measurement and accountability instruments. Much depends on the purchasers' sources of revenue. If funded by fixed revenue, purchasers may have an incentive to contain costs by limiting the benefits package, even for services that are cost-effective from a societal perspective, unless adequate information and accountability arrangements are in place. If funded by capitation payments, purchasers may offer fashionable services that attract patients in order to secure their capitation payment. However, they may still have an incentive to skimp

Box 5.1 Factor and product markets: contestability and measurability

Health care goods and services can be categorized on a continuum from high-contestability and high-measurability services to low-contestability and low-measurability services, and significant information asymmetry, as illustrated in Figure 5.1. (Preker & Harding, 2000).

The production of consumable items and the retail of drugs, medical supplies and other consumables would be the best example of highly contestable goods where outputs are also easy to measure. Many companies usually jostle for a share of the market, and barriers to entry are few (the initial investment capital is modest and there are few requirements for specialized licensing or skills). Unskilled labour also belongs in this category. As we move across the first row, a number of factors begin to contribute to raising the barriers to entry, thereby reducing the contestability of the goods or services in question. Investment cost (sunk cost), increasing technical specifications and the increasing tendency for larger suppliers such as retailers and wholesalers of pharmaceuticals to command more and more market power making them quasi monopolies and giving them the ability to extract rents by setting prices above those which a competitive market would support. As we move to the second row, measurement of the outputs and outcomes become more problematic. Outputs and outcomes can be measured but it is more difficult than in the case of activities in the first row.

Interventions and services can also be categorized along a similar continuum from high contestability and high measurability through to interventions and other outputs with low contestability, low measurability and significant information asymmetry. Whereas reduced contestability due to market concentration is one of the main problems encountered in factor markets (production of inputs), a key problem with interventions and other outputs (product markets) has to do with difficulties in specifying and measuring outputs and outcomes. In addition to difficulties in measuring output and outcomes, most clinical interventions are characterized by an additional constraint of information asymmetry. At times, information may be readily apparent to patients for example, the quality of 'hotel services' such as courtesy of clinical staff, the length of waiting periods, the cleanliness of linen, the palatability of food, and privacy. Health insurance and purchasing arrangements are somewhere in the middle of this grid. Outputs such as treatment in clinics and hospitals are much less tangible and much more difficult to measure.

Based on the above discussion, it is now easy to map the goods and services that can be bought by purchasing arrangements, those where coordination is enough, and those that are better produced inhouse. The size of the 'make' of the inhouse production area will depend largely on the effectiveness of policy instruments to deal with contestability and measurability problems (Preker *et al.*, 2000).

	High contestability	Medium contestability	Low contestability

High measurability	**Type I**
	• Production of consumables
	• Retail of
	  • Drugs & equipment
	  • Other consumables
	• Unskilled labour
		Type II
		• Production of equipment
		• Wholesale
		  • Drugs & equipment
		  • Other consumables
		• Small capital stock
			Type III
			• Production
			  • Pharmaceuticals
			  • High technology
			• Large capital stock

Medium measurability	**Type IV** • Non-clinical activities • Management support • Laundry & catering • Routine diagnostics	**Type V** • Basic training • Skilled labour • Clinical interventions • High tech diagnostics	**Type VI** • Research • Knowledge • Higher education • High skilled labour
Low measurability	**Type VII** • Ambulatory care • Medical • Nursing • Dental	**Type VIII** • Public health interventions • Inter-sectoral action • Inpatient care	**Type IX** • Policy making • Monitoring/evaluation

Figure 5.1   Health care services: from whom to buy?

on many services that do not affect demand for insurance. On the other hand, if revenue is dependent on activity then purchasers have an incentive to stimulate demand artificially.

Transaction costs

The principal–agent problems in health care can give rise to substantial transaction costs, in the form of specifying and monitoring contracts. Competitive purchasing can give rise to especially high transaction costs, particularly when patients are free to choose providers. Markets give rise to demanding information and auditing requirements and may impose substantial delivery costs on providers, for example in the use of different clinical guidelines or copayments for patients covered by different health insurers.

There are other potentially undesirable features of market activity. Considerable resources will be diverted to marketing and promotion. Markets are dynamic entities that can exhibit instability as participants exit and enter. The mass entrance and subsequent exodus of managed care plans in the competitive United States Medicare programme is a case in point. Powerful purchasers may seek to erect barriers to entry, or to capture the regulatory regime. In order to retain competitive advantage, market participants may seek to keep secret many aspects of corporate behaviour, compromising accountability and comparability.

In a purely competitive system, older, sicker individuals are likely to pay higher premiums, unrelated to ability to pay. Many may therefore find it impossible to secure insurance, or may have to settle for a severely circumscribed package of care. Moreover, insurers may offer a menu of alternative plans to attract different types of clients. Variations might include differences in the package of care offered, and in the levels of copayments. Under these circumstances, there is a strong incentive for purchasers to seek out detailed information on members and potential members in order to offer competitively optimal premiums and exclusions. In practice, the poor and the sick would be particularly disadvantaged by a pure competitive system, which fails to address many equity objectives (Keen *et al.*, 2001).

If an insurer cannot distinguish between good and bad risks it must charge a single premium that reflects the average costs of health care. But individuals may be able to judge more accurately than the insurer whether their own risk is above average (the sick) or below average (the healthy). If such private information exists, the sick may purchase the insurance, the healthy may not, a phenomenon known as adverse selection. If the healthy can take their business elsewhere, the insurance pool in time becomes less healthy, leading to increased premiums and in turn withdrawal of the comparatively healthy members of the remaining pool. The insurance function therefore breaks down.

Policy responses

Any one of the problems sketched in the preceding paragraphs can give rise to substantial market failure. One can of course still have competition and markets with market failure, and in some systems they may even offer advantages over any alternative organization of purchasers, but markets are unlikely to operate effectively unless they are carefully managed. If they are not, purchasers may be able to pursue profits through stratagems such as risk selection, quality shaving, service skimping, cost shifting and monopoly pricing from market niches, rather than being pressed by the invisible hand of competition to increase cost-effectiveness. Therefore, whatever system of purchasers is in place, the role of stewardship is to put in place the institutions, regulation and legislation that maximizes the effectiveness of the chosen market structure.

The market rules deployed to ensure that purchaser markets address society's health system objectives include the following:

- the degree to which some sort of insurance (in the form of membership of a health fund) is mandatory for all citizens;
- the degree to which the health fund can select the level of premiums and copayments;
- the degree to which the health fund can vary premiums, copayments or terms and conditions according to the perceived risk rating of the individual or group;
- the degree to which premiums and copayments are related to ability to pay;
- the degree to which the health fund can refuse applications for membership;
- the degree to which the health fund must be financially self-reliant, or whether there are subsidies or mechanisms for transfers between funds;
- the extent to which other risk sharing arrangements exist;
- the degree of regulation over the package of care offered;
- the extent to which funds are able to insist that members make use of preferred providers.

Each of these introduces important incentives and protections for purchasers and patients.

Mandatory insurance

If insurance is mandatory for all citizens, and yet insurers are free to set risk-rated premiums and reject applications from 'bad' risks, then some citizens will not be able to secure coverage from the market and there will be a need for an insurer of last resort, probably in the form of a government purchaser. Such an arrangement exists in Lebanon.

Fixed revenue

If insurers have no power to vary levels of premiums or copayments then they must effectively operate within a fixed budget, determined either by the level of premiums collected or by an externally determined limit. This is the system under which national tax-based health care systems usually operate. For example, United Kingdom purchasers received a fixed budget from the national government under the internal market. Insurers with fixed revenues can compete only on the package of care offered and its quality and responsiveness and not on patient payments.

Risk-rated premiums

If insurers are not permitted to vary premiums according to an individual's perceived risk status, and there is no compensation for covering less healthy patients, then they may seek to 'cream skim' relatively healthy members. That is, within a particular risk category, insurers may use a number of direct and indirect techniques to select low risks, select out high risks, increase revenues for the latter or reduce claims paid out (Van de Ven & Ellis, 2000). To do this, they may invest heavily in a search for individual-level data. They may then use devices such as charging higher premiums, excluding coverage for pre-existing conditions, higher deductibles and copayments, not covering unprofitable services, setting caps on services or payments and refusing to sell policies at all. Regulators will usually wish to prohibit cream skimming. They will also in general need to compensate purchasers for taking on high-risk patients.

Payments based on ability to pay

In many systems, premiums must be community rated, based on indicators of ability to pay (such as income) rather than health status. Under these circumstances, if insurers receive no compensation for covering poorer patients, then – as well as the difficulties noted under *risk-rated premiums* – they would also wish to recruit rich rather than poor citizens, other things being equal, as these yield higher revenue for identical needs. The equalization of purchasers' revenue bases can be achieved through financial transfers, as described below.

Membership refusal

If purchasers are prohibited from refusing coverage to those they perceive to be bad risks or low financial contributors then they may have an incentive to adopt indirect methods of deterring unwanted members (and encouraging profitable members) such as careful attention to marketing, withdrawing from the market in certain geographical areas, or offering poor quality service to unprofitable members. Again, financial transfers can be designed to counter this incentive.

Transfers between purchasers

If community-rated premiums are used, financial transfers between funds to compensate for variations in clinical risk and income base may be required (Van de Ven & Ellis, 2000). Although the need for such mechanisms is undisputed, the practical design of risk adjustment methods is highly contentious (Rice & Smith, 2001). Purchasers have a strong incentive to seek to influence the choice of method by political means. For example, in Switzerland, health funds with relatively healthy enrolees have been prepared to challenge in court the adoption of risk adjustment methods that would disadvantage them financially. In Germany, several health funds and even some state governments have filed lawsuits against the process and outcome of the risk adjustment mechanism. Some Spanish regions successfully delayed implementation of any meaningful risk adjustment system. In practice, the limitations of current risk adjustment procedures mean that risk selection appears to be a far easier mechanism for generating purchaser profits than seeking out quality or efficiency improvements.

Risk sharing

There may exist other reinsurance mechanisms whereby the liabilities of a purchaser are shared with another agency. For example, as in Israel, costs associated with certain conditions might be paid by the national government. Or annual costs on an individual in excess of some threshold might be reinsured, as in the Netherlands. An extreme case is the periodic financial rescue of regional purchasers by the national government in countries such as Portugal. Other examples are Belgium, where deficits are partially compensated by *ad hoc* government subsidies, and Switzerland, where the cantons may provide resources for hospitals and premium subsidies. Clearly, any such cost sharing arrangement offers a potential for cost shifting and gaming on the part of the purchaser.

Package of care

The package of care offered is a crucial determinant of purchaser behaviour. Many systems seek to offer 'comprehensive' health care but there is usually great scope for variations in interpretation, particularly regarding mental health, certain pharmaceuticals and chronic care. This has led to what, in the

United Kingdom, is referred to as 'postcode rationing', as different purchasers offering nominally the same package come to different interpretations as to its contents. One policy prescription is to seek to promulgate explicit national guidance on what is and is not covered, a process implemented in England through the development of National Service Frameworks and the National Institute for Clinical Excellence (Smith, 2002). Where ambiguity exists there is scope on the part of purchasers for cost shifting to patients or other agencies (Keen *et al.*, 2001).

Choice of providers

If patients remain free to use any provider, then purchasers may have to reimburse providers on a fee-for-service basis, and exert little effective purchasing power over providers. The scope for securing a quality or cost advantage over competitors is then limited to employing efficient administrative systems. Some insurers have therefore found it advantageous to seek out competitive advantage by insisting that their members use preferred providers who have agreed to discounted fees and, possibly, to certain quality standards. For example, in Switzerland some insurers offer a discounted premium to members who agree to use preferred providers.

Some of the incentives created by purchaser markets are intended and beneficial (for example, attention to consumer preferences, seeking out cost-effective providers). Some are unintended and adverse (for example, cream skimming, leading to inequitable outcomes and transaction costs). The operational details of the regulatory regime may profoundly modify the strength and nature of these incentives, so the outcome for the effectiveness of the health care system depends crucially on careful design and implementation. Moreover, whether the introduction of stronger market forces is beneficial depends also on how strongly the current system is performing and the nature of the health system's objectives.

The market in providers

Although the subject of this chapter is the market in purchasers, system outcomes are likely to be highly dependent on the nature of the market in health care providers to which purchasers have access (Dranove & Satterthwaite, 2000). Indeed, participants at a conference convened to compare international experience with competition in health care 'tended to agree that markets had a much stronger role – and potential to improve social welfare – in the delivery than in the financing of health care' (Rice *et al.*, 2000).

At one extreme, if there is no effective competition in provision, it is unlikely that the purchasing function in itself will secure appreciable improvements in the cost-effectiveness of health care, whatever the extent of competition between purchasers. Without a competitive provider market, purchasers will be restricted to seeking competitive advantage through strategies not directly related to health care, such as cutting their own administrative costs, designing novel insurance plans, marketing and deterring unprofitable membership.

A highly competitive provider market may enable purchasers to 'shop around' for advantageous contracts with providers (based on aspects such as quality and price). This might offer a powerful engine for cost-effectiveness if purchasers are able to insist that their members use only preferred providers with which the purchaser has negotiated a contract. Again, the strength of the effect will depend on the market in purchasers. A single purchaser could in principle exert strong monopsony power on a competitive provider market but may not have a great incentive to do so. Competitive purchasers will individually have less market power and may have to settle for being price and quality takers. Their actions alone will have little influence on providers, so they will have little incentive to be active health care purchasers. A possible implication is, therefore, that active purchasing will be encouraged most in a market with a small number of competing purchasers.

An alternative scenario is that, in the absence of careful purchasing and outcome measurement, a competitive provider market might fuel a 'race to the bottom', such as has occurred in mental health service in the United States (Schreter *et al.*, 1994; Morrisey, 1999; Schlesinger & Gray, 1999; Bazelon Center for Mental Health Law, 2002; McFarland, 2002; Wang *et al.*, 2002). Providers compete through skimping on quality and erecting barriers to access. Such possibilities emphasize the need for agreed treatment protocols and good measures of quality with which to support the purchasing function.

Furthermore, the market in providers will often be strongly influenced by the economies of scale and scope found in the hospital sector. Hospital services therefore become natural monopolies in many geographical settings, leading to a need for countervailing instruments. Introducing a contestable market for hospital management teams may be one such possibility.

Health care purchaser markets in practice

This section summarizes some of the salient features of competitive purchasing in practice. It first discusses the nature of competition between purchasers, noting that competition exists even in nominally non-competitive systems. It then summarizes efforts to introduce competition in Europe. The section concludes with a summary of evidence on the effectiveness of competitive purchasing arrangements, gleaned largely from the American experience.

Collective purchasing of health care at the macro level is often characterized rather starkly as competitive or non-competitive. In Europe, competitive systems, in which citizens have some degree of choice over which insurer organizes their health care, include the reformed systems of social insurance found in Germany, Switzerland, Israel, Belgium and the Netherlands. Examples of non-competitive systems, in which citizens are assigned to a purchaser on the basis of characteristics such as geographical area of residence or sector of employment, include the Scandinavian systems of local government and the centralized United Kingdom National Health Service (geography) and the French system of social insurance (employment).

In practice almost all health systems exhibit some element of competitive pressure. Even in non-competitive systems, local administrations may differ in priorities, efficiency and available resources. Therefore, some citizens, particularly those with certain chronic conditions, may migrate to areas offering a preferred pattern of services and good support networks, even though the price paid for health care is uniform across the country, suggesting an implicit element of consumer choice and competition. Moreover, some non-competitive systems may allow citizens to take out supplementary private health care insurance, or even to opt out of the public insurance system, again implying an element of choice for those with adequate means.

In systems based on local government, the decision as to where to reside may for some citizens be influenced by variations in local tax rates and the level of copayments, as well as the package of health care offered. Citizens may in any case be free to use facilities outside their home jurisdiction. In the same way, it is possible that, in a non-competitive system of sickness insurance, based on employment, sickness insurance premium levels and packages of care may influence the employment decisions of some citizens. The economic consequences of implicit competition between local jurisdictions were set out by Tiebout (1956), and have been explored in an extensive literature on fiscal federalism (Oates, 1999), although the extent to which these models are applicable to health care has not been widely explored.

Apparently uncompetitive purchasing arrangements, such as local government systems, may also exhibit strong elements of pseudo-competition if the management or strategic control of the purchaser is contestable. For example, publication of comparative performance may induce voters to throw out a poorly performing local administration, or a national health service might sack local management teams that are deemed to be performing inadequately.

Conversely, many nominally competitive systems in practice offer consumers little in the way of competition or choice. For example, in the competitive United States market, employers have progressively reduced choice so that by 2001 about 50% of employees were offered only one plan, and 15% offered two (Trude, 2002). Furthermore, evidence from the United States suggests that insurance choices in such a system are only weakly influenced by formally reported quality, and that informal perceptions and price are the most important influences on patient choice.

Systems of competitive purchasing in Europe reflect the principle of solidarity, which regards the outcome of the purely competitive system as unacceptable. Full details can be found in the European Observatory series of reports on health systems in transition (http://www.observatory.dk). In most European social insurance systems, full insurance is mandatory for all citizens, although there may be exclusions (such as the self-employed in Belgium, those above a certain income level in the Netherlands, and civil servants in Germany). In general, insurers cannot refuse membership to any applicant. Uniform packages of care can be found (with minor exceptions) in Germany, Switzerland, France, Austria, the Czech Republic, Luxembourg, Belgium (where there is a uniform package of care within compulsory insurance, although competing health funds offer additional non-health-related services) and the Netherlands (for health fund insurance). Contributions are set according only to income in most countries (Belgium, Germany, Netherlands health funds, France, Austria, Luxembourg, Czech Republic), and at a flat per capita rate within each Swiss canton.

Risk-adjusted capitation seeks to establish a 'fair' market in insurance in which health funds compete on a level playing field. The most rudimentary risk adjustment systems (such as Switzerland) consider only age and sex. The German mechanism has evolved to consider age, sex, disability status, and participation in disease-management programmes. Regulations for high-risk patients are found in the Netherlands (private insurance) and in Germany. In Belgium, the allocation of funds was traditionally based on retrospective costs and is gradually being transformed into prospective payments based on a risk-adjusted capitation formula. In the Czech Republic, 60% of the revenues of the health funds are distributed according to age (under 60/60+).

Cream skimming continues to be a central concern of many designers of competitive purchasing systems, and strenuous efforts are being made to improve the design of inter-fund transfers in order to reduce the incentive to cream skim. However, even the best risk adjustment schemes account for no more than 12% of the variance in individual health care expenditure. Therefore, without additional arrangements such as reinsurance of high-cost patients, there remains substantial scope for health funds to seek out private information – such as historical utilization data – to determine whether the revenues associated with an individual are expected to exceed health care costs.

Historically, many purchasers in European health care systems have been passive insurers. Access to health care is liberal and choice of provider is left to the patient. Providers have typically been reimbursed on a fixed-fee basis. There has been only modest interest in seeking to influence the actions of patients or providers, in the form of utilization, quality or costs. Notable exceptions are the Netherlands and the Czech Republic, where primary care physicians act as gate-keepers for medical care. Selective contracting is possible in some countries (such as the Czech Republic and the Netherlands) but is only rarely used. In Switzerland, some insurers contract with Health Maintenance Organizations (HMOs) or networks of gatekeeping primary care physicians and have established new mechanisms of reimbursement such as capitation. In Germany, experiments with selective contracting have not yet reached maturity. The emphasis to date has been on creating satisfactory risk adjustment mechanisms designed to deter risk-selective behaviour on the part of insurance companies. As a result, there remains in most social insurance systems considerable scope for overconsumption of health care caused by supplier-induced demand (provision of unnecessary or even harmful clinical services) on the part of providers.

The United Kingdom experimented from 1991 to 1997 with a 'quasi-market' in which general practitioners could opt to become fundholders with certain purchasing powers. However, this was never an effective competitive market in purchasing organizations, as consumers exercised little realistic choice over general practitioner. Moreover, the introduction of the quasi market was never subjected to rigorous evaluation (Light, 1997, 2001; Le Grand et al., 1998). However, some research evidence is available. Fundholding by GPs did appear to result in large increases in management costs, most especially in the writing, management and monitoring of contracts (Audit Commission, 1996). Patients of GP fundholders secured favourable waiting times in comparison with patients of non-fundholders (Propper et al., 2002). And fundholders succeeded in reducing use of non-emergency secondary care by about 5% compared with their non-fundholding counterparts (Dusheiko et al., 2003).

In contrast with the European experience, in the United States numerous managerial tools have been deployed by competitive insurers to curb excessive supply under the general banner of managed care (Robinson & Steiner, 1998; Glied, 2000). Under prospective payment, purchasers reimburse providers on the basis of fixed-fee schedules based on (say) capitation, negotiated budgets or the diagnosis-related group (DRG) categories of patients. The choice of reimbursement method has profound implications for incentives and risk sharing between purchaser and provider. For example, a modest transfer of risk from purchaser to provider occurs when a fixed price per case (in the form of a DRG payment, for example) is substituted for fee-for-service. The risk associated with the diagnosis of a case remains with the purchaser. However, the risk associated with variations in treatment costs is transferred to the provider.

A more radical transfer of risk from purchaser to provider occurs using capitation, under which the provider is required to manage all health care needs of a patient population within a fixed (usually annual) budget. This arrangement, often referred to as a block contract, effectively transfers the responsibility for managing uncertain costs to the provider and transfers the locus of responsibility for controlling costs and quality to the provider. It may lead to vertical integration of purchaser and provider. Capitation is common in United States managed care, but the consequences have proved unpopular with many consumers. Equally, however, American purchasers of health care insurance seem to be very sensitive to price. There may therefore be a case for competitive insurers offering consumers a choice of either a low premium and a managed care contract, or a higher premium with fee for service. Of course, the consequent plethora of plans may be administratively complex to manage for both purchaser and provider, and may lead to unequal treatment of otherwise identical patients (for example, fee-for-service patients may enjoy lower waiting times for surgery).

In an attempt to control quality and costs, there has been widespread experimentation in the United States with independent scrutiny of the actions of participating providers under systems such as utilization review. The intention is to ensure that patients receive health care in accordance with an agreed protocol. It has analogies with European arrangements, such as the best practice guidelines encompassed in United Kingdom National Service Frameworks and the quality registers used in Sweden (Rehnqvist, 2002). If integrated properly with economic notions of cost-effectiveness, there is some prospect that such principles could lead to a clearer definition of the package of care to which patients are entitled, and act as a basis for monitoring physician compliance. Again, under purchaser competition, a problem encountered by American providers is the wide variety of protocols and guidelines under which patients from different plans should be treated.

Managed care mechanisms failed to slow down cost escalation in the United States during the 1980s, largely because providers found ways to 'work' them so that they were paid even more than before. The lesson is that applying these tools is not straightforward and can have unanticipated effects. More stringent measures in the second half of the 1990s seemed to slow down cost increases. However, these strong measures by the purchasers of managed care led to a patient and clinician backlash, which has forced purchasers to pull back and has created a climate of mistrust in both purchasers and providers. Mistrust undermines all efforts at cost containment, even efforts to eliminate unnecessary services, and is hard to extinguish (Light, 2000).

Conclusion

There are strongly diverging views among commentators as to the merits or otherwise of increasing competitive pressures among health care purchasers. Some observers have concluded that strong, well informed purchasers, rather than purchaser competition, are the key to efficiency and effectiveness. Others see heightened purchaser competition as the only means of dealing with entrenched interests, waste and inefficiency. In practice, the preoccupations of policy makers, and the urgency of making reforms, vary greatly between systems, depending on the existing institutions, objectives, performance and culture. There are, furthermore, numerous design issues that policy makers must address when introducing increased competitive pressures.

In summary, our discussion suggests that, if properly implemented, a market in purchasers might yield benefits such as:

- purchasers becoming more responsive to the preferences of citizens;
- purchasers promoting the search for innovation and new modes of care;
- citizens being able to choose from a menu of insurance packages, varying in coverage, quality of care, premiums and copayments;
- dominant parties such as governments and provider groups having greater difficulty 'capturing' purchasers;
- competition stimulating the drive for higher quality information.

On the other hand, heightening competition between purchasers brings distinct perils, such as:

- providers having to deal with numerous purchasers, offering different packages of care, leading to administrative complexity and bureaucracy costs;
- patient choice being reduced, as they are permitted to use only services contracted by their purchaser;
- equity objectives being compromised;
- purchasers 'cream skimming' preferred patient groups, leaving the disadvantaged with little effective choice;
- the provider market becoming unstable without a dominant purchaser, leading to underinvestment and market failure;
- the health care system becoming fragmented and uncoordinated;
- the market power of a single purchaser being lost;
- managerial costs increasing.

Irrespective of the purchasing arrangement used to transfer funds from the collection/pooling subfunctions to providers, governments have a stewardship responsibility in ensuring that broad policy objectives such as maximizing health, assuring financial protection, reducing inequalities and enhancing consumer satisfaction are achieved subject to the chosen level of resources. This stewardship function is the essence of good government, and is treated in Chapter 8. This chapter has indicated that – if a market approach to purchasing is being considered – key stewardship issues on market structure include:

- What should be subject to competition?
- Who can buy and sell?
- How will transactions take place?
- How much risk is to be borne by which parties?
- How good is the market information on product, quality and price?
- How transparent are the market transactions?
- What regulation and sanctions should there be for breaches of contract?
- What role should patient and citizen preferences play?
- What are the major externalities not taken into account?
- Who should be accountable to whom and for what?
- How should a fair market be constructed?
- How should market reforms be implemented?

The choices made on these and related issues will define the incentive structure within which patients, purchasers and providers operate.

Furthermore, within any market or non-market structure, information is a key stewardship issue. Elements of competition between purchasers can be secured through mechanisms such as yardstick competition, benchmarking and contestability (Shleifer, 1985). For example, some countries are experimenting with various forms of public reporting of performance. In England this has taken the form of a system of 'star ratings' under which both purchasers and providers are ranked on a four-point scale (Smith, 2002). Implementation of robust information systems is a prerequisite of a properly functioning market in purchasers. Many countries have been experimenting with greater use of provider performance information to improve collective purchasing decisions. Increasingly, insurers are seeking to include criteria such as clinical quality, efficiency, consumer satisfaction and financial risk into their purchasing decisions, necessitating a major development of information resources (Mello *et al.*, 2003).

Even apparently non-competitive systems exhibit important elements of purchaser competition. Contestability is an underdeveloped notion in health care purchasing, but could take the form of elected management (as in local government systems of health care) or franchised management, which must periodically submit itself to reappointment. Where implementation of a conventional market in purchasers is deemed infeasible, such mechanisms may introduce beneficial competitive elements into the purchasing function.

In conclusion, we would note the poor evidence base for offering policy advice in this area. The complexity of the issues discussed in this chapter makes it imperative that – to the extent that it is possible – any reforms should be implemented and evaluated with great care, and commissioning relevant research should be considered a key element of the stewardship function.

References

Audit Commission (1996) *What the doctor ordered: a study of GP fund-holders in England and Wales.* London, HMSO.

Bazelon Center for Mental Health Law (2002) *Disintegrating systems: the state of states' public mental health systems.* Washington, D.C., Bazelon Center for Mental Health Law.

Cutler, D. and Zeckhauser, R. (2000) The anatomy of health insurance. *In*: Newhouse P.J. and Culyer, A.J., eds. *Handbook of health economics.* Amsterdam, Elsevier.

Dranove, D. and Satterthwaite, M. (2000) The industrial organization of health care markets. *In*: Newhouse, P.J. and Culyer, A.J., eds. *Handbook of health economics.* Amsterdam, Elsevier.

Dusheiko, M. *et al.* (2003) The effect of budgets on doctor behaviour: evidence from a natural experiment. Discussion Paper 03/04.

Eatwell, J., Milgate, M. and Newman, P. (1989) *Allocation, information and markets.* New York, Macmillan.

Evans, R.G. (1997) Going for the gold: the redistributive agenda behind market-based health care reform. *Journal of health politics, policy and law,* **22**: 427–466.

Glied, S. (2000) Managed care. *In*: Newhouse, P.J. and Culyer, A.J., eds. *Handbook of health economics.* Amsterdam, Elsevier.

Grembowski, D., Diehr, R. and Novak, L. (2000) Measuring the 'managedness' and covered benefits of health plans. *Health services research,* **35**: 707–734.

Keen, J., Light, D. and Mays, N. (2001) *Public–private relations in health care.* London, The King's Fund.

Kirzner, I. (1973) *Competition and entrepreneurship.* Chicago, University of Chicago Press.

Le Grand, J., Mays, N. and Mulligan, J. (1998) *Learning from the NHS internal market.* London, King's Fund Institute.

Light, D. (1992) The practice and ethics of risk-rated health insurance. *Journal of the American Medical Association,* **267**: 2503–2508.

Light, D. (1994) Escaping the traps of postwar Western medicine. *European journal of public health,* **3**: 281–289.

Light, D. (1997) From managed competition to managed co-operation: theory and lessons from the British experience. *Milbank quarterly,* **75**(3): 297–341.

Light, D. (2001) Managed competition, governmentality and institutional response in the United Kingdom. *Social science and medicine,* **52**: 1167–1181.

McFarland, B. (2002) Cause for concern. *Behavioral health care tomorrow,* **11**: 22–31.

Mello, M., Studdert, D. and Brennan, D. (2003) The leapfrog standards: ready to jump from marketplace to courtroom? *Health affairs,* **22**(2): 46–59.

Morrisey, J. (1999) Integrating service delivery systems for persons with a severe mental illness. *In*: Horwitz, A. and Scheid, T., eds. *A handbook for the study of mental health.* Cambridge, Cambridge University Press.

Myles, G. (1995) *Public economics.* Cambridge, Cambridge University Press.

Normand, C. and Busse, R. (2002) Social health insurance financing. *In*: Mossialos, E. *et al.*, eds. *Funding health care: options for Europe.* Buckingham, Open University Press.

Oates, W.W. (1999) An essay on fiscal federalism. *Journal of economic literature,* **37**(3): 1120–1149.

Ormerod, P. (1984) *The death of economics.* London, Faber and Faber.

Preker, A. and Harding, A. (2000). *The economics of public and private roles in health care: Insights from institutional economics and organizational theory.* HNP discussion paper. Washington, D.C., World Bank.

Preker, A., Harding, A. and Travis, P. (2000) Make or buy decisions in the production of health care goods and services: new insights from institutional economics and organizational theory. *Bulletin of the World Health Organization,* **78**(6): 779–790.

Propper, C., Croxson, B. and Shearer, A. (2002) Waiting times for hospital admissions: the impact of GP fund-holding. *Journal of health economics*, **21**: 227–252.

Rehnqvist, N. (2002) Improving accountability in a decentralised system. In: Smith P., ed. *Measuring up: improving health systems performance in OECD countries*. Paris, OECD.

Reinhardt, U.E. (1996) A social contract for 21st-century American health care: three-tier health care with bounty hunting. *Health economics*, **5**(6): 479–499.

Rice, N. and Smith, P. (2001) Capitation and risk adjustment in health care financing: an international progress report. *Milbank quarterly*, **79**(1): 81ff.

Rice, T. (2002) *The economics of health care reconsidered*. Chicago, Health Administration Press.

Rice, T. *et al.* (2000) Reconsidering the role of competition in health care markets: introduction. *Journal of health politics, policy and law*, **25**(5): 863–873.

Roberts, J. (1987) Perfectly and imperfectly competitive markets. In: Eatwell, J., Milgate, M. and Newman, P., eds. *The new Palgrave: a dictionary of economics*. New York, Macmillan.

Robinson, R. and Steiner, A. (1998) *Managed health care: US evidence and lessons for the NHS*. Buckingham, Open University Press.

Saltman, R., Busse, R. and Figueras, J., eds. (2004) *Social health insurance systems in Western Europe*. European Observatory on Health Systems and Policies Series. Maidenhead, Open University Press.

Schlesinger, M. and Gray, B. (1999) Institution change and its consequences for the delivery of mental health services. In: Horwitz, A. and Scheid, T., eds. *A handbook for the study of mental health*. Cambridge, Cambridge University Press.

Schreter, R. and Sharfstein, S. (1994) *Allies and adversaries: the impact of managed care on mental health services*. Washington, D.C., American Psychiatric Association.

Shleifer, A. (1985) A theory of yardstick competition. *Rand journal of economics*, **16**(3): 319–327.

Smelser, N. and Swedberg, R. (1998) The sociological perspective on the economy. In: Smelser, N. and Swedberg, R., eds. *The handbook of economic sociology*. Princeton, NJ, Princeton University Press.

Smith, P.C. (2002) Performance management in British health care: will it deliver? *Health affairs*, **21**(3): 103–115.

Tiebout, C.M. (1956) A pure theory of local expenditures. *Journal of political economy*, **64**: 416–424.

Trude, S. (2002) *Who has a choice of health plans?* Issue Brief 27. Washington, D.C., Center for Studying Health System Change.

Van de Ven, W. and Ellis, R. (2000) Risk adjustment in competitive health plan markets. In: Newhouse, J.P. and Culyer, A.J., eds. *Handbook of health economics*. Amsterdam, Elsevier.

Wallis, J. and Dollery, B. (1999) *Market failure, government failure, leadership and public policy*. New York, Palgrave Macmillan.

Wang, P., Demler, O. and Kessler, R. (2002) Adequacy of treatment for serious mental illness in the United States. *American journal of public health*, **92**: 92–98.

chapter SiX

Purchasers as the public's agent

Andre P. den Exter

Introduction: the roles of citizens

The patient–purchaser relationship is a subset of the third-party relationship that dominates health care, wherein the third party acts as the patient's agent, assuming the decision-making power in the purchase of health services (Smith *et al.*, 1997).

In recent years, the patient–purchaser relationship has become more prominent and the subject of debate. Developments such as increased 'marketization' of the health care sector and consequent 'patient empowerment' movements have led to patients asserting more influence on purchasers' decision making. Such developments can be expected to affect the role of the purchaser as the public's agent. For instance, acting as a prudent agent for the patient means that purchasers are increasingly held accountable for contracting decisions by supervisory authorities and, more recently, also by the insured party or taxpayer. Moreover, 'patient empowerment' reinforces patients' involvement in decision making about medical treatment, choice of provider and purchaser, election of health authorities and control over budget and service allocations (Saltman, 1994).

The citizens' role in purchasing decision making can be examined from two perspectives. First, one may consider collective and individual *influences* on purchasing decisions. Collective influence is exercised, for example, when consumers influence the package of care and benefit coverage. Individual influence refers to the power of an individual consumer to influence the purchase and receipt of care on his or her behalf.

The second perspective looks at the *mechanisms* available to citizens to influence purchasing decisions. These can be grouped following Hirschman's notions on organizational behaviour into 'voice' and 'exit'. Voice is essentially a political or administrative category, whereas exit is market-based. Voice mechanisms include: information; consultation and assessment of public views; advocacy groups; formal representation; and patients' rights. Exit revolves around consumer choice (Hirschman, 1970).

This two-dimensional approach aims to characterize the roles of individuals as patients, consumers and members of the public. It indicates the level of citizen participation in purchasing decision making, clarifies the quality and manner of involvement and brings out the distinction between the individual and collective levels. This chapter is primarily structured according to the second dimension, mechanisms to influence purchasing decisions, but it also considers whether this influence is exercised collectively or individually.

Voice mechanisms

Information, consultation and assessment of public views

Providing information, consulting the public and assessing public views constitute one aspect of consumer participation in collective purchasing decisions that set health care priorities and define the basic package of care. Although the effects of such approaches are limited in some cases, they can be quite effective in involving the public and measuring its preferences. One such initiative was the establishment of citizens' juries in the United Kingdom (see Box 6.1). Other countries could learn from these experiences, although the model would clearly need to be adjusted to take account of local needs (Lenaghan, 1999).

Box 6.1   Citizens' juries in rationing decisions in the United Kingdom

A group of broadly representative jurors is recruited from the community, with a primarily advisory role. The members address important questions about policy and planning, and their recommendations are meant to supplement existing democratic decision-making processes (Lenaghan, 1999). Since 1996, a number of citizens' juries have been set up to enhance public involvement in the allocation of finite health care resources (Harrison & Mort, 1998). They appear to be useful tools for enabling the public – as citizens rather than individual consumers – to define values or criteria for rationing decisions (Lenaghan, 1999).

Another, more recent, initiative in the United Kingdom is led by the National Institute of Clinical Excellence – the official body charged with assembling and disseminating scientific evidence on the clinical and cost effectiveness of health care technologies – which has established a citizens' panel to provide input in its deliberations.

Apart from citizens' juries and panels, the use of surveys is a useful instrument for acquiring information to be used in the development of national standards for core services to be purchased. The current United Kingdom government has formulated such standards in the National Service Frameworks (NSFs), which primarily implement guidelines and protocols on best practice, albeit with a strong element of prioritization (Robinson, 2001).

Many other countries have also made use of patient surveys and consultation techniques to assess public views. A well known example is the Dunning Report (Ministry of Welfare, Health and Cultural Affairs, 1992) from the Netherlands, whose guidelines on priority setting were based on consumer consultations, *inter alia*. The Swedish Parliamentary Priorities Commission has also developed a set of guidelines, whereby managers consider the needs of the population as a whole (derived from citizen consultations), whereas doctors consider the needs of individual patients (Swedish Parliamentary Priorities Commission, 1995). At the moment, one of the leading institutions carrying out patient surveys in Sweden is the Picker Institute (mostly inpatient surveys in Scandinavia). Its questionnaires include issues such as variations in quality, availability of medical personnel, waiting lists and accountability, and provide valuable data to support performance comparisons and evidence-based decision making.

Advocacy groups

Patient advocacy groups can also constitute a key mechanism for citizens to influence purchasing decision making. There is a wide variety of advocacy groups, ranging from general consumer platforms to specific disease associations, each with particular characteristics – organizational structure, membership, degree of professionalism, and so forth – that may influence purchasers. This is particularly the case for consumer and patient groups whose supporters may have different agendas.

These organizations may indirectly affect political decisions on collective purchasing by active lobbying. The extent of their influence varies from country to country, depending on the local traditions and degree of activism. The case of the Netherlands is one of relative success by consumers in influencing the public debate on priority setting. In France, patients' associations have played an important role in fuelling public debate on health care issues (Box 6.2). The role of user groups is also growing in Italy, where consumer associations have taken part in monitoring the quality of care provided in both the private and public sectors, although they do not have an institutional role in health care planning and monitoring (Donatini, forthcoming).

In many countries, particularly among the CEE and CIS, there is little tradition of consumer groups and patient associations. In some countries, however, their roles are increasing. For instance, in the Czech Republic, patient organizations are invited to participate in negotiations between health insurance funds and providers on the list of services. In some cases (for example Alzheimer's disease, diabetes) patient organizations advocate full reimbursement of drug costs, and their power is increasing (Hava & Dlouhy, 2002). Nonetheless, consumer advocacy groups have relatively limited influence on the benefits packages. These countries usually have statutory laws or derived legal norms controlling decisions on the basic benefits packages. Social (health insurance) law defines the nature and scope of statutory entitlements and procedures

Box 6.2   Role of consumer associations in the Netherlands and France

In the Netherlands in 1995, the Dutch Consumers Association asked for an evaluation of the rule excluding dental care for adults from basic health insurance. After discussion in Parliament, dentures for adults were returned to the package. The main argument prompting the decision was that private insurers offered insufficient supplementary policies. In addition, people in need of dentures (1.9 million insured by the sickness funds are supplied with dentures) had insufficient private insurance to cover dental prosthesis and it was felt that this coverage could not be left to individual responsibility. Ultimately, the Dutch Cabinet decided to include dental prosthesis in both the sickness fund and standard (private) package up to a maximum reimbursement of 75% of the total costs, with the remaining 25% to be paid by the insured (Hermans & den Exter, 1998).

In recent years in France, patient associations have changed their traditional roles, shifting from fundraising for medical research towards influencing research choices and promoting the role of patients as active agents in their own health care. There has been a simultaneous reinforcement of consumer organizations: recently, health care associations have regrouped to form a collective unit, *Collectif inter-associatif sur la santé* (CISS), which has exerted pressure to strengthen the voice of consumers in various levels of the health system (Polton, 2001).

and in most cases the relevant tariffs as well. Decisions on the *nature* of the benefits package are predominantly a parliamentary or governmental task, decided by the Ministry of Health (Israel, Poland, Hungary), or delegated to public bodies, such as the Board for Health Care Insurance in the Netherlands.

Formal representation

Citizens can also influence purchaser decision making through formal representation. Traditional models of formal citizen representation include governments (national and regional), parliament, health insurance boards, regional or district health authorities and even the judiciary.

In many national health service countries the central government, in theory, representing the public, has a considerable impact on regional purchasing of health services through the allocation of health care resources. See Box 6.3, for instance, for a brief account of the role of the central government in Italy. Also, in some CEE countries, decisions on the nature of the basic benefits package are predominantly a parliamentary or governmental task, decided by the Minister of Health (for example, in Poland, Hungary), or delegated to public bodies. See Chapter 8 for a detailed account of the stewardship role of the government in steering purchasers.

Box 6.3 The central government's role in Italy

Italy introduced the principle of a common package of benefits in the 1994 National Health Plan. Additional regulatory measures to influence health purchasing in the regions include the introduction of fiscal federalism in financing health care and the planned introduction of a monitoring system to evaluate the extent to which regions guarantee the basic benefits package (Donatini, forthcoming).

Virtually all countries with social health insurance systems have created a legal basis for citizen representation in the management of health insurance organizations. In these systems, statutory law regulates the underlying principles of health insurance, including mandatory social insurance, the principle of solidarity, entitlements to health care or reimbursement of health services, premium payment, and formal representation (the rights of consultative voting). These formal rights provide a means of consumer participation in purchaser decision making. Good examples of the rights of the insured are provided by the German Social Code Book (Box 6.4) and the similar Austrian code (Theurl, 1999).

Box 6.4 The German Social Code Book

The German Social Code Book (SGB V) regulates the structure of most health funds, including the executive management and the assembly of delegates who decide on bylaws and other regulations, pass the budget, set the contribution rate and elect the executive board. Usually, the assembly includes representatives of both the insured and employers. The assembly in substitute funds, however, includes only representatives of the insured. The representatives of the insured and the employers are democratically elected every six years. Many representatives are linked to trade unions or employers' associations (European Observatory, 2002a).

The formal role of Dutch insured is, however, less clear. Although the Sickness Fund Act entitles the Minister of Health to make rules for the participation of the insured on the fund board, such rules have not been made. In 1994, the former Dutch Sickness Fund Council advised that the interests of the insured should be protected by 'a reasonable amount of influence' on the board. This was generally interpreted as an equal share of board seats, but the funds found this unacceptable. Instead, most funds established a Council of the Insured (*ledenraad*), and some representatives of the insured also participate on the supervisory board (Box 6.5).

Box 6.5 The Council of the Insured in the Netherlands

The competencies of the Council of the Insured may include appointment of board members, amendment of statutory laws and approval of the budget and annual accounts. Other issues being discussed include the internal organization and the fund's general policy, external policy, collaboration and merger, premiums and service package, and complaint procedures. In a way, the institutionalization of the Council restored the influence of the insured on purchasing decision making. Others consider it as part and parcel of 'corporate governance', which also covers the influence of shareholders or its members. A major advantage of the Council's role is functioning as a platform to assess new ideas from the managerial board. Despite its formal role, however, both the insured and the funds considered the Council's actual influence to be limited. Only in certain cases has the Council functioned as more than a sounding board by overruling specific managerial decisions, such as the planned merger of two sickness funds (College voor Zorgverzekeringen, 2002).

In France, the management of health insurance funds by labour unions was originally thought to assure representation of patients' interests. Reforms in 1996, however, shifted part of this responsibility to the National Assembly. Recently, there has been growing interest in finding alternative ways of involving users in health care system decision making and increasing accountability. Current initiatives include increased consultations with local residents in regional hospital planning (Polton, 2001).

Despite differences in legal status, newly established social health insurance funds in Central and Eastern Europe also include citizen participation in purchaser decision making. Health insurance legislation formally stipulates the role of citizens in managerial decision-making structures in Bulgaria, the Czech Republic, Hungary and Poland, for example. Formal representatives in the region have developed a new approach for influencing purchaser decision making by mobilizing the judiciary. On several occasions, members of parliament in the Czech Republic (Box 6.6), Hungary and Estonia have used the judiciary to influence decision making on the introduction of copayments in the social health insurance system. They have initiated complaints at newly established Constitutional Courts, challenging the constitutionality of such governmental decisions. Although the role of the judiciary is limited to incidental cases, these examples show that court rulings may impinge upon administrative decisions.

Baltic health insurance systems, on the other hand, are oriented more towards Scandinavian models, with elected representatives on health councils. In these countries, the different organizational structures mean that the citizens' formal role in purchasing decisions is stronger than in other CEE countries. However, some commentators argue that, in practice, citizens in these countries have had limited influence on purchasers due to the highly politicized setting (den Exter, 2002).

Box 6.6 The role of the judiciary in the Czech Republic

> The Czech court ruled that ministerial regulations introducing patients'
> copayment for basic health care services violated the constitutional right
> to health care, forcing the government to reverse its decision and include
> a statutory list of health care benefits in the Public Health Insurance Act
> (den Exter, 2000).

The Israeli National Health Insurance Act 1994 guarantees consumer representation in two statutory decision-making bodies, namely, the directorate councils of the health insurance funds, and the National Health Insurance Council, which advises the Minister of Health on changes to the benefits package. In practice, however, views of elected consumer representatives tend to be dominated by special interests, whereas the Health Insurance Council's discussions are dominated by the agenda of the Ministry of Health (Chinitz, 2000).

Patients' rights

Another means of enhancing the role of consumers in purchaser decision making and accountability is to stipulate their rights and the responsibilities of purchasers. The first two parts of this section emphasize patients' rights as defined in international and national law respectively. The third part deals with complaint procedures as mechanisms to enable patients to realize their rights. Finally, it addresses the figure of the ombudsperson to support patients.

Patients' rights are subject to numerous international and regional declarations and conventions. These legal standards reflect a trend towards strengthening the rights of patients in the purchaser–provider relationship. The increasing complexity of the health care sector, the technological developments in medicine and the introduction of market elements in the health care system have increased the need to guarantee patients' rights by law. Although some commentators have questioned the emphasis on the legal approaches to patients' rights (Barolin, 1996; Angell, 2000), an explicit consideration of the patient's perspective fits well with a general democratic evolution in many countries (Reiser, 1993).

The concept of patients' rights is moving from a focus on individual rights – that is, restricting state intervention in the individual's right to life and privacy – to a focus on the collective right to health care. In addition to ensuring access to health services, the right to health care has also been interpreted as including consumer participation via procedural mechanisms to implement their preferences, for example ILO Convention 130, or the European Social Code. The World Health Organization took up the subject of citizen participation and collective rights as early as 1994, in its Declaration on the Promotion of Patients' Rights in Europe, stating that 'patients have a collective right to some form of representation at each level of the health care system in matters pertaining to the planning and evaluation of services, including the range, quality and functioning of the care provided'.

Patients' rights at European level

The Council of Europe has played a key role in the promotion and protection of human rights in health care (Box 6.7). A landmark was the establishment of the Biomedicine Convention (1997), the first legally binding treaty harmonizing biomedical values, currently in force in 13 of 31 signatory countries. The Council has also defined citizen participation and representation in the health care system as a fundamental right.

Box 6.7   The Council of Europe and citizens' rights

The Council of Europe recommends that governments of member states:

- ensure citizens' participation in all aspects of health care systems, at all levels, honoured by all health care system operators, including professionals, insurers and regulators;
- take steps to reflect the document's guidelines in legislation;
- create legal structures and policies to promote citizen participation and patients' rights, if these do not already exist (Council of Europe, 2001).

The Council has elaborated proposals for mechanisms of participation, from the legal foundation and support of cooperative efforts to their institutional implementation. This constitutes the first comprehensive political programme of citizens' participation at European level (Hart, 2001).

The harmonization of values by the Council of Europe is being strengthened by the requirements of the European Union's single market. Its charter emphasized the rights of citizens in establishing a single market in the Community (1989). The Maastricht and Amsterdam amendments of the EC Treaty (1993 and 1997) are even more explicit, stipulating community competencies in public health issues. Subsequent policies have strengthened health-related rights (for example, occupational health, and consumer protection). In addition, the internal market principles play a key role in defining patients' rights to access health care across borders. The European Court of Justice, based on the free movement provisions, has in many instances ruled in favour of patient mobility and access to health care abroad.

Undoubtedly, the application of European principles by the Court has strengthened the concept of cross-border care (Box 6.8). However, at present the actual numbers of patients crossing borders to obtain medical services is still very low, such that cross-border health care takes only a marginal amount – between 0.3% and 0.5% – of the total health budget (Palm *et al.*, 2000). Nonetheless, the Court's approach to judgments on health care has created uncertainties and major difficulties for health care policy making in the member

Box 6.8 European Court decisions

In decisions such as Decker and Kohll, Smits-Peerbooms[1] and Müller-Fauré,[2] the Court simplified and extended access to cross-border, inpatient health care, notably in the case of waiting lists. Second, it said that member states should apply the communally justified limitation procedure consistently, and that patients cannot be denied health care abroad arbitrarily. For patients entitled to benefit-in-kind services, this means that it should be just as easy to receive not-contracted non-hospital medical treatment in a visited country as in the country of insurance. Further principles from the Court's decisions reinforce the notion of non-discrimination among nationals (Ferlini).[3]

states. Although the Court explicitly acknowledged individual member states' competencies in defining the benefits package, for example, the Court allowed citizens in certain cases to claim reimbursement for effective and appropriate services available in another member state, thus setting a possible precedent for interfering with the national prerogative of defining the package.

In order to minimize these conflicts and ambiguities, several policy experts have called for the development of an explicit European health policy that should be embedded in the new treaty (Mossialos, 2002).

Strengthening patients' rights at national level

Aside from European norms, statutes at the national level are indispensable to assuring patients' rights. Most countries have developed patients' rights legislation, whereas others have developed so-called patients' charters or ethical codes. Although such declared rights are not legally enforceable and leave no recourse to the courts in the event of non-performance, they have had a major impact on public awareness of the performance of health care providers and purchasers. These charters stipulate what people can expect of their purchasers, for instance in terms of access and treatment from the publicly financed system. Furthermore, they set out the patients' responsibilities and what they can expect from their providers. Thus, rights codified either by law or Charter inform patients of their rights and expectations, and may encourage purchasers (possibly by means of financial incentives) to negotiate higher standards. Nonetheless, the advantage of legal rights over charter rights is that the former are generally stronger and enforceable in court in the event of failure to implement them.

The recognition of patients' rights in national law, although important, is only a first step to empowering patients and consumers in health care. These rights must also be implemented and safeguarded in daily practice. This is, however, a major problem confronting countries, requiring the involvement of all relevant stakeholders (Fallberg, 2000). Health professionals and patients must be educated about their rights and duties and patients must be involved in health care decision making at all levels, including planning and management. Patient rights legislation has also played a key role in stimulating patient participation and increased representation – see also the section above on formal representation. One example of increased patient and public participation is the introduction of patients' forums in the United Kingdom (Box 6.9).

Box 6.9   Patients' forums in the United Kingdom

In the United Kingdom, patients' forums will be set up in every NHS trust and primary care trust as independent statutory bodies. They will have a key role of monitoring and reviewing services and informing management decision making in their trust. The forums will have one elected seat on the trust board, thereby directly making the local NHS more responsive to what local patients actually want. In addition, newly established organizations called 'Voice' will ensure that the views of the public are built into local authorities' health-related planning decisions (Department of Health, 2001a).

Critics of the provisions for lay participation in the NHS have, however, been fairly pessimistic about the law's role in promoting citizens' involvement in the health care system (Harrington, 2001). For instance, doubts have been raised concerning the independence of the Patient Advocacy and Liaison Services (PALS) on the grounds that they are staffed and funded entirely by the NHS trusts in which they are to operate. Patient forums have been criticized as 'little more than talking shops, owing to their probable lack of any significant statutory powers' (Harrington, 2001).

Complaint mechanisms

Complaint mechanisms are also part of the patients' rights concept. The use of voice, notably through formal complaint procedures, can be particularly effective in health insurance systems, leading to influence over individual purchasing decisions. Dissatisfied patients can actively raise their voice by formal complaint procedures, established by law. Complaints may concern both the patient–purchaser relationship and the patient–provider relationship. However, the majority of complaints focus on statutory entitlements, registration and membership, and therefore concentrate on the patient–purchaser relationship. Due to the contractual relationship in social health insurance models, these complaints are raised before the civil or administrative courts or in quasi-judicial bodies, such as the office of the ombudsperson or disciplinary committees. Although the outcomes of court procedures may be diverse, experiences in countries with comparable health insurance systems, such as Germany and Switzerland, confirm the importance of the complaint mechanism in enforcing social health insurance claims.

The majority of complaints by insured concern funds' refusal of reimbursement of health care entitlements. Other cases have dealt with failures to contract health services (in the case of waiting lists) or update the service package, denials of free choice of provider, and failures to provide medical information. Disputes focusing on technologies excluded from benefit packages have attracted a good deal of attention and have raised accusations of judicial interference with administrative decisions on the scope of insurance coverage. In general, however, the courts have respected the administrative authority to define the benefit package, but have imposed more rational decision making, based on objective, evidence-based criteria, that excludes discrimination.[4] More problematic in this respect is the use of medical guidelines.

Box 6.10   Court decisions in the Netherlands

On several occasions, courts in the Netherlands have ruled on the denial of services by purchasers on the basis of clinical guidelines.[5] Since budget restrictions play a key role in purchasing decisions, patients are increasingly resorting to the courts to assert their rights. According to the courts, contractual agreements made between sickness funds and providers may contain limitations on the volume of purchased care. Such limitations, however, may not frustrate the realization of the statutory entitlements of the insured, except in cases of *force majeure*. In cases involving inadequate resources, the courts have decided that the government could be held responsible, meaning that individual plaintiffs can claim their statutory entitlements.[6]

The absence of formal contracts and legally enforceable entitlements in national health service-based models reduces the scope for consumers to assert health claims. This does not, however, mean that citizens cannot influence purchaser decision making. The NHS complaint system in the United Kingdom, for instance, provides dissatisfied patients with several methods to lodge complaints. The current procedure has two stages: local appeal to the service provider, followed, if necessary, by independent review. Recent reforms have also introduced additional measures to help complainants, including independent advocacy services and patients' advice and liaison services.

Box 6.11   Complaint advocacy services in the United Kingdom

These monitor the service delivery from a patient's perspective and should promote public and patient involvement in the NHS. Evaluation of the complaint procedures showed that the main causes of dissatisfaction among the complainants are operational failures: unprofessional attitude of NHS staff, poor communication, and lack of information and support (Department of Health, 2001b). To improve performance, it was recommended that the board of every NHS organization be held accountable for handling complaints and ensuring that serious mistakes are not repeated.

The ombudsperson

Many countries have introduced an ombudsperson not only to address consumer complaints but also to assist the enforcement of patient rights. In the United Kingdom, for example, if NHS complainants are not satisfied, they may refer the case to the Health Service Commissioner (Box 6.12).

Box 6.12 The Health Service Commissioner in the United Kingdom

The Health Service Commissioner is independent of the NHS and can investigate any aspect of care provided by the NHS. The Commissioner has played a vital role in drawing attention to shortcomings in the NHS, regularly reporting on investigations and making recommendations to correct injustices and improve the system. Nevertheless, the Commissioner has no power of enforcement (Harpwood, 1996).

Scandinavian health care systems also make use of ombudspersons. In fact, Finland was the first country to introduce an ombudsperson by law, in 1993. Recently introduced patients' rights reforms in Central and Eastern Europe mean that most of those countries (such as Hungary, Poland and the Czech Republic) have ombudsperson offices. Sometimes, however, there is a difference between the patient ombudsperson and the national or parliamentary ombudsperson, who does not generally deal with health benefit complaints, although the situation is changing. In Hungary, for example, the Parliamentary Commissioner of Human Rights is increasingly investigating health insurance complaints. In addition, new legislation has introduced a more informal and decentralized figure: independent patients' advocates, located in hospitals and acting primarily as mediators but also informing patients of their rights. In Poland the ombudsperson also plays a key role in protecting citizens' rights (Box 6.13). These examples make clear that the use of judicial 'voice' is viewed as an important influence on individual purchasing decisions and as a means of improving accountability to consumers.

Box 6.13 The ombudsperson in Poland

The ombudsperson office in Poland has been strongly influenced by the Scandinavian model. The office of the parliamentary commissioner was established in 1987, to function as an independent institution accountable to Parliament. It has frequently acted as patients' advocate in individual complaints. In health care, most complaints deal with violations of citizens' rights of access to health care in public institutions, often related to 'voluntary donations' for surgical activities. The ombudsperson produces annual reports to Parliament and to government, and has developed an 'early warning system' to identify violations of citizens' rights and recommend action for improvement.

Mechanisms of consumer choice and exit

In recent years, several ways have emerged through which consumers can influence or take responsibility for purchasing decisions by exercising the right to choose purchasers and providers. The concept of choice constitutes an important element of libertarian values and of consumer sovereignty. At the same time, greater choice may create competitive pressures on providers and purchasers to improve efficiency and quality (Saltman & Von Otter, 1989), on the assumption that informed consumers will seek the best service. For this system to function, good information is vital in order to weigh options, select a provider or health insurance package, and evaluate quality and price service (Øvretveit, 1996).

Consumers in most countries have the right to choose general practitioners. In social health insurance countries they can also choose hospitals, whereas this choice is more restricted in national health service systems, although in Sweden one can choose to be treated in a hospital outside the county of residence. Also in Denmark and Norway, patients have some degree of choice about the hospitals at which they are treated. In the same way, the English NHS has plans to increase patient choice of hospitals.

Box 6.14   Patient choice of hospitals in Norway

Patients in Norway have a right to choose among public hospitals at the same level of care. This is a means of raising hospital utilization and reducing waiting time, as it is assumed that patients will seek the shortest waiting lists. The right of choice is expected to increase the flow of patients treated at hospitals outside their home county, which will continue to be responsible for the payment. Adjustments will be made to remove incentives that make out-of-county patients more or, in some cases, less valuable than in-county patients (European Observatory, 2000b).

More recently, several countries have introduced an individual financing mechanism, a voucher system, which enables consumers to choose between different care arrangements and effectively become the purchasers for a limited set of services. The introduction of vouchers is meant to enhance demand and self-management. An example of particular interest is the personal budget system (PGB) in the Netherlands (Box 6.15).

The Dutch PGB system differs from equivalent experiences in Germany (personal budgets based on the *Pflegeversicherung*) and the United Kingdom (direct payments for chronic problems under the Community Care Act), in that needs are determined by independent regional indication committees, whose aim is to indicate functional needs based on objective protocols. Thus, health providers will be stimulated to satisfy patient demands. When needs assessment is carried out by sickness funds, as in Germany, there is a danger that patients will be wrongfully classified into cheaper categories of care in order to maintain costs.

Box 6.15   The Dutch personal budget voucher

In the Netherlands, the personal budgets (*persoonsgebonden budget*) were introduced for specific types of care (home, elderly, and ambulatory psychiatric). Patients may choose between entitlements in kind or opt for a personal budget enabling them to purchase care from individuals or institutions. Patients' associations are highly supportive of the idea of PGBs both in the cure and care sectors, and it is expected that, given its success, this system of individual budgets will increase in importance in the near future.

In addition to the free choice of provider and individual purchasing by patients, several countries have also introduced a free choice of insurer (for example, Switzerland (Box 6.16), Germany and the Netherlands).

Box 6.16   Free choice of insurer in Switzerland

In 1996, the Swiss Health Insurance Law (LAMal) introduced a mechanism of free choice of basic health coverage and free movement among insurers. This combined a free choice of insurer with standardized health benefits, some form of risk compensation, and requirements for information disclosure to the public. However, it appears that in competitive health insurance markets few people seem to take advantage of the opportunity to switch freely among sickness funds. Switching behaviour seems to be linked with age, health status and region (Colombo, 2001).

Evidence on whether the free choice of insurer enhances consumers' capacity to choose and increases efficiency is rather disappointing. It suggests that the choice of insurer might not function well for all, particularly for bad risks, and that the information is not always adequate to support informed choices. Moreover, consumer reluctance to switch insurers means that exit has not yet strengthened competition among insurers (Colombo, 2001). There has been little increase in the quality of health services because the funds either lack instruments to do so, as in Germany, or do not use the available instruments, such as selective contracting in the Netherlands (Gress *et al.*, 2002). By contrast, however, other authors, such as Busse, conclude that, generally speaking, the introduction of individual free choice of insurer in Germany was a success, because it raised accountability of the funds and stimulated their development from payers to more active purchasers (Busse, 2001).

Despite the increased emphasis on choice in the United Kingdom, the NHS continues to place far more emphasis on voice than on exit. Consumers have no choice as to their purchaser of public-funded health care services. Patients may only move between primary care trusts (PCTs) when they relocate to an area covered by a different PCT. Therefore, consumers rely primarily upon the voice mechanism to influence purchasing decisions. Before the current government's reforms, there was some possibility of exit for the GP fundholder, who could act on the patients' behalf in the purchase of services, but since the creation of large primary care trusts, this mechanism creates significant agency problems and trusts are probably less responsive to individuals' preferences than are GP fundholders (Flood, 2000).

Conclusions: towards a purchaser–patient partnership

As stated previously, there are several mechanisms through which citizens can influence purchaser decision making, both collectively and individually. Following Hirschman's theory on organizational behaviour, these may be viewed as either voice or exit mechanisms. They include information, consultation and assessment of public views; advocacy groups; formal representation; patients' rights; and consumer choice. These mechanisms influence purchaser decisions differently. For instance, informing, consulting and assessing public views and advocacy groups affect purchasers' decision making indirectly and are collective activities. This level of influence is rather limited but important. Certainly collective experiences in France, the Czech Republic and the Netherlands make clear that organized advocacy groups may have considerable impact on purchaser decisions, including the package of care made available.

On an individual level, the patients' rights developments have resulted in effective tools for influencing purchaser decision making, particularly when legally codified. These developments may incur increased costs, threatening solidarity and financial stability, but they are a consequence of a democratic evolutionary process in many health care systems and cannot be ignored. Furthermore, it is possible to argue that emphasis on the individual level compensates for the deficit of consumer participation and accountability on the collective level. Therefore, in order to minimize the negative consequences of enhancing patients' rights, countries should empower the currently weak collective participation by consumers and accountability mechanisms. This requires an active partnership among users, purchasers and providers, aimed at balancing their respective powers. Such a strategy creates a more interactive relationship between the public and purchasers.

These measures could be strengthened by the adoption of guidelines on 'good purchaser practice' as a counterpart to 'good clinical practice'. These guidelines would take into consideration ethical, economic and legal aspects of the patient–purchaser relationship in each country. While they would help to inform and educate the public, their main aim would be to promote 'good purchasing practice', by strengthening the position of the patient and outlining the respective parties' obligations. By making purchasing decisions more rational and transparent, they may also increase efficiency and contribute to cost containment in health care. The success of such guidelines would depend not just on their quality, but also on their implementation in daily practice. To encourage implementation, sanctions for non-compliance should be considered. Also, these guidelines might need to acquire a binding character by incorporating them in a contract or statutory law.

Initiatives designed to promote good purchasing practice are similar to the proposals formulated in the Council of Europe's recommendation on enhancing citizen involvement. Purchasing guidelines could therefore easily work alongside these recommendations and deal with matters pertaining to participation and representation. Such guidelines could, for instance, specify the kinds of collective participation (informational, procedural, advisory or decision-making) and at what level (national, regional or local). Such guidelines could further integrate a concept of collective rights, further promoting citizen participation (Hart, 2001). Implementing guidelines in daily practice would mean that citizens would have a say in the allocation of resources, choice of services, contracting policy and different aspects of the organization, including complaint mechanisms and internal assessment. Thus, purchasing guidelines may contribute to real development in the partnership between the users, purchasers and providers.

Notes

1 ECJ Case 157/99 Geraets-Smits/Stichting Ziekenfonds VGZ and Peerbooms/Stichting CZ Groep Ziekenfonds, 12 July 2001, para 108; ECJ Case C–385/99, Müller-Fauré v Onderlinge Waarborgmaatschappij OZ Zorgverzekeringen and Van Riet v Onderlinge Waarborgmaatschappij ZAO Zorgverzekeringen, 13 May 2003, para 109.
2 ECJ Case 368/98, Vanbraekel v Alliance nationale des mutualités chrétiennes (ANMC), 12 July 2001.
3 ECJ Case C–411/98, Angelo Ferlini v Centre hospitalier de Luxembourg, 3 October 2000.
4 For example, German Federal Social Court, *Bundessozialgericht* (BSG), B 1 KR 2/99, R-R v Barmer Ersatzkasse, 11 May 2000; Swiss Federal Insurance Court (EVG), KV 90, 9 July 1999; EVG KV 87, 14 June 1999, para 4b; Belgium Labour Court, Brussels, 8 January 1997; *Rechtskundig Weekblad* no. 18, 2 January 1999: 605–608.
5 For example, Regional Court of Rotterdam, 31 August 1994, RZA No. 1994/146; Central Appeals Board 17 December 1997. USZ 1997/37.
6 Court of Appeal Hertogenbosch, 24 February 1959, RZA 1987; 87/26; Regional Court of The Hague, 18 June 1987, RZA 87/185; Regional Court of Zwolle, 14 February 2000, no. 53325 KG ZA 00–45; Regional Court of Maastricht, 15 September 2000, no. 00/1077.

References

Angell, M. (2000) Patients' rights bills and other futile gestures. *New England journal of medicine*, **342**(22): 1663–1664.
Barolin, G. (1996) Patient rights alone are not enough, too many rights can also be harmful. *Wiener Medizinische Wochenschrift*, **146**(4): 79–84.
Busse, R. (2001) Risk structure compensation in Germany's statutory health insurance. *European journal of public health*, **11**(2): 174–177.
Chinitz, D. (2000) Regulated competition and citizen participation: lessons from Israel. *Health expectations*, **3**: 90–96.
College voor Zorgverzekeringen (Health Care Insurance Board) (2002) *Influence of insured on the management of health insurance funds*. Amstelveen, College voor Zorgverzekeringen.

Colombo, F. (2001) *Labour market and social policy. Towards more choice in social protection? Individual choice in insurer in basic mandatory health insurance in Switzerland.* OECD occasional paper no. 53. Paris, OECD.

Coulter, A. and Ham, C. eds. (2000) *The global challenge of health care rationing.* Buckingham, Open University Press.

Council of Europe (1999) Criteria for the management of waiting lists and waiting times in health care. Report and recommendation No. R(99) 21. Strasbourg, Council of Europe.

Council of Europe (2001) Recommendation No. R(2000) 5 of the Committee of Ministers to Member States on the development of structures for citizens' participation in the decision-making process affecting health care. *European journal of health law,* **8**: 268–271.

Davis, H. and Daly, G. (1999) Achieving democratic potential in the NHS. *Public money and management,* **19**(3): 59–61.

den Exter, A.P. (2000) Health legal reforms in the Czech Republic and Hungary. In: Krizova, E. and Simec, J., eds. *Health care reforms in Central and Eastern Europe: Outcomes and challenges.* Prague, Charles University Press.

den Exter, A.P. (2002) *Health care law-making in Central and Eastern Europe. Review of a legal-theoretical model.* Antwerp: Intersentia.

Department of Health (2001a) *Involving patients and the public in health: a discussion document.* London, DoH.

Department of Health (2001b) *Reforming the NHS complaints procedure: a listening document.* London, DoH.

Donatini, A. (forthcoming) Case study on Italy. In: Figueras, J., Robinson R. and Jakubowski, E., eds. *Purchasing to improve health systems performance: Case studies in European countries.* Copenhagen, European Observatory on Health Systems and Policies, World Health Organization.

Dunning, A.J. (1992) *Government committee on choices in health care.* Rijswijk, Netherlands, Ministry of Welfare, Health and Cultural Affairs.

European Health Management Association (EHMA) (2000) *The impact of market forces on health systems. Scientific evaluation of the introduction of market forces into health systems.* Final report. Dublin, EHMA.

European Observatory on Health Care Systems (2002a) *Health care systems in transition: Germany.* Copenhagen, European Observatory on Health Care Systems.

European Observatory on Health Care Systems (2002b) *Health care systems in transition: Norway.* Copenhagen, European Observatory on Health Care Systems.

Fallberg, L. (2000) Patients' rights in Europe: where do we stand and where do we go? *European journal of health law,* **7**(1): 1–3.

Flood, C.M. (2000) *International health care reforms – a legal, economic, and political analysis.* London: Routledge.

Gress, S., Groenewegen, P., Kerssens, J., Braun, B. and Wasem, J. (2002) Free choice of sickness funds in regulated competition: evidence from Germany and the Netherlands. *Health policy,* **60**(3): 235–254.

Harpwood, V. (1996) The Health Service Commissioner: an extended role in the new NHS. *European journal of health law,* **3**: 207–229.

Harrington, J.A. (2001) Citizen participation in the United Kingdom health care system: the role of the law. *European journal of health law,* **8**: 243–256.

Harrison, S. and Mort, M. (1998) Which champions? Which people? Public and user involvement in health care as a technology of legitimation. *Social policy and administration,* **32**(1): 60–70.

Hart, G. (2001) Recommendation No. R(2000) 5 of the Committee of Ministers to Member States on the development of structures for citizen and patient participation in the decision-making process affecting health care. *European journal of health law,* **8**: 265–271.

Hava, P. and Dlouhy, M. (2001) *Purchasing questionnaire, Czech Republic.* Copenhagen, European Observatory.

Hermans, H. and den Exter, A.P. (1998) Priorities and priority-setting in health care in the Netherlands. *Croatian medical journal,* **39**(3): 346–355.

Hirschman, A.O. (1970) *Voice, exit and loyalty.* Cambridge, MA, Harvard University Press.

Lenaghan, J. (1999) Involving the public in rationing decisions. The experience of citizens' juries. *Health policy,* **49**: 45–61.

Ministry of Welfare, Health and Cultural Affairs (1992) Government Committee on Choices in Health Care Report (the Dunning Report), Rijswijk, Netherlands.

Mossialos, E. and McKee, M. (2002) *EU law and the social character of health care.* Brussels, Peter Lang.

Øvretveit, J. (1996) Informed choice? Health service quality and outcome information for patients. *Health policy,* **37**: 75–90.

Palm, W. *et al.* (2000) *Implications of recent jurisprudence on the co-ordination of health care protection systems.* Report produced for the European Commission, Directorate-General for Employment and Social Affairs. Brussels, Association Internationale de la Mutualité.

Polton, D. (2001) *Purchasing questionnaire: France.* Copenhagen, European Observatory.

Reiser, S.J. (1993) The era of the patient. Using the experience of illness in shaping the missions of health care. *Journal of the American Medical Association,* **269**(8): 1012–1017.

Richards, S. (2001) *Purchasing questionnaire.* Germany, European Observatory.

Robinson, R. (2001) *Purchasing questionnaire.* United Kingdom, European Observatory.

Saltman, R.B. (1994) Patient choice and patient empowerment in northern European health systems: a conceptual framework. *International journal of health services,* **24**(2): 201–229.

Saltman, R.B. and Von Otter, C. (1989) Public competition versus mixed markets: an analytical comparison. *Health policy,* **11**: 43–55.

Smith, P.C. *et al.* (1997) Principal–agent problems in health care systems: an international perspective. *Health policy,* **41**: 37–60.

Swedish Parliamentary Priorities Commission (1998) *Priorities in health care.* Stockholm: Ministry of Health and Social Affairs.

Theurl, E. (1999) Some aspects of the reform of the health care systems in Austria, Germany and Switzerland. *Health care analysis,* **7**: 331–354.

seven

Purchasing to promote population health

Martin McKee and Helmut Brand

Introduction

While there may still be considerable controversy about how to measure them, there is a growing consensus that the goals of health systems include improvement in population health, responsiveness to legitimate public expectations, and fairness of financing (World Health Organization, 2000). This chapter examines the first of these goals, improvement in population health, and the contribution that strategic purchasing of health care can make to achieve it.

At the outset it is necessary to recognize, as previous chapters have indicated, that the concept of *strategic* purchasing to improve health is still far from the agenda of health policy makers in many countries. The two limbs of the triple agency relationship, linking purchasers with public and providers, are often well established, especially in countries with funding through social insurance, but the role of purchasers in these relationships has largely been confined to acting as a means of collecting, pooling and paying the funds required to provide health care (Busse *et al.*, 2002). The question of what that health care should consist of has largely been defined by a combination of aggregate popular demand (in other words, the sum of thousands of individual decisions to seek care) and opinions of health care providers about what to offer and to whom. Traditionally, purchasers may have taken a view on the total amount that they spend, or on the general boundaries of the package that they fund, such as what is considered health and what social care, or what is considered mainstream and what alternative care, but with a few exceptions they have been content to take a passive role.

This is not entirely surprising. Until the twentieth century, health care could offer little apart from a place of sanctuary. The risk of infection made surgery an intervention of last choice (Porter, 1997). Consequently, many of the organizations that we now consider as potential purchasers of care would, at that time, have placed a much greater priority on their other tasks such as the provision of financial support for the afflicted and their families. Clearly this situation has now changed beyond recognition. Modern health care can cure many previously fatal disorders and, where cure is impossible, allow those with chronic diseases to lead a normal life (McKee, 1999a). For example, the discovery of insulin transformed juvenile-onset diabetes from an acute, rapidly fatal disease of childhood into a chronic, lifelong disorder affecting many body systems whose management requires the integrated skills of a broad range of specialists. With diabetes, as with many chronic diseases, the issue of integration is crucial, as can be seen from the much worse outcomes in the fragmented American health care system compared with the more integrated models in some European countries (Leggetter *et al.*, 2002).

Advances in health care account for about half of the improvement in life expectancy in Western Europe in the past three decades (Mackenbach *et al.*, 1988), but these advances have not benefited everyone to the same extent. There are still many people who die unnecessarily, either from conditions that are treatable or from the adverse effects of treatment. Although less easy to identify, it seems likely that there are also many people with non-fatal disease who are being treated inappropriately so that the benefits they achieve from treatment are less than optimal. Importantly, these differences are not random. Wherever it has been looked for, death from causes that are preventable with timely and effective health care is more common among the poor and among marginalized populations (Marshall *et al.*, 1993). In the next section we examine why this is so, and what implications it holds for strategic purchasing.

Need or demand?

The traditional model of health care provision, based on a principal–agent relationship between the public and providers, with purchasers simply acting as financial intermediaries, is based on the concept that providers should respond to demand for health care, voiced by individual members of the public and their families.

But what happens when those in need are unable to express their need as demand? Traditionally there are two areas where this has been an issue, and, in both, governments have felt it necessary to put in place alternative arrangements. These are communicable disease and mental health. Leaving aside any spirit of altruism (Dowie, 1985), in both cases society has an interest in ensuring that those in need are treated (or if treatment is not possible, then confined). In the first case this is because of the risk of contagion. In the second it is the risk to the orderly conduct of society. Yet in both cases there will be people in need of care who are either unable or unwilling to demand it. Indeed, they may demand *not* to be treated. Consequently, health care systems have traditionally created separate systems to deal with these issues, often in adjacent facilities, such as the large fever and psychiatric hospitals on the outskirts of many European cities (Lomax, 1994; Freeman, 1995). These facilities often have had, and in some cases still have, separate funding streams. Where mainstream care has been funded from social insurance, local or central government has typically paid for such facilities.

There are many other situations in which individuals are unable effectively to express their need for health care as demand. In some cases they will be unaware of their need. This is especially true in relation to screening programmes. Simply making a service available does not ensure that it is taken up. Indeed, it may widen health inequalities as those in most need are often least likely to use it as they face a variety of real and perceived barriers. This is especially likely with cervical cancer, which is more common among the poor but who are least likely to use screening services, even when provided free at point of use (Gillam, 1991). However, it is also true for many other conditions that individuals may have difficulty distinguishing from the normal ageing process (Sarkisian *et al.*, 2001). Again this is often socially patterned, with the least well off least likely to seek help. In other cases they will recognize their need but be unable to express it as demand. This is especially likely among those from minority populations (Shaukat *et al.*, 1993; Stronks *et al.*, 2001), and especially illegal migrants, but it is also true of many other groups whose marginalization is less but is still present, such as the disabled. Yet even when need can be expressed as demand it does not necessarily mean that the demand will be met.

A second question is whether health care providers respond to need. There are many factors that motivate health professionals to provide services. One is financial, but this is not the only factor. Health care is more likely to be provided if it is interesting and involves interactions that are perceived as emotionally rewarding by the provider. As the technical challenges increase, so the willingness to spend time on the routine diminishes. It is therefore unsurprising that waiting times for established procedures tend to be greater than for those introduced more recently (Pope *et al.*, 1991). Similarly, all else being equal, there is likely to be a reluctance to work in settings that are perceived as especially difficult, such as deprived inner city areas.

Furthermore, even if need is met, it cannot be assumed that it is met in the most appropriate way. The relationship between the patient and the health professional is characterized by asymmetry of information. The patient is certainly able to judge the quality of many non-clinical aspects of care, but he or she is disadvantaged in relation to many clinical matters. Clearly, the growth in access to information via the Internet can redress this imbalance to some extent, at least in relation to choice of treatment, but it does little to ensure that those providing treatment have adequate knowledge and skills and are using them effectively. It also does little to ensure that full opportunity is being taken to go beyond meeting the immediate need of the individual patient during an episode of illness, in particular to anticipate their future needs by means of health promotion.

Thus, a major justification for strategic purchasing is that the traditional principal–agent relationship between the public and providers fails. Specifically, in addition to the widely recognized asymmetry of information between citizens and providers, there is also an asymmetry of information between providers and purchasers. Each has information not available to the other. The providers have additional knowledge of the patients seeking their help. The purchasers have knowledge of the broader population, including those who do not seek help. The next section explores this issue in more detail, focusing on the propensity of providers to respond to expressed demand for care.

The implications for purchasing

The issues raised in the preceding paragraphs effectively determine a framework for action by organizations that are engaged in strategic purchasing and seek to enhance the health of their populations. This framework is cyclical, reflecting the standard model used widely in quality assurance within provider organizations, where the goal is also to ensure that optimal care is provided (Figure 7.1).

Ideally they would engage in a series of linked activities, each embedded within an overall strategy to improve health. The first step is to assess health needs, and in particular those that are less likely to be voiced as demand. The second is to determine how those needs might best be met, drawing on evidence of effectiveness, not just in relation to individual interventions but also in relation to organizational structures and configurations that are most likely to deliver effective care. The third is to purchase care that complies with this specification, employing the model of contracting appropriate for their situation. The fourth is to monitor the impact of this process, seeking to ensure that effective care is now in place. Finally, as health needs are continually changing, the assessment of health needs would be revisited.

The reality is, inevitably, far from the ideal. Each of the steps involves complex and often difficult processes. These will be examined below. However, it is necessary to emphasize that this stylized model rests on one fundamental assumption. This is that the purchasing of health care is taking place as part of an agreed strategy, in which the key stakeholders in the health system (and beyond it) have signed up to programmes that have clearly defined objectives to improve health. Thus, health strategies are one manifestation of the third limb of the triple agency relationship underpinning this book. It might be expected that such strategies would be common, given that all countries have signed up to initiatives such as the WHO 'Health 21' strategy and, before that, to 'Health for All (HFA) by the Year 2000' (WHO Regional Office for Europe, 1985). But what has happened in practice? The next section reviews the current state of health strategies within Europe.

Health strategies

One of the most extensive sources of information on national health strategies in Europe is that looking at the use of health targets conducted by Van Herten and Van de Water. It reflects the situation in 1998 (Van Herten & Van de Water,

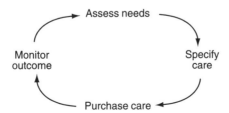

Figure 7.1 Schematic overview of the purchasing process.

2000), although the situation in individual countries with strategies has been updated in a subsequent publication in 2002 (Marinker, 2002). While many countries have a written policy document promoting health, most 'express the desirable rather than the actual situation'. Most policies are inspirational rather than managerial or technical tools to achieve change, indicated by the relative paucity of quantitative health targets or specification of ways to achieve them.

A national health policy produced by Sweden, in 2000, illustrates the inspirational nature of many targets, which in this case included 'strong solidarity and communal spirit', 'good working conditions', 'safe sex' and 'improved health orientation in health care' (Örtendahl, 2002). Yet the situation is changing, in part as a consequence of the active exchange of experiences within Europe. Several countries, and regions within countries, have recently gone beyond the inspirational to develop quantitative health targets. In 1998, Italy published a national health plan containing five priority areas with 100 targets. Many were still inspirational, such as to 'improve quality of life', but others defined the extent of change aimed at, such as reducing mortality from heart disease and stroke by at least 10% (France, 2002). In 2001, Finland adopted a new intersectoral health programme, building on its earlier ones. It had previously rejected the concept of health targets, citing its experience in the 1980s when targets had failed to stimulate effective action. This time, drawing on a careful analysis of successes and failures elsewhere, it has included eight main targets, such as a decrease in accidental and violent deaths of one-third among young adult men, by 2015 (Koskinen & Melkas, 2002). Also in 2001, Ireland adopted a detailed health strategy encompassing a wide range of issues, with clearly defined targets linked to timescales and designation of responsibilities for action (Department of Health and Children, 2001).

Yet the impact of many of these strategies has been disappointing, for several reasons. Few have achieved a sense of ownership among key stakeholders. Krasnik has noted how an attempt to develop a health strategy in Denmark elicited the response from the medical profession that 'health for all should be left to Africans and to nurses' (Krasnik, 2000). The Italian strategy has been weakened by the inability to engage the regions, which are increasingly important players in the health sector. In some countries, such as Spain, progress towards agreed health strategies has been complicated by political changes (Alvarez Dardet, 2002). Yet there are exceptions, although these have often emerged at subnational level.

Since 1991 the regional health department in Catalonia has published a series of health plans, developed through a process of wide consultation and disseminated extensively among key stakeholders. These have fed into a further consultative process involving health providers and professionals, the pharmaceutical industry, and non-governmental organizations that had sought to generate a consensus on effective interventions to meet the needs identified in the plans (Tresserras et al., 2000). The results were used to develop guidance of models of care, including strengthening of preventive activities, which were then incorporated into contracts with providers.

Also in Spain, a strategy developed in the Canary Islands achieved wide public participation. In Sweden, the county of Östergötland worked closely with municipal authorities and professional associations to develop policies based on widespread consensus and which formed the basis for effective partnerships (Hansson, 2000). In North-Rhine-Westphalia, initially in the face of the traditional German opposition to an extension of the role of government in the health care system, a State Health Conference has been established bringing together a wide range of stakeholders, including the sickness funds, chambers of physicians and other professions, employers and trade unions (Weihrauch, 2002). This has progressively refined a regional health strategy incorporating quantitative health targets. Ireland's health strategy sets broad national targets but establishes a system by which regional health boards can adapt them to local circumstances.

Another reason explaining the limited success has been the weak evidence base on which many strategies are established, both in terms of defining targets (determining what is achievable but challenging) and establishing what interventions are likely to be effective in particular circumstances. Again there are exceptions. For example, each of the Finnish targets is based on a detailed epidemiological analysis and supported by a series of intermediate goals and by evidence-based policy guidance on how these might be achieved.

Often this weak technical base reflects inadequacies in systems of health monitoring. Recent European Union initiatives have highlighted the many barriers that exist to assessing the health of the population of Europe. As a consequence, health strategies in many countries have been accompanied by measures to enhance health information systems. In the United Kingdom each of the constituent parts of the country (England, Scotland, Wales and Northern Ireland) has developed its own strategy, although all are broadly similar. The earlier English strategy 'Health of the Nation' is one of the few to have been subject to a comprehensive evaluation (Fulop *et al.*, 2000), a process that has provided important insights into the challenges of implementing a comprehensive health strategy. To set these insights in context it may be helpful to provide some brief details of what the British strategies involved, using the English 'Health of the Nation' strategy as an example.

The strategy was based on five key areas: coronary heart disease and stroke, cancers, mental health, sexual health and accidents. These were chosen on the grounds that they were major causes of premature death and disability, effective policies existed that could reduce them, and measurable targets could be set. Each key area generated a series of specific, time-defined targets, such as 'to reduce the death rate from lung cancer by at least 30% in men and 15% in women by 2010'. While recognizing that progress required action in many sectors, local health authorities, which were responsible for purchasing health care as well as for wider public health activities, were designated as the focal point for coordination and implementation. Action was supported by detailed guidance on the effectiveness of potential local policies and a regular national health survey was established to track progress towards achieving the targets. Importantly, the evaluation of the strategy found evidence that many elements were being incorporated into purchasing contracts.

This experience yields important lessons. Strategies should not conflict with existing systems of accountability. Although England has a well-developed system of performance management, at all levels of the National Health Service, managers were judged on the basis of their ability to meet financial and waiting list targets rather than those relating to health attainment, which, as a consequence, was often given a low priority. The corollary of this is that performance can only be achieved if necessary resources are made available. Second, targets should be credible and should reflect both national and local issues. One target, a reduction in suicides, was widely criticized because it was far from clear how it might be achieved. Third, the policies of those involved in delivering the strategy should be consistent and credible. Commitment to the Health of the Nation strategy, launched by a Conservative government, was diminished because of the refusal by government to address, or even to mention, the term 'health inequalities', preferring the euphemism 'health variations'. The subsequent Labour government's 'Our Healthier Nation' strategy was similarly tarnished by controversy involving a political donation linked to tobacco advertising.

While these findings are important, a note of caution is required. England is among the most centralized of the industrialized countries. In particular, there is a clear chain of accountability from the Secretary of State (Minister) for Health to individual physicians that simply does not exist in most other European countries. Health authorities, as both purchasers of care and bodies accountable for implementing the health strategy, were uniquely well positioned to bring the two strands together. This is also the case in Spain, where Catalonia was able to adopt a similar approach. In contrast, in Germany, North-Rhine-Westphalia established a new body, bringing together the key stakeholders, to try to achieve the same goals. The implication is that, where responsibilities for purchasing care and implementing health strategies are not combined, mechanisms are needed that will bring them together.

However, the limitations of existing health strategies have important implications for strategic purchasing. Effective purchasing for health gain requires that the third limb of the triple agency relationship, between the state and purchasers, should be underpinned by such a strategy. In practice this relationship is often dominated by concerns about containing costs, as part of the state's responsibility to ensure macro-economic stability. Yet in the absence of an agreed health strategy, regardless of who has developed it, it is difficult to envisage how strategic purchasing can take place.

Assessing health needs

Health strategies provide a broad framework within which purchasing can take place, but strategic purchasers must also be informed by the health needs of the populations for which they are responsible if they are to act effectively on their behalf. For the reasons stated earlier, need does not simply equate to demand. It is not sufficient to wait for all those in need of care to turn up at the door of a health facility. Instead it is necessary to take active steps to assess needs (Gillam, 1991), defined as the ability to benefit from health care and in particular where need is least likely to be voiced as demand. It is also important to look not only where need is not being met, but also where it is inappropriately met, for example where individuals are receiving interventions that are inappropriate for them and so do not gain health benefits. Assessing need is therefore inextricably linked with the issue of clinical effectiveness.

At the very least, information should be obtained, where possible, from the growing number of national and local health reports (http://www.eva-phr.nrw.de/), describing patterns of mortality, morbidity and other health-related measures. For example, successive health plans in Catalonia have been linked closely to the process of purchasing, as have the new regional health plans in France. In addition, the French Health Ministry has begun to produce annual health reports (*Haut Comité de la Santé Publique*, 2002), which, by highlighting issues that have otherwise received little attention, are having a gradual impact on regional strategies.

Perhaps the best known model of needs assessment is that developed by Stevens and Raftery (Box 7.1), which overlaps with the next section, on specifying care models. This has been used as a framework to bring together the evidence required for comprehensive assessments of need for a large number of common conditions. The subjects covered include diabetes, coronary heart disease, stroke, and various cancers, as well as most common surgical procedures.

Box 7.1   Framework for assessing need

1. Statement of the context of the problem.
2. Subcategories.
3. Prevalence and incidence.
4. Services available.
5. Effectiveness and cost-effectiveness of services.
6. Models of care.
7. Outcomes and targets.

Source: Stevens & Raftery (1994).

Health needs assessment is, prima facie, a means of increasing the probability that the health gain achieved for a given investment of resources will be maximized. Although the principles of assessing need are now well understood there is little evidence that purchasers (except in the United Kingdom and in some parts of Spain) have, to any significant extent, developed explicit mechanisms that involve links to purchasing.

It is always difficult to say why something does not happen. However, a few observations concerning the United Kingdom may be pertinent. The prominence given to needs assessment is a direct consequence of the establishment of a purchaser–provider split in 1990 when health authorities were made responsible for the health (and not just the health care) of a defined population. This degree of responsibility is rare in Europe, especially in systems with social insurance where there is no geographically defined population. The scope to assess need was considerable because of the extensive data on population health, and in particular on inequalities in health and access to health care by social class and ethnicity, as well as data from a virtually monopolistic provider of care, again a situation that did not apply in many other countries. Finally, the United Kingdom has a very strong public health community, with many public health professionals employed in the National Health Service. It was almost inevitable that they would be called upon to use their epidemiological skills once the idea of a purchaser–provider split was conceived.

The corollary is that several of these factors are not present in some other systems, so even if the intention to develop needs assessment linked to purchasing exists, it may be more difficult to implement.

Specifying care models

Having assessed the health needs of the population on whose behalf care is being purchased, the next, and inextricably linked, step is to define the models of care that should be provided. This activity has its origins in the technology assessment and evidence-based health care movements. In the 1960s and 1970s it became clear that the effectiveness of many health interventions had been inadequately evaluated. Researchers identified numerous examples of variation in use of interventions that were attributed to uncertainty about the indications for using them (McPherson *et al.*, 1982). At the same time, the growth in medical technology and concerns about the safety of ever more powerful drugs were stimulating a reassessment of the ability of existing evaluative and regulatory regimes to both ensure safety and reduce unnecessary costs.

In part these problems reflected weaknesses in the evidence base on which decision makers could draw. They also reflected weaknesses in the decision-making process.

Initiatives such as the Cochrane Collaboration contributed to major methodological advances (Sheldon & Chalmers, 1994), in particular the principles of systematic literature review and meta-analysis. This work has highlighted issues such as publication bias, lack of internal and external validity in many of the studies used to inform policy (Britton *et al.*, 1999), and simply a shortage of evaluative research.

At the same time, governments have established mechanisms that can draw on this evidence to decide on what interventions are effective, and in what circumstances. Most Western European countries now have some form of technology assessment programme (Banta, 1994), although the situation in CEE is less well developed and capacity is almost non-existent in most parts of CIS.

In many cases programmes were established primarily to decide on whether complex and expensive interventions should be funded, with the primary goal of containing health care costs. Indeed, in many books, technology assessment is listed as a means of cost containment, despite the considerable evidence that, when the appropriate questions are asked, it often uncovers unmet need. However, the main issue is that discrete interventions, such as a particular type of scan or a surgical procedure, are only one part of the integrated package of care that an individual will receive. Fewer technology assessment programmes have taken the next step, to look at these entire packages, including both the interventions and the organization of services to deliver them. There is, however, a growing volume of research on the effectiveness of different models of organization. In what can seem like an echo of the past, when the early work on technology assessment identified wide variations in outcomes from different interventions, it is now becoming clear that the way in which services are organized can also be important. For example, the outcome of treatment of many cancers is better in specialized centres (Karjalainen, 1990; Kehoe *et al.*, 1994). Hospitals that have supportive organizational cultures achieve lower inpatient mortality (Aiken *et al.*, 1994). Thirty-day mortality in AIDS units is lower where there are specialized physicians and a high nurse-to-patient ratio (Aiken *et al.*, 1999). Yet research findings are often context dependent. For example, trauma centres achieve improved outcomes in the United States, with its very high level of firearms injuries, but much less so in the United Kingdom (Nicholl & Turner, 1997). Helicopter ambulances are cost-effective among the fjords of northern Norway but not in London (Snooks *et al.*, 1996).

In other cases, differences in outcomes are recognized but inadequately understood. Cancer survival varies considerably within Europe (Sant *et al.*, 2001). Some of this variation can be explained by differences in resources but it is also likely that factors influencing speed of referral and intensity and nature of treatment play a part. These are largely determined by how cancer care is organized. Survival of young diabetics is very much higher in the United Kingdom and Finland than in the United States or Japan, which is also likely to reflect differences in how care is organized (Matsushima *et al.*, 1997; Laing *et al.*, 1999).

Unfortunately, there is still very little research that can provide the information that is needed by purchasers when deciding what type of care they wish to buy. As this information is a classic public good, it will be underproduced if not paid for by governments but few governments seem to have made it a priority. Two rare exceptions are the Institute of Health Services and Policy Research in the Canadian Institutes of Health Research and the Health Service Delivery and Organization Programme, within the United Kingdom National Health Service Research and Development Programme (http://www.lshtm.ac.uk/php/hsru/sdo/).

While the outputs of research on health care interventions and organizational structures are an important prerequisite, a further step is necessary to create models of care. Again there are relatively few examples. An exception is the series of National Service Frameworks (NSFs) produced by the English National Institute for Clinical Excellence (http://www.doh.gov.uk/nsf/about.htm). At the time of writing, eight have been published (and it is planned to produce approximately one each year, while updating those already prepared): Cancer, Coronary Heart Disease, Diabetes, Mental Health, Older People, Paediatric Intensive Care, Renal Services and Children (see Box 7.2).

As well as combining research evidence on both interventions and methods of service delivery, NSFs take account of existing practice, the potential for, and likely timescale of change, and the resources required, both in terms of money and other inputs, such as staff and equipment. They take a broad view of health improvement, encompassing primary and secondary prevention, diagnosis and treatment, and rehabilitation. For example, the coronary heart disease NSF identifies as immediate priorities the establishment of smoking cessation clinics, rapid access diagnostic facilities for patients with chest pain, quantified improvements in the speed of thrombolysis for those with myocardial infarctions, and enhanced use of drugs such as beta-blockers and statins in those recovering from an infarction.

Box 7.2 National Health Service Frameworks (United Kingdom)

- Cancer
- Coronary Heart Disease
- Diabetes
- Mental Health
- Older People
- Paediatric Intensive Care
- Renal Services
- Children

The NSF model appears to have much strength as a basis for purchasing for health gain, in particular its breadth of coverage, drawing together the various elements of care in an integrated fashion and linking aspirations to quantifiable goals.

A caveat is, however, required. The intrinsic uncertainty in much clinical practice means that it is unwise to be overprescriptive (McKee & Clarke, 1995). It is important that this process does not undermine legitimate clinical judgement and lead to deprofessionalization of health care professionals, with long-term adverse consequences for the provision of health care.

Finally, it is important to recognize that purchasing can contribute to population health by encouraging health care providers to place more emphasis on health promotion. Health care settings offer many opportunities to promote health (McKee, 1999b). Thus, on average one of every 35 people advised by a physician to stop smoking will do so, a success rate that is doubled if linked to use of nicotine replacement therapy. Making health facilities smoke free sends out a powerful message about the dangers of second-hand smoke. And health facilities are also major employers, so creation of a healthy environment for their staff will have wider population benefits.

Consideration of the process of specifying care models raises many questions, the answers to which are likely to be highly contextual. Who should develop the evidence? To what extent can evidence developed in one setting be applied in another? How can this evidence best be incorporated into purchasing? The existence of these unanswered questions highlights once again the importance of developing national programmes of research on the organization and delivery of health care.

Purchasing care

Having defined the health needs for which care is to be purchased and the models of care that are sought, the next step is to purchase it. As this activity is examined in detail in other parts of this book it is not necessary to repeat it here, although an important issue affecting the ability of purchasers to focus on health gain is whether they are allowed to contract selectively. Thus, in the Netherlands, sickness funds must contract with all accredited institutions. In Germany, contracts for disease management programmes have been developed within a regional framework, involving negotiations between associations of sickness funds, physicians and hospitals, that made it impossible to deviate from rather general conditions and, in particular, to develop contracts that span different levels in the system, such as inpatient and ambulatory care. Although such contracts became possible in 2000, they are only now being used. Where they have been employed, they have, however, made possible a range of innovative developments, including integrated care pathways. These developments will be of increasing importance in the future with the growth of chronic diseases that, coupled with the potential offered by new technology and research on innovative organizational responses, will demand ever more complex models of care. This will create very considerable challenges for many existing purchasing arrangements that are often based on an increasingly outdated model of care being provided in the framework of an isolated encounter between an individual patient and an individual physician.

For the present purposes, the key issue is that purchasing, if it is to ensure optimal health care, and thus maximize health gain, should be embedded within a broader strategy to ensure availability of high quality inputs. Thus, there appear to be benefits from having systems where planning, contracting and capital funding are at least coordinated. Since 1998, the newly created regional hospital agencies (ARH) in France have assumed much of the responsibility for purchasing previously undertaken by the sickness funds. Their position is strengthened as they combine planning, contracting and, for public hospitals, funding responsibilities. Although experience is still quite limited, several have shown how they can combine these functions effectively to bring about changes in the configuration of, and working of, hospitals that align them much more closely with population health needs (McKee & Healy, 2002). This model is of particular interest because it is so different from that in many other countries with funding through social insurance, such as Germany, where hospital planning and revenue funding are quite separate. It is, however, somewhat similar to the model adopted for the regional health authorities in Italy, in 1999, working within a tax-financed system (Donatini *et al.*, 2001).

The key issue is that purchasing can only work if there is something to purchase, yet the failings of the market are all too apparent. As noted above, many of the inputs to health services, such as research on effectiveness, are public goods and will be underproduced in the absence of action by the state or those acting on its behalf. With some inputs, such as trained staff, the process of production is long, over 10 years in the case of a specialist physician. Thus, any signals generated by the market cannot possibly produce an effective response within a reasonable timeframe. For others, such as health facilities, the return on investment available in the cash-limited public sector may be lower than can be achieved in other sectors, thus leading to underinvestment.

For these and other reasons an ideal strategy will therefore address production of the major inputs necessary to provide health care: people, facilities and knowledge. This is clearly a task that goes well beyond purchasers. Governments have a key role to play, but so do universities, professional associations, industry and many others.

Yet high quality inputs are not, in themselves, sufficient. Purchasing must also be embedded in a system to ensure that quality is maintained. Again this should take account of people, facilities and knowledge. In many cases an individual provider will have relationships with multiple purchasers. Consequently there is a strong case for having national or regional mechanisms that can ensure that agreed minimum standards are met. Of course, some such mechanisms are already ubiquitous, such as the maintenance of a register of physicians, membership of which implies completion of a specified training programme. Similarly, pharmaceuticals are everywhere subject to licensing regimes that are designed to ensure product safety. However, when one goes beyond these universal systems it becomes clear that there is widespread variation in the approaches that countries have taken. These have been described in detail by Scrivens (2002). While there are many terms used to describe these activities, they can be thought of as falling at different points on two dimensions (Figure 7.2).

Perhaps the best known review mechanism is the American Joint Commission on Accreditation of Health-care Organizations (JCAHO), although similar organizations also exist in Canada and Australia. These models have often attracted interest in Europe, although this has usually been short-lived or on a small scale. Thus, from time to time, small groups of hospitals have participated in a process of accreditation, but on a voluntary basis. In part this is because of

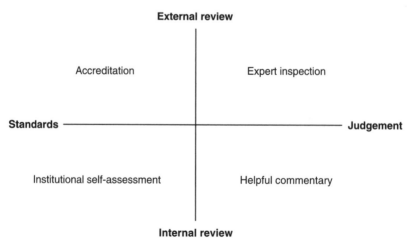

Figure 7.2 Mechanisms to ensure quality.

Source: Scrivens (2002).

the very different situation in the United States, where there were many small private hospitals subject to none of the checks and balances that have existed in more regulated European systems.

The few examples of established accreditation systems in Europe have mostly arisen in settings where many of the hospitals are privately owned. Thus, in 1987, Belgium introduced a system of certification of hospitals. This had the immediate effect of reclassifying many small hospitals as nursing homes and so absolving sickness funds of the requirement to contract with them for hospital services. In 1996, France established the *Agence Nationale d'Accréditation et d'Evaluation en Santé* (ANAES) to develop and implement standards for health care facilities (ANAES, 1999). The United Kingdom has established the Commission on Health Improvement, a body that sets standards and combines regular inspections with publication of measures of performance, such as waiting times (http://ww.chi.nhs.uk/).

Other countries have rejected the model based on external inspection, instead requiring health care providers to demonstrate that they are engaged in internal quality assurance activities. Examples include Germany, in 1991, and the Netherlands in 1997. The United Kingdom has also adopted this system, in a series of activities termed 'clinical governance', which make continued registration as a physician contingent on having participated in such activities. Of course there are many quality assurance activities in other countries but most involve enthusiastic groups of individuals acting on their own initiative.

It is not easy to get these mechanisms right, and there are many pitfalls. They often fall outside the triple agency relationship, as the bodies often depend for their credibility on being independent of government and purchasers yet they are required to reflect the priorities of both. This is a difficult balancing act. While explicit standards have the benefit of promoting consistency they may also stifle initiative, deflect efforts to meeting measurable standards rather than less visible, but more important goals, and promote opportunistic behaviour. Even when failings are identified it may not be clear who is responsible. Is it the provider management or is it the purchaser, who has provided inadequate funding? There is also a delicate balance between allocating blame and providing support to change practices. They are, however, an important element of strategic purchasing to improve health.

Purchasing need not, of course, be limited to health care. It is also possible to purchase interventions that are aimed at promoting health by other means. Thus, in the United Kingdom, some health authorities have purchased smoke alarms or cycle helmets to be distributed in poorer areas. Clearly, whether this is appropriate will depend to a considerable extent on the organizational features of the purchasing structure.

Monitoring outcomes

While appropriate structures and processes are important prerequisites for high quality care, it is also necessary for strategic purchasers to assure themselves that the care they are purchasing is leading to optimal outcomes. This task is extremely challenging and, at present, there are no perfect solutions. There are several fundamental problems. One is the difficulty in attributing health outcomes to specific health interventions. Outcomes reflect not only the technical quality of care but also the initial condition of the patient, the choices that the patient makes in relation to his or her treatment and, when small numbers of events are considered, the play of chance (McKee & Hunter, 1995). A second is the possibility that a focus on outcomes that are measurable may deflect attention from others that are less easily identifiable, but perhaps more important for the patient (Smith, 1995).

So far, attention has focused most on measures of performance based on routinely collected data, either from existing data systems or, increasingly, enhanced systems providing additional information on, for example, severity of illness. Most experience has been obtained from the United States, where several states publish the mortality rates achieved by individual hospitals, or in some cases, by individual surgeons (Hannan *et al.*, 1994).

Clearly the provision of health care involves many different activities, and some will be more amenable to performance measurement than others. Wilson has produced a useful framework (Figure 7.3) within which to think about the potential strategies that can be used for different activities (Wilson, 1991). A hospital laboratory might be considered as one of his production organizations where standard output measures are easily quantifiable; although it is important to be aware that quality may be less easy to measure. However, most of the work of health care providers will fall into his category of procedural organizations, which implies that emphasis is likely to be on having clear operating rules and a strong professional focus. For this reason, monitoring of process measures is likely to be especially informative. For example, the largest French sickness fund

	Activities observable? Yes	No
Results Yes	**Production organizations** Postal service Tax collection	**Craft organizations** Army at war
No	**Procedural organizations** Army in peacetime	**Coping organizations** Police work

Figure 7.3 A framework for understanding performance management in the public sector.

Source: Wilson (1991).

made imaginative use of process data to study adherence to the guidelines for care of diabetes, developed by ANAES (Weill *et al.*, 2000). It identified widespread variations in the care provided and, as a consequence, it developed a programme to improve adherence.

There is now an extensive body of research on the use of performance measures, not only in the health sector but also in areas such as education, the environment and policing (Fitz-Gibbon, 1996; Goddard *et al.*, 2000). These experiences have been described in detail elsewhere. In brief, the key findings from research on this topic are as follows. First, except in some highly specialized areas, such as intensive care, where large amounts of very detailed data are routinely collected, it is extremely difficult to adjust adequately for differences in severity of patients, and thus to be certain that observed differences are really due to variations in quality of care. Second, it is often only possible to know the outcome of care a long time after that care was given. For example, cancer survival is typically measured at five years post-treatment, which, allowing for delays in collecting and processing data, means that data are likely to relate to care provided at least seven years previously. Third, for many conditions the number of cases that an individual provider will treat will be few so results will be subject to considerable random fluctuation. Fourth, publication of performance measures will often lead to unintended behaviour, such as an aversion to operate on patients at especially high risk (Green & Wintfeld, 1995). An important additional caveat in some European countries, such as Germany and Spain, is that laws on data protection and privacy may preclude the use of some techniques developed elsewhere. Thus, the requirement to obtain consent from patients whose diseases were recorded by the Hamburg cancer registry reduced its coverage by 70%, effectively precluding its use for public health purposes (Verity & Nicoll, 2002).

The implication of this analysis is that monitoring performance by health care providers in respect of health improvement is extremely complex. It is likely to involve an iterative approach combining different methods. Thus, concerns raised in analysis of routine data might be investigated further using more detailed examination of case records or site visits. This, in turn, implies a need for high-level evaluative skills within purchaser organizations.

The English performance management framework provides an example of how this might be done (http://www.doh.gov.uk/nhsperformanceindicators/2002/index.html). Routinely collected data are used to create a series of performance indicators, based on six key issues: fair access, effective delivery of appropriate care, health improvement, patient/carer experience, efficiency, and health outcomes. For example, measures of health outcomes include deaths in hospital following emergency surgery, or following a fractured hip or myocardial infarction. Unexpected results on these measures should generate further investigation and the findings are used to inform both the regular inspections by the Commission for Health Improvement and purchasers during the contracting process.

The initial choice of measures in England was criticized on a number of grounds, including the quality of the data used to generate them, the difficulty in attributing results to aspects of health care, and in some cases the use of composite indicators whose interpretation is not especially meaningful (McKee &

Sheldon, 1998). They have, however, undergone a process of refinement, and while there is little evidence of public interest in them, they do provide an opportunity to begin to explore otherwise unexplained variations. However, caution is required. They have also provided a wealth of empirical evidence on the unintended consequences of performance monitoring (Chapman, 2002). As the English experience shows, intelligent use of information can be valuable but an oversimplistic approach is not only useless but frequently harmful.

Screening: a litmus test?

The fundamental arguments underpinning this chapter are that strategic purchasing is necessary because, in its absence, health needs that are not expressed as demand may not be met and appropriateness of the care provided cannot be ensured. The examples cited have drawn predominantly on a few countries that have been especially active in developing the institutional components of a strategic purchasing policy. However, it is possible that other countries have not needed to develop these components, as their routine systems are adequate to identify unmet need and develop integrated care packages. This is a hypothesis that can easily be tested by looking at population screening. For some types of screening, such as mammography and cervical screening, there is a consensus that need exists but it may not always be expressed. In particular, there is considerable evidence that uptake is systematically lower among disadvantaged populations, even when services are free at the point of use (Sutton *et al.*, 1994). There is also good evidence that outcomes are better where screening is seen not as an end in itself but as part of an integrated system of early diagnosis and treatment, which includes ensuring the quality of all stages of the screening process as well as mechanisms for referral for further investigation, treatment and follow-up (Hakama *et al.*, 1985). There is also evidence, for breast screening, that radiologists who read most films have higher detection rates (Esserman *et al.*, 2002) and that large screening centres obtain better results than smaller ones (Blanks *et al.*, 2002), both arguments for organizing specialized programmes. An ideal purchaser would wish to pay for integrated programmes that monitored uptake among different groups in the population and provided a coordinated package of care. For other types of screening, such as routine ultrasonography in pregnancy or prostate-specific antigen (PSA) testing, there is either no evidence of effectiveness or evidence of ineffectiveness. In these cases an ideal purchaser would not, at present, pay for these interventions.

An important source of information on these issues is a recent volume of the *International Journal of Technology Assessment in Health Care*, which brings together a series of national case studies examining the operation of mammography, PSA screening, and ultrasonography in pregnancy in selected Western European countries. For the present purposes these have been supplemented by other published papers, including material from the International Breast Cancer Screening Network (http://appliedresearch.cancer.gov/ibsn/), the European Network of Reference Centres for Breast Cancer Screening (http://home.hetnet.nl/%7Emartinth/index.html) as well as by a survey of key informants in selected countries undertaken to inform this chapter. The case studies confirm that there is wide variation between countries (Klabunde *et al.*, 2001). Taking breast cancer screening (the choice of words is deliberate as mammography is only one element of a screening programme) as an example, a few countries, such as the United Kingdom (http://www.doh.gov.uk/public/sb0201.htm), the Netherlands, Luxembourg (Autier *et al.*, 2002), Iceland (Sigfusson & Hallgrimsson, 1990) and Finland (Dean & Pamilo, 1999) have managed to develop integrated policies based on population registers and overseen by quality assurance systems. Similar local programmes have been implemented, with varying degrees of success, in some parts of other countries, such as the Flemish community in Belgium (Vermeulen *et al.*, 2001), the cantons of Geneva, Valais and Vaud in Switzerland (Faisst *et al.*, 2001), the city of Vienna, and in several regions of France, Italy, Spain and Sweden. There are, however, only a few published evaluations of these subnational programmes and those that exist often report low levels of uptake (Ganry *et al.*, 1999) and give little information on other measures such as recall rates or stage at diagnosis.

Where successful, programmes have involved creation of new institutional entities, which can take various forms. Thus, in the United Kingdom, breast cancer screening is undertaken within the National Health Service but as a separately managed programme. It manages the population registers on which invitations are based (derived from lists of women registered with general practitioners), monitors uptake (and takes action where this is low, either in general or in particular groups within the population), provides purpose-built screening centres (both fixed and mobile), and monitors a range of performance measures. It also maintains close links with other parts of the National Health Service, in particular surgical facilities and general practitioners, to ensure that the process of care is integrated.

Other solutions are required in more pluralistic systems. For example, the Dutch system is based on a network of regional cooperatives involving municipal public health offices and cancer centres. Luxembourg, which has also achieved good results within a social insurance system, also established a separate programme backed up by the refusal by sickness funds to reimburse screening mammograms outside the screening programme (Autier *et al.*, 2002).

Elsewhere, however, screening is largely opportunistic. The challenges are especially great in countries with multiple sickness funds. In these countries, state health authorities have often taken responsibility for the other common collective intervention, immunization, as it has proved difficult to achieve high uptake rates simply by reimbursing private physicians. In Germany, for example, it is not even possible to obtain timely information on uptake, which is only obtained at school entry at age six. Immunization is, however, a fairly straightforward, discrete intervention. The problems are even greater for the much more complex process of cancer screening, with its requirement for integration of a population-based element, including monitoring of equity of uptake, with rapid referral to curative care where appropriate. For example, in Germany, although large numbers of mammograms are undertaken, the reduction in breast cancer mortality seen in countries such as the United Kingdom has not occurred (Figure 7.4). The challenges of implementing such programmes in countries where purchasers serve populations that are not defined

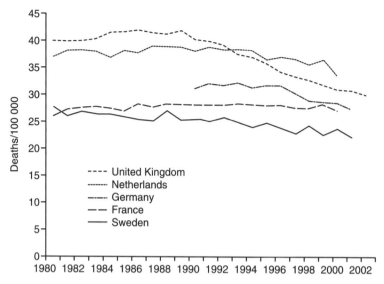

Figure 7.4 Trends in death from breast cancer in selected countries.

by geography are explored in more detail in a companion volume in the European Observatory series (Saltman *et al.*, 2004).

Taking PSA screening as an example of a test that has not been shown to be effective, the United Kingdom was the only one where guidance that it should not be offered has both been produced and been relatively effective. In conclusion, if the nature of screening activities can be considered a tool to assess the scope and nature of strategic purchasing in Europe, it would appear that developments have been extremely uneven.

Conclusions

This chapter suggests a major contradiction between the health system goal to improve health, set out in the *World Health Report 2000* and endorsed by all European governments, and the reality in most European health systems. The evidence presented suggests that the third limb of the triple agency relationship is frequently very limited, at least with regard to improving health. One response is that we have failed to recognize a vast amount of work that takes place routinely but, as it is so commonplace, it is not recorded. We dispute this. In preparation for writing this chapter the initial review of published and unpublished literature, as well as the relevant sections of the Health Systems in Transition reports (www.observatory.dk) was supplemented by a detailed questionnaire that was sent to key informants in most Western European countries and the conclusions were supported by the participants at the workshop during which the chapters of this book were discussed.

If we do believe that achieving health gain should be a central goal of health purchasing, what are the implications? Perhaps the most important one, which is often overlooked, is that purchasing must take account of the changing nature of disease and the responses to it. As we have noted above, in many health systems the organizational and financing structures imply that health care consists of brief, clearly defined interactions between patients and providers. A typical example might be an acute respiratory infection or a cataract extraction. Yet a combination of ageing populations and new therapeutic opportunities means that an increasingly large volume of health care will be for chronic disorders, requiring coordinated interventions by different professionals and specialists over a prolonged period of time. However, many reforms of health services, such as the introduction of diagnosis-related groups, go in the opposite direction, seeking to package health care into isolated, homogeneous interventions. In reality, it is becoming increasingly difficult to define precisely what the product of health care really is.

The information asymmetry between informed purchasers and providers, with the former knowing more about unmet need, means that, unless purchasers intervene actively, treatment will often be suboptimal, especially for those already disadvantaged.

This chapter has identified a series of functions that should take place if improvements in population health are to be achieved. They are development of a health strategy, assessment of needs, design of effective packages of interventions, ensuring that the elements required to deliver these packages are available, and monitoring outcome. The question is then, who should do these things? Specifically, which functions fall within the purchasing role, undertaken by health authorities and sickness funds, and which fall within the stewardship role (see Chapter 8), undertaken by government or agencies acting on its behalf?

In some cases the answer is relatively clear but for others it will depend on the context. Effective health strategies combine both technical and political elements, with the latter including the need for ownership and accountability. They are an intrinsic part of the concept of stewardship and, as such, will inevitably require a major role by government. Stewardship also includes many of the elements required to provide a high quality service, such as regulation of professionals, design standards for facilities, ensuring safety of drugs and equipment, and the generation of knowledge through targeted research programmes. While some of these can be delegated to para-state bodies, they remain the responsibility of governments. Indeed, within the European Union, competition law may preclude purchasers from developing a regulatory role in some circumstances (Mossialos & McKee, 2002).

On the other hand, tasks such as assessment of need, negotiation of contracts for appropriate models of care, and assessment of outcome are more appropriately the rules of purchasers, as they will usually be closer to their populations. However, a note of caution is required. In countries with multiple social insurance funds it may be difficult to know who the population is, as is illustrated by the earlier example of screening.

For other functions, such as the definition of packages of care, the most appropriate location will depend on several circumstances. In many cases there will be economies of scale so that it will be more efficient for guidance to be developed nationally or even internationally. While recognizing the need to respect national differences, there is considerable scope for shared learning here. For example, the Spanish Ministry of Health has adapted and translated some of the English National Service Frameworks.

There is, however, one important message that transcends all of these issues. It is the need for a major investment in the skills available to governments, acting as stewards, and purchasing organizations. Health care purchasing is different from purchasing in many other sectors. The needs are less obvious and the services purchased are more complex. Furthermore, without active involvement by purchasers to support coordination by providers, it is unlikely that the services required will be available for purchase. This means that both governments and purchasers must enhance their skills in the many disciplines that fall within the remit of public health and health service research. It seems likely that it is the relative lack of this expertise that will be the main constraint on the development of effective strategic purchasing in many countries.

References

Agence Nationale d'Accreditation et d'Evaluation en Santé (1999) *Préparer et conduire votre Démarche d'Accreditation*. Paris, ANAES.

Aiken, L.H., Smith, H.L. and Lake, E.T. (1994) Lower medicare mortality among a set of hospitals known for good nursing care. *Medical care*, **32**: 771–787.

Aiken, L.H. *et al.* (1999) Organization and outcomes of inpatient AIDS care. *Medical care*, **37**: 760–772.

Alvarez Dardet, C. (2002) Spain. *In*: Marinka, M., ed. *Health targets in Europe: polity, progress and promise*. London, BMJ Publications.

Autier, P. *et al.* (2002) A breast cancer screening programme operating in a liberal health care system: the Luxembourg Mammography Programme, 1992–1997, *International journal of cancer*, **97**: 828–832.

Banta, H.D. (1994) Health care technology as a policy issue. *Health policy*, **30**: 1–21.

Blanks, R.G. *et al.* (2002) Does individual programme size affect screening performance? Results from the United Kingdom NHS breast screening programme. *Journal of medical screening*, **9**: 11–14.

Britton, A. *et al.* (1999) Threats to applicability of randomised trials: exclusions and selective participation. *Journal of health services research and policy*, **4**: 112–121.

Busse, R., Van der Grinten, T. and Svensson, P.-G. (2002) Regulating entrepreneurial behaviour in hospitals: theory and practice. *In*: Saltman, B.R. and Mossialos, E., eds. *Regulating entrepreneurial behaviour in European health care systems*. Buckingham, Open University Press.

Chapman, J. (2002) *System failure*. London: Demos.

Dean, P.B. and Pamilo, M. (1999) Screening mammography in Finland – 1.5 million examinations with 97 percent specificity. Mammography Working Group, Radiological Society of Finland, *Acta oncologica*, **38**(Suppl. 13): 47–54.

Department of Health and Children (2001) *Quality and fairness: a health system for you*. Dublin, Department of Health and Children.

Donatini, A. *et al.* (2001) *Health care systems in transition: Italy*. Copenhagen, European Observatory on Health Care Systems.

Dowie, J. (1985) The political economy of the NHS: individualist justifications of collective action, *Social science and medicine*, **20**: 1041–1048.

Esserman, L. *et al.* (2002) Improving the accuracy of mammography: volume and outcome relationships, *Journal of the National Cancer Institute*, **94**: 369–375.

Faisst, K., Schilling, J. and Koch, P. (2001) Health technology assessment of three screening methods in Switzerland. *International journal of technological assessment in health care*, **17**: 389–399.

Fitz-Gibbon, C.T. (1996) *Monitoring education: indicators, quality and effectiveness*. London, Cassell.

France, G. (2002) Italy. In: Marinker, M., ed. *Health targets in Europe: polity, progress and promise*. London, BMJ Publications.

Freeman, H.L. (1995) The general hospital and mental health care: a British perspective. *Milbank quarterly*, **73**: 653–676.

Fulop, N. *et al.* (2000) Lessons for health strategies in Europe: the evaluation of a national health strategy in England. *European journal of public health*, **10**: 11–17.

Ganry, O., Peng, J. and Dubreuil, A. (1999) Evaluation of mass screening for breast cancer in the Somme district (France) between 1990 and 1996. *Revue d'épidémiologie et de santé publique*, **47**: 335–341.

Gillam, S.J. (1991) Understanding the uptake of cervical cancer screening: the contribution of the health belief model. *British journal of general practice*, **41**: 510–513.

Goddard, M., Mannion, R. and Smith, P. (2000) Enhancing performance in health care: a theoretical perspective on agency and the role of information. *Health economics*, **9**: 95–107.

Green, J. and Wintfeld, N. (1995) Report cards on cardiac surgeons. Assessing New York State's approach, *New England journal of medicine*, **332**: 1229–1232.

Hakama, M. *et al.* (1985) Evaluation of screening programmes for gynaecological cancer. *British journal of cancer*, **52**: 669–673.

Hannan, E.L. *et al.* (1994) New York state's cardiac surgery reporting system: four years later. *Annals of thoracic surgery*, **58**: 1852–1857.

Hansson, L.R. (2000) Targets for health: a regional participatory approach in Sweden, *European journal of public health*, **10**: 30–33.

Haute Comité de la Santé Publique (2002) *La santé en France*. Paris, Haute Comité de la Santé Publique.

Karjalainen, S. (1990) Geographical variation in cancer patient survival in Finland: chance, confounding, or effect of treatment? *Journal of epidemiology and community health*, **44**: 210–214.

Kehoe, S. *et al.* (1994) The influence of the operating surgeon's specialization on patient survival in ovarian carcinoma. *British journal of cancer*, **70**: 1014–1017.

Klabunde, C. *et al.* (2001) Quality assurance for screening mammography: an international comparison. *Journal of epidemiology and community health*, **55**: 204–212.

Koskinen, S.V. and Melkas, T.A. (2002) Finland. In: Marinker, M., ed. *Health targets in Europe: polity, progress and promise*. London, BMJ Publications.

Krasnik, A. (2000) Targets for health: the learning curve. *European journal of public health*, **10**(4S): 17–19.

Laing, S.P. *et al.* (1999) The British Diabetic Association cohort study, I: all-cause mortality in patients with insulin-treated diabetes mellitus. *Diabetic medicine*, **16**: 459–465.

Leggetter, S. *et al.* (2002) Ethnicity and risk of diabetes-related lower extremity amputation: a population-based, case-control study of African Caribbeans and Europeans in the United Kingdom. *Archives of internal medicine*, **162**: 73–78.

Lomax, E. (1994) The control of contagious disease in nineteenth-century British paediatric hospitals. *Social history of medicine*, **7**: 383–400.

Mackenbach, J.P. *et al.* (1988) Post-1950 mortality trends and medical care: gains in life expectancy due to declines in mortality from conditions amenable to medical intervention in the Netherlands. *Social science and medicine*, **27**: 889–894.

Marinker, M. (2002) *Health targets in Europe: polity, progress and promise*. London, BMJ Books.

Marshall, S.W. *et al.* (1993) Social class differences in mortality from diseases amenable to medical intervention in New Zealand. *International journal of epidemiology,* **22**: 255–261.

Matsushima, M. *et al.* (1997) Geographic variation in mortality among individuals with youth-onset diabetes mellitus across the world. DERI Mortality Study Group, Diabetes Epidemiology Research International. *Diabetologia,* **40**: 212–216.

McKee, M. (1999a) For debate – does health care save lives? *Croatian medical journal,* **40**: 123–128.

McKee, M. (1999b) Settings 3: health promotion in the health care sector. *In:* European Commission *The evidence of health promotion effectiveness: shaping public health in a new Europe.* Luxembourg, European Commission.

McKee, M. and Clarke, A. (1995) Guidelines, enthusiasms, uncertainty, and the limits to purchasing. *BMJ,* **310**: 101–104.

McKee, M. and Healy, J. (2002) Réorganisation des systèmes hospitaliers: leçons tirées de l'Europe de l'Ouest. *Revue médicale de l'assurance maladie,* **33**: 31–36.

McKee, M. and Hunter, D. (1995) Mortality league tables: do they inform or mislead? *Quality in health care,* **4**: 5–12.

McKee, M. and Sheldon, T. (1998) Measuring performance in the NHS: good that it's moved beyond money and activity but many problems remain. *BMJ,* **316**: 322.

McPherson, K. *et al.* (1982) Small-area variations in the use of common surgical procedures: an international comparison of New England, England, and Norway. *New England journal of medicine,* **307**: 1310–1314.

Mossialos, E. and McKee, M. (2002) *EU Law and the social character of health care.* Brussels, Peter Lang.

Nicholl, J. and Turner, J. (1997) Effectiveness of a regional trauma system in reducing mortality from major trauma: before and after study. *BMJ,* **315**: 1349–1354.

Örtendahl, C. (2002) Sweden. *In:* Marinker, M., ed. *Health targets in Europe: polity, progress and promise.* London, BMJ Publications.

Pope, C.J., Roberts, J.A. and Black, N.A. (1991) Dissecting a waiting list. *Health services management research,* **4**: 112–119.

Porter, R. (1997) *The greatest benefit to mankind.* London: HarperCollins.

Saltman, R., Busse, R. and Figueras, J., eds. (2004) *Social health insurance systems in Western Europe.* European Observatory on Health Systems and Policies Series. Maidenhead, Open University Press.

Sant, M. *et al.* (2001) Cancer survival increases in Europe, but international differences remain wide. *European journal of cancer,* **37**: 1659–1667.

Sarkisian, C.A. *et al.* (2001) Expectations regarding ageing among older adults and physicians who care for older adults. *Medical care,* **39**: 1025–1036.

Scrivens, E. (2002) Accreditation and the regulation of quality in health services. *In:* Saltman, R.B., Busse, R. and Mossialos E., eds. *Regulating entrepreneurial behaviour in European health care systems.* Buckingham, Open University Press.

Shaukat, N., De Bono, D.P. and Cruikshank, J.K. (1993) Clinical features, risk factors, and referral delay in British patients of Indian and European origin with angina matched for age and extent of coronary atheroma. *BMJ,* **307**: 717–718.

Sheldon, T. and Chalmers, I. (1994) The United Kingdom Cochrane Centre and the NHS Centre for reviews and dissemination: respective roles within the information systems strategy of the NHS RandD programme, coordination and principles underlying collaboration. *Health economics,* **3**: 201–203.

Sigfusson, B.F. and Hallgrimsson, P. (1990) Breast cancer screening in Iceland: preliminary results. *Recent results in cancer research,* **119**: 94–99.

Smith, P. (1995) On the unintended consequences of publishing performance data in the public sector. *International journal of public administration,* **18**: 277–310.

Snooks, H.A. *et al.* (1996) The costs and benefits of helicopter emergency ambulance services in England and Wales. *Journal of public health medicine*, **18**: 67–77.

Stevens, A. and Raftery, J. (1994) *Health care needs assessment: volume 1*. Oxford, Radcliffe Medical Press.

Stronks, K., Ravelli, A.C. and Reijneveld, S.A. (2001) Immigrants in the Netherlands: equal access for equal needs? *Journal of epidemiology and community health*, **55**: 701–707.

Sutton, S. *et al.* (1994) Prospective study of predictors of attendance for breast screening in inner London. *Journal of epidemiology and community health*, **48**: 65–73.

Tresserras, R. *et al.* (2000) Health targets and priorities in Catalonia, Spain. *European journal of public health*, **10**(4S): 51–56.

Van Herten, L.M. and Van de Water, H.P.A. (2000) Health policies on target? Review on health target setting in 18 countries, *European journal of public health*, **10**(4S): 11–16.

Verity, C. and Nicoll, A. (2002) Consent, confidentiality, and the threat to public health surveillance. *BMJ*, **324**: 1210–1213.

Vermeulen, V., Coppens, K. and Kesteloot, K. (2001) Impact of health technology assessment on preventive screening in Belgium: case studies of mammography in breast cancer, PSA screening in prostate cancer, and ultrasound in normal pregnancy. *International journal of technological assessment in health care*, **17**: 316–328.

Weihrauch, B. (2002) North-Rhine-Westphalia. *In*: Marinker, M., ed. *Health targets in Europe: polity, progress and promise*. London, BMJ Publications.

Weill, A., *et al.* (2000) Modalities of follow-up on non-insulin treated diabetics treated in metropolitan France in 1998. *Diabetes metabolism research and reviews*, **26**(Suppl. 6): 39–48.

Wilson, J.Q. (1991) *Bureaucracy*. New York, Basic Books.

World Health Organization (2000) *The world health report 2000. Health systems: improving performance*. Geneva, WHO.

World Health Organization Regional Office for Europe (1985) *Targets for health for all: targets in support of the European strategy for health for all*. Copenhagen, WHO.

eight

Steering the purchaser: stewardship and government

David J. Hunter, Sergey Shishkin and
Francesco Taroni

Introduction

Stewardship remains a comparatively new term in the lexicon of health policy. Indeed, it has yet to be translated into all languages in Europe. In Germany, for instance, the term has no translation but is used in its English version. But what does stewardship mean? And why has it assumed greater importance in the context of health system reform?

In its *World Health Report 2000*, the World Health Organization (WHO) defined stewardship as 'the careful and responsible management of the well-being of the population' and as constituting 'the very essence of good government' (World Health Organization, 2000). It identified stewardship as 'arguably the most important' health system function, ranking above health service delivery, input production and financing. The reason for this is that 'the ultimate responsibility for the overall performance of a country's health system must always lie with government.' In this respect, stewardship has similarities to the notion of public governance, although there are important distinctions to be made (Travis *et al.*, 2002). Whereas governance includes many actions unconnected with improving health, the actions of stewardship are all about improving health. Therefore, 'stewardship, as one of the core functions of the health system, is a distinct entity' (Travis *et al.*, 2002). It is also inevitably, given its importance and centrality to the operation of a health care system, an intensely political activity because how it is performed and the goals it pursues, either explicitly or implicitly, involve paying attention to particular values and ignoring, or devoting less attention to, others.

According to WHO, stewardship embraces three core tasks undertaken by government and its agents, primarily by the health ministry charged with overseeing and guiding the working and development of the nation's health actions on the government's behalf. The three tasks are:

- formulating health policy – defining the vision and strategic direction;
- exerting influence – including approaches to regulation;
- generating and using intelligence.

In their discussion of stewardship, Travis *et al.* (2002) elaborate on these tasks and produce an augmented set of domains, which include ensuring tools for implementation, coalition/partnership building, a fit between policy objectives and organizational structures and culture, and accountability. At the heart of the concept is the notion that resources – both human and financial – for health care must be used for the benefit of all. These resources do not 'belong' to those exercising stewardship; they have been entrusted to them to act on in the best interests of society. Stewardship is therefore about *collective* rather than *individual* responsibility.

The theme of this chapter is government's stewardship role in health systems with regard to purchasing. This is a recent notion and we shall consider what it means for government to perform a stewardship function in purchasing and provide a conceptual framework for understanding it. We shall detail the core tasks of stewardship, using examples drawn from European health systems and the case studies of purchasing arrangements derived from 11 countries and specially prepared for this project (Figueras *et al.*, forthcoming) and consider what constitutes good stewardship and the barriers to its attainment. Again, the points are illustrated with examples from European experience. A final section identifies some practical guidance for policy makers in respect of the stewardship function and the principles and mechanisms that need to be in place to ensure its effective operation.

We should point out that in examining stewardship across Europe there are strict limits on how far it is possible to generalize because its application in practice is highly context specific. Good stewardship depends on both the type of health care system in place and the type of government, decentralized or centralized. Among the health systems to be found in Europe there is 'a plethora of complex administrative and clinical arrangements under which patients obtain health care' (European Commission, 2001). These systems have evolved over a long period of time and are based on very different organizational patterns and principles. Often a mix of models adds to the complexity of health care systems. Moreover, many health care systems are in a constant state of flux, so there is dynamic movement between models with different combinations emerging. Such diversity and constant change make understanding the stewardship of purchasing a complex and incomplete endeavour.

Government as steward

Why has the notion of government as steward become an issue for health policy makers and organizations like WHO? The rise of big government following the Second World War was a consequence in part of introducing welfare systems in many European countries, coupled with the increasing complexity of tasks in which governments unavoidably became engaged. In recent years, there has been a move to encourage governments to 'row less and steer more'. Steering is akin to stewardship and involves making strategic policy decisions and establishing the vision, whereas rowing is about operational service delivery and implementing the vision (Osborne & Gaebler, 1993). Separating the steering and rowing tasks is aimed at allowing governments more scope and space to focus on setting the strategic vision without becoming distracted by, or preoccupied with, delivery and operational concerns.

For all the public cynicism about government and its perceived inability to deliver effective public services, there is no self-evident or viable alternative to effective government involvement in shaping the strategic direction of health systems, ensuring equity, deciding priorities and financing care. As Travis *et al.* (2002) point out, 'a country's government, through its Ministry of Health, remains the "steward of stewards" for the health system, with a responsibility to ensure that they collectively provide effective stewardship.'

If governments are to stand back and steer more while rowing less and become enablers rather than doers, major changes will be needed in the way they have traditionally functioned, especially in centralized and highly politicized health systems. There may be a need for some structural changes, but much more important is the need for a change in mindset and in ways of conducting business. Unfortunately, when it comes to health policy, most governments, in the shape of ministries of health and other central departments, are ill equipped to act as effective steering organizations. As Osborne and Gaebler point out, when governments separate policy management from service delivery they often find that they have no real policy management capacity or the appropriate skills to hand; they have to be acquired or invented. Whatever their pretensions to the contrary, government departments often become embroiled in service delivery or micro-management with the consequence that policy management at a strategic level is done poorly or not at all. The case studies of European health systems, upon which we have drawn to illustrate our arguments, tend to support this conclusion.

Stewardship in the context of purchasing

The theoretical perspective adopted in this book is that purchasers are the government's agents and are expected to fulfil the principal's (the government's) objectives. In a purchasing-based model of health care, government entrusts some stakeholders (for example, 'hived off' agencies, health authorities, regional governments, health funds, local governments, primary care organizations) operating at some level in the system (macro, meso or micro) to purchase a range of health care services on its behalf for the population. Public funds are entrusted to purchasers either through a direct transfer from its central funds or by ensuring mandatory insurance contributions by employers and employees. But government does not have complete information about the allocation of funds by purchasers or about their actions in regard to the delivery of health care services needed by the population and reflected in health priorities. Therefore, exercising leadership, regulation and the acquisition of intelligence become important features of stewardship (see below).

Stewardship as accountability

Another way of conceptualizing stewardship is to view it as a form of accountability. Travis *et al.* (2002) consider accountability a stewardship responsibility since it is about ensuring that all those engaged in health systems, including purchasers, are held to account for their actions. There are many types of accountability (Day & Klein, 1987). Two are important for this discussion. First, there is *accountability for performance*, according to which governments are held to account, at least in democratic theory, by their populations for the successful implementation of their policies, including those health policies for which they are responsible and about which they have been explicit. This type of top-down accountability complements other forms that might be more bottom-up in character and are reviewed elsewhere (see Chapter 6). Much of the discussion about regulation has a bearing on this type of accountability (see below). In the context of purchasing, meeting targets and managing the performance of those organizations operating on behalf of the principal would represent important ways of ensuring accountability. Second, there is *accountability for reasonableness* (Daniels, 1998), which is associated with procedural justice, that is, with how decisions are reached. The process of decision making is therefore as important as the actual substantive decision. Even in cases where the outcome of the decision-making process is contested, if the process of arriving at it is transparent and defensible then this may be said to constitute good stewardship.

Stewardship and levels of government

The exercise of stewardship with respect to the purchasing function occurs in a variety of ways, including: centralized governmental arrangements, devolved governmental arrangements and non-governmental arrangements that might operate centrally and/or locally. In centralized systems, governments can mandate health care organizations to meet specified standards. In decentralized systems, issues of divided responsibility give rise to additional complexity and may produce tensions between national and local levels.

Most European countries have devolved health systems although there are marked variations between the freedoms and powers enjoyed by the various subnational bodies when it comes to purchasing health care. Even countries like the United Kingdom, with a strong tradition of centralization, are attempting to move in the direction of devolving power and responsibility as evidenced by the devolution of political power to elected assemblies in Wales and Northern Ireland and to an elected parliament in Scotland. Regional government in England remains a possibility in the not too distant future. Many other European countries, such as Spain and Italy, have recently gone much further, and some, such as Germany, have long histories of decentralized government.

In decentralized systems there are two forms of accountability. The first involves traditional public accountability where federal and regional governments report separately to their respective constituencies and give an account of the results of their policies and programmes – in the case of health, the extent to which they have delivered on agreed targets and policy goals. The second involves regional governments accounting to the federal government in exchange for resources or because the federal government is the guardian of citizens' rights either through adherence to general principles, as in Sweden, or to specific entitlements, as in Germany, or to both, as in Italy.

Devolving responsibility is not a neutral act and may carry profound consequences for the government's strategic vision and stated policy goals (Hunter *et al.*, 1998). In the case of the purchasing function in health, there is a major tension between striving for uniformity on the one hand and encouraging diversity, and choice on the other. Many European countries have decided in favour of diversity, and the grip of central government over the health system is weak or restricted to fiscal regulation.

Devolution is intended to increase accountability and responsiveness to local communities, and provide appropriate incentives for efficient and high quality public services sensitive to individual preferences. Devolving responsibility to local organizations, however, creates a tension insofar as they may wish to use their freedoms and purchasing power to diverge from the national policy agenda and do things differently to meet what they consider to be more important local needs and circumstances. However, central governments may have other motives. Devolution may be a convenient way of absolving responsibility and diffusing and deflecting blame when/if things go wrong (Klein, 1995). In this way, central government can divest itself of any effective stewardship role and blame the periphery for getting it wrong.

There are therefore sound reasons for the concern expressed by some observers that health care systems displaying principles of universalism and solidarity might be adversely affected by devolving responsibilities for the financing and/or purchasing of health care to subnational governments. Devolution in health systems means trading off local autonomy with national policy commitments to equity and public financing. Almost by definition, greater local responsibility, power and control are likely to result in difference and a widening of variations as local concerns and priorities jostle with national ones. However, many would argue that encouraging variation and diversity, or at the very least tolerating it, is the whole point of devolution, provided that minimum standards exist to ensure adherence to an acceptable level of quality and performance.

Multilevelled governance inevitably makes the stewardship function in purchasing health care more complex and less clear. The evidence across Europe is that countries have either devolved responsibilities over the planning and regulation of health policy to regional bodies or are in the process of doing so. But these are dynamic developments and in countries as diverse as Hungary and the United Kingdom there are pressures operating to ensure that central government retains overall control over what happens at subnational levels. As we shall consider below, the growth of regulation can be a means through which central government can reassert itself and restore its weakened influence and power. The relationship between central government and subnational levels is therefore one that has constantly to be renegotiated as circumstances change.

Formulating health policy

The first task of stewardship lies in formulating the direction of health policy. Government has the task of formulating a strategic vision for the health system as a whole within which the activities of purchasers are expected to occur but its ability to influence purchasing through such means can be problematic. The attempt to formulate a vision usually occurs in policy statements and strategic plans in many countries, and can take many forms. It might focus on health gain/outcomes or on the functioning of the health care system, and direct purchasers to emphasize cost containment or result in structural changes in health care delivery – for example, a shift from secondary to primary care or from inpatient to outpatient treatment – or to the application of clinically effective and efficient procedures such as evidence-based medicine.

Many governments seek to address both means (the amount of resources allocated to health care, or numbers of doctors and nurses, and so forth) and ends (health gain, narrowing the health gap between social groups) although there is sometimes a tendency for the means to overshadow the ends, or even become ends in themselves. There can also be questions about the link between ends and means insofar as it is not at all clear that simply putting more resources into health care services will lead to an improvement in health (Lewis *et al.*, 2000).

Having an explicit health policy can serve several purposes. At a purely symbolic level it provides a rallying point for those seeking to change the health system as well as for those striving to maintain traditional principles. It can point the way forward to a different future and act as a route map for getting there and, by doing so, make the clash of values explicit – witness the debate over creeping privatization of the British NHS and the Italian SSN in the early 1990s. It can also be a means of prioritizing the objectives of a health system. Health policy is, therefore, an important instrument of governments and, in WHO's terms, 'an important role of governance'.

When health policy focuses on health gain, it is common practice for countries to produce eloquent and usually highly ambitious strategies. These are often of an aspirational nature – long on rhetoric and good intentions but short on delivery. There are many reasons for this, including the absence of ownership of the strategies by those charged with their implementation. A good example of the fate that can often befall grandiose strategies can be found in the United Kingdom at the time of the first health strategy in England, *The Health of the Nation*, which existed from 1992 to 1997. Though welcomed by those who sought to strengthen a commitment to health rather than simply health care, the strategy largely went unimplemented. It ceased to matter as the attention of ministers and their officials continued to centre almost exclusively on the health care delivery system and its performance (Department of Health, 1998; Hunter, 2003a).

Italy adopted a similar strategy based on health targets in 1998 with its National Health Plan. The strategy covered five key areas of population health (promoting healthy behaviour and lifestyles; combating major diseases; improving the environment; protecting disadvantaged people; upgrading the system to European standards) and set 100 national targets for each of these.

The task of implementing the new agenda for health, possibly the most ambitious and challenging set by any Italian government, failed miserably, mainly because of political and institutional problems (France & Taroni, 2000) (see Box 8.1). The 'whole health approach' means that action at the national, regional and local levels must be coordinated, and that no single agency at any level owns the targets. Policy integration requires the different agents to form a 'seamless' health policy, in stark contrast to decades of intergovernmental conflicts marked by the erosion of mutual trust and respect.

Box 8.1 National Health Plan in Italy

In Italy, the central government failed to have its National Health Plan 1998–2001 implemented and the new health strategy remained trapped in complex negotiations between the national government, parliament and the regions. The shift to market solutions in the early 1990s led to a new conception of the role of the state. It was restricted to establishing and safeguarding the basic principles for health services and controlling global spending through appropriate framework legislation. Further reform in 1999 implied a departure from the market model and a shift in the style of state intervention, including a strengthening of the planning responsibilities of the management bodies at regional level. The three-year National Health Plan mentioned above set out objectives translated into a set of targets. Regional and local plans reflect these targets and set out how they will be achieved. The Ministry of Health is responsible for assessing implementation of the National Health Plan, but with the move to decentralization since the early 1990s, the controls available to the Ministry are limited. Most powers have been devolved to the regional health departments and local health units.

Some European countries have issued no health policy statement or strategy and, even where one exists, its influence on health system outputs and outcomes is often limited. For example, in the Czech Republic, the Ministry of Health is responsible for health policy but this is simply a description of regulatory measures and legislative plans and there is no vision for health that is related to, for example, the WHO's 'Health 21'. Government representatives are members of the boards of directors of the health insurance funds. These boards set the strategic direction for purchasing health services but the focus is more on maintaining financial stability than on undertaking strategic purchasing. The government has limited power to control the quality or volume of services. Similarly, in Estonia, the role of government in setting the strategic direction has been minimal, although the regulatory powers of the central health insurance fund are increasing. Public health programmes are reflected in the plan of the national fund.

In Germany, the government's role has centred on regulation rather than on producing a clear health policy vision in relation to the purchasing functions of the health funds and their ability to control patterns of service provision. As a result, there is no integration of public health priorities into purchasing decisions. Progress has not occurred because the issue goes to the heart of the German health system and the balance of power between physicians and their autonomy versus the interests of the health funds to control costs.

In countries like Spain and Italy with weak central government departments and powerful regions, the stewardship role of central government is shared with regional governments. In Spain, despite the central government's intention to exercise stewardship through its central health plan, which lays down the general framework of the health system and sets priority areas for action in accordance with the regional plans, there has been difficulty in approving plans to perform these functions.

Producing the vision or strategy is often the easy part. As the examples above have shown, ensuring effective implementation is much more problematic because it involves time-consuming alliance building among many potentially competing interests. Governments must rely for success in meeting their policy goals on the compliance of those providing services on the front line. Often this is not forthcoming, particularly when those front-line practitioners have no sense of ownership of a policy they perceive to be largely imposed on them and suspect government of being motivated by political considerations rather than by what might be in the best interests of those working in, and receiving, health care. As a consequence, many countries suffer from an 'implementation gap' when it comes to realizing their policy goals. Moreover, effective stewardship demands high standards of probity and a high-trust environment if those agencies charged with implementing government policy (and the public) are to comply with government demands. In countries like Hungary, for instance, there is a general distrust of government which serves as a major impediment to effective stewardship. Such distrust is a growing feature of all governments and may, paradoxically, result in part from the growing advance of the regulatory state (see next section).

It would appear from the above discussion that influencing the direction of health systems through health policy has, despite some brave attempts to change direction, largely been a failure. Limited success has occurred in producing impressive policy statements and in attempts by some governments to focus on health improvement, but they have not been accompanied by a similar commitment to action or ensuring effective and sustainable implementation of policy objectives. Perhaps it is the persistence of implementation failure that has encouraged governments to pay greater attention to the regulatory function.

Exerting influence through regulation

Regulation is a key component of stewardship and, in particular, of ensuring that those charged with purchasing succeed in achieving the desired policy goals. It entails putting in place appropriate institutional arrangements consistent with the vision and capable of monitoring the activities of the purchasers in carrying out their functions. It has been defined as 'sustained and focused control exercised by a public agency over activities which are valued by a community' (Selznick, 1985). In the main, and regardless of how or by whom it is conducted, regulation in most European countries centres on cost control or on ensuring that the books are balanced and bottom lines are respected. It tends not to be overly concerned with strategic issues of a particular health system's vision or with quality considerations. Even where quality factors do figure, the suspicion remains that cost issues are critical as far as politicians are concerned.

With the move in the late 1980s/early 1990s from an integrated model of health service finance and provision to a contract model, regulation has assumed greater importance as a key component of stewardship (Ham, 1996; European Health Management Association, 2000). The growing complexity, diversity and plurality of health systems poses particular challenges in adopting the optimal regulatory framework and equipping the regulators with the appropriate understanding and skills to be able to execute their task effectively. Regulation has therefore become a growing preoccupation of governments as they seek not only to control the cost of health systems but also to ensure their quality and responsiveness to patients and public. It goes beyond the narrow economic concern of remedying market failure as it can be an instrument to achieve wider social goals such as equity or social solidarity as well as to hold powerful professional and/or corporate interests to account (Walshe, 2002). As governments seek to avoid, or withdraw from, direct micromanagement of the health system at subnational levels by ministries of health or other central departments – the so-called 'age of steering' – regulatory arrangements assume greater importance as the means of exercising control over the periphery (Moran, 2001). A separate volume in the Observatory series provides an in-depth analysis of government efforts to regulate entrepreneurial behaviour in European health care systems (Saltman *et al.*, 2002).

Despite moves to devolve powers to purchasing/paying organizations, most national governments remain in overall charge and retain a social responsibility for health service delivery according to the needs of the population. They have an influencing rather than controlling role over the actions of purchasers. In the case of France, for instance, a great deal of regulation continues to be conducted at a national level by the government despite efforts to strengthen the regional level. In contrast, in Estonia the regulatory role of government has been mini-mal, although a new health insurance bill before the parliament providing more direct regulation over purchasing could change the situation. In Italy, too, the role of central government has become less relevant as responsibility for the functioning, effectiveness and efficiency of health agencies has been devolved to regional governments.

In Hungary, health insurance funds are independent, legally constituted institutions. The government can regulate these funds in a variety of ways. First, government representatives from the Ministries of Finance and Health partici-pate on the board of directors and supervisory boards of the health insurance fund. Second, the government approves decisions coming out of negotiations among insurers, providers and professional chambers on coverage, prices and conditions for delivering care. Third, the government is entitled to make decisions on coverage and so on if decisions cannot be reached through negotiations between the funds and providers. On several occasions, the Minis-try of Health has set fees. Despite these powers, the government has limited tools to control quality or volume of services. In the Russian Federation, the enforcement of the federal regulation of purchasers is weak, with most regulation carried out at the regional level. In Germany, regulation is a multilayered endeavour involving self-regulatory institutions, the government and the social courts.

Within national governments, the regulatory role may be split between separate departments or ministries. In Spain, for instance, the Ministries of Health, Labour and Social Affairs, Economy, Finance, and Public Administration all have a regulatory function in the health system.

Regulation can take two basic forms – deterrence or compliance (Walshe, 2002). The deterrence model is akin to the form of regulation criticized by O'Neill (2002) as it assumes that those being regulated are 'amoral calculators' who put profit or other motivations before the public good. Lack of trust is almost built into the model. Demanding standards and tough enforcement are therefore required to ensure that stated goals are met. The compliance model, on the other hand, assumes that those being regulated are fundamentally well meaning and would do the right thing if they could. Regulators therefore provide support and advice and are forgiving if lapses occur.

Regulatory mechanisms

With respect to stewardship, governments must decide which form of regulation they wish to support to achieve effective policies and services. Structural arrangements and mechanisms put in place by governments to regulate purchasing include:

- setting health benefits package;
- strategic health planning;
- regulation of purchasers' budgets and risk compensation;
- framework and rules for contracting;
- participation on boards of purchasers;
- regulation of consumer information and participation; and
- setting requirements for purchasers' reports.

Setting health benefits packages

Governments often set some requirements that determine the structure, volume, quality and cost of health care services that might, or should, be purchased for the eligible population. The health benefits package is the principal tool used to set such requirements in many countries. Some countries have set universal national packages that include the types of care and/or positive lists of services guaranteed for all citizens or insured persons. Such packages have been adopted in, for example, Armenia, the Czech Republic, Estonia, Germany, the Russian Federation, Slovakia, Slovenia, Spain and Switzerland. A very different approach from setting a health benefits package is to establish negative lists of medical services that are excluded from public funding. Such lists are evident in, for instance, Finland, Latvia, Lithuania and Italy (see Box 8.2 for details of the basic benefits package in Italy). Yet another approach, as found in Sweden, involves setting guidelines and priorities for purchasers.

Box 8.2 Basic benefits package in Italy

In Italy, the national government and the regions reached an agreement over the basic benefits package (*livelli essenziali di assistenza*) that was supposed to define the appropriate level of health service coverage the regions must ensure under the comprehensiveness principle of the SSN. A negative list approach was adopted implicitly, assuming that comprehensiveness means 'what doctors and hospitals do' (and is paid for from the public purse). A few marginal procedures were excluded from public coverage, with a limited impact on the financial outlay of the SSN, including cosmetic surgery and alternative medicine. Benefits excluded from public funding can, however, be covered either through additional regional resources or complementary private insurance. For both technical reasons, such as limited evidence of effectiveness, and matters of political priorities, the basic benefits package does not provide a positive list of citizens' entitlements but defines instead a relatively high financial floor of public expenditure for health care. However, the lack of a positive list also leaves the central government without the teeth to enforce its national standards of coverage which remain open to interpretation and negotiation.

The setting of explicit lists, both positive and negative, raises the question of whether purchasers might have some freedom to alter established packages of benefits and in particular to offer additional benefits over and above these under private or complementary insurance arrangements. The general view is that such freedom is undesirable because the possible variations among purchasers in the benefits packages available would have negative consequences on risk-selection processes. This issue is perhaps best illustrated by developments in Germany, where the minimum services covered by social health insurance are set out in the Social Code Book, article 3, in generic terms: prevention of disease; screening for disease; treatment of disease (ambulatory medical care, dental care, drugs, non-physician care, medical devices, inpatient/hospital care, nursing care at home, and certain areas of rehabilitative care); transportation, and so on. The reform proposal to make some benefits (spa treatment, rehabilitative services, short-term nursing care, non-emergency ambulance transportation and physiotherapy) optional for insurers was considered in 1996. The intention was to allow individual health funds to decide upon inclusion of these services in their benefits catalogue. However, the reform proposal failed because of the threat of cream skimming, that is, the removal by some health funds of the additional benefits from their package and the offer of lower contribution rates to attract a healthier clientele. At the same time, expenditure of other health funds for voluntary benefits would have been outside the risk compensation mechanism operating among the funds. This would have had the effect of forcing generous insurance funds out of the market.

Strategic health planning

A number of European countries have used strategic health plans as reference guides for purchasers. Hospital planning is a traditional tool available to governments in most countries. But its content has evolved in recent years in those countries where the conception of stewardship has been developed. For example, in France, hospital planning used to define targets in terms of bed/population ratios or equipment/population ratios in geographical areas. Such plans were used for the authorization of proposals to establish new beds or change the use of existing ones, whether in public or private hospitals. However, since the mid-1990s, strategic planning has evolved towards a more qualitative and output-based planning of services. These plans are based on a general framework for regional action and priorities. They resemble the National Service Frameworks introduced into the NHS in the United Kingdom, which cover cancer, coronary heart disease, care for elderly people, mental health and diabetes. See Box 8.3 on regional planning in France.

Box 8.3   Regional planning in France

In France, the regional strategic health plans set out the goals for the direction of regional provision of hospital care over a five-year period. The plans permit the regional hospital agencies to act as purchasers, giving them responsibility to grant authorizations, approve proposals submitted by the providers, and negotiate contracts with hospitals. In turn, the regional strategic health plans are influenced by national strategic health planning. The French government has issued policy frameworks to define national programmes for priority health action. Cancer, diabetes, mental health, control of pain, and tobacco addiction are among the current national priorities, with both preventive and curative objectives. These priorities constitute a general framework for regional action and are translated into regional health programmes and hospital plans.

In some countries, governments regulate the activities of purchasers by setting plans and defining the volume of health care services that should be available to the eligible population. The example of the Russian Federation is illustrated in Box 8.4.

Regulation of purchasers' budgets and risk compensation

In most European countries, governments have put in place mechanisms to regulate the size of the budget and ensure redistribution of financial resources among purchasers according to population. There are three main ways to regulate purchasers' budgets:

• Approval of a purchaser's budget in cases where the purchaser is a public organization. The approved budget may consist of spending ceilings for different kinds of health care. For instance, in Hungary each year, parliament

Box 8.4 Programme of state guarantees in the Russian Federation

In the Russian Federation, the government annually approves the Programme of State Guarantees for Free Health Care for the Citizens of the Russian Federation, setting the volume of outpatient, inpatient and ambulance care per 1000 population that should be delivered free to the citizens and funded from public sources. This programme obliges the state to provide specified medical care to the population and at the same time it is a tool to push structural changes in the health care system. Regional governments approve their own territorial programmes of state guarantees on the basis of the federal programme. The territorial programme includes a set of corresponding local programmes. These programmes are used as framework plans for the purchasers of health care services (territorial mandatory health insurance funds and their branches, health insurance companies, regional and local governments).

determines the size of the budget of the National Health Insurance Fund Administration for acute and chronic inpatient care, outpatient specialist services and primary care. It is not allowed to transfer money between them.
- Setting a projected ceiling or soft budget for a purchaser. In France, the National Assembly approves the ceiling for health insurance expenditure for the coming year in the annual act on the financing of social security. This is a target, not a cash-limited budget.
- Setting the rules for the distribution of funds among purchasers. For instance, in the Netherlands the Minister of Health establishes the rules governing the allocation of public funds by the Board for Health Care Insurance among purchasers.

In most mandatory health insurance systems governments introduce a financing mechanism to compensate for differences in the risk structure of different purchasers. For example, in Germany a risk structure compensation mechanism is in place to provide all health funds with an equal starting position or a level playing field for competition aimed at equalizing contribution rates (due to varying income levels) and expenditure (taking into account the age and sex of the enrolled population). In the Netherlands, a much more complex process aims at defining a risk adjustment formula taking into account as many demographic and clinical factors as possible in order to prevent selection among the health funds (Van de Ven *et al.*, 1994; Van de Ven & Ellis, 2000). The compensatory mechanism includes the risk compensation scheme among health funds, which are required to provide or receive compensation for the differences in their contributory incomes as well as in average expenditures and morbidity.

Framework and rules for contracting

A widespread form of purchasing regulation involves a framework contract with purchasers, providers and professional chambers. For example, in France the framework contract concerning the budget ceiling is agreed between the state and the national fund organization that manages the general health insurance scheme. In Slovenia, the sectoral framework contracts are negotiated by the Ministry of Health, the National Health Insurance Institute and each relevant provider association. Framework contracts determine the selective contracts that the insurance fund signs with health care providers.

In some countries the government either directly participates in contracting among purchasers and providers or approves such contracts. For example, in the Czech Republic the government approves agreements negotiated among the insurers, providers and professional chambers on coverage, prices and conditions for delivering care, and the Ministry of Finance issues the decisions as an order. The government is also entitled to make these decisions if they cannot be reached through negotiation between funds and providers. In France, the Ministry of Health approves the national agreements signed between the health insurance funds and the organizations representing the health care professionals in private practice.

Contracting procedures can also be subject to regulation. In Germany, the government regulates through the Social Code Book, which defines the goals and scope of negotiations between the sickness funds and providers of health care. In France, the government regulates the procedures governing litigation between health professionals and the insurance funds. In Italy, an accreditation process has been introduced whereby all public and private facilities must satisfy specific criteria in order to be contracted by the SSN.

Participation on boards of purchasers

A principal tool for regulating the management of purchaser organizations is the participation of government representatives on boards of health insurance funds. For example, in the Czech Republic representatives of the national government are members of the board of directors of the national health insurance fund as one of three stakeholders. Such governmental participation on boards of mandatory health insurance funds raises questions about who exactly should be represented on the boards. The Estonian experience highlights some problems arising from the participation of local government representatives on the advisory boards of regional health funds. As owners of the local hospitals, the representatives often defend those hospitals' interests rather than protecting the interests of the insured, especially in those cases where treatment is only available outside the region.

Regulation of consumer information and participation

Many countries, particularly those with social health insurance systems, have also put in place regulation to ensure citizen participation on purchaser boards (see Chapter 6). Moreover, regulatory arrangements are in place to improve the information given by purchasers to consumers. This kind of regulation is evident in France. According to the law enacted in 2003, health funds, as well as complementary insurers, set up call centres to give advice to the insured on professionals and facilities (for example, the prices of services offered by physicians who are allowed to charge fees in excess of the standard negotiated tariff).

Setting requirements for purchasers' reports

Finally, governments can also regulate purchasing by setting the formal criteria for standardized reports of purchasers. However, these reports are sometimes limited in scope. For example, in the Czech Republic the health insurance funds have to issue annual reports and annual accounts according to strict requirements. The reports have to be approved by the parliament. In practice, though, the only criteria for approval are the financial stability of the system (for example, no catastrophic losses for funds or providers), and the political balance in the health sector, to wit, no explicit dissatisfaction from physicians or the public. The quality or volume of services are given little emphasis in the approval process.

Using intelligence

Good intelligence, or what is sometimes referred to as knowledge management, is an essential component of modern health systems. These have become more complex and involve numerous interactions and relationships between multiple professional groups and organizations both public and private (profit and not-for-profit) not to mention growing involvement by patients and consumer associations. Understanding their respective values and cultures and how they work is essential to ensure optimal joint working (Degeling et al., 2001; Hunter, 2002). Good stewardship in respect of effective purchasing requires sound intelligence in order to show the extent to which government health policy is being achieved and the constraints that hinder implementation. Such knowledge is necessary to inform policy and perhaps modify it in the light of experience.

Intelligence is broader than information. As Travis et al. (2002) explain, 'it implies identifying and interpreting essential knowledge for making decisions from a range of formal and informal sources – routine information, research, the media, opinion polls, pressure groups etc.'

Intelligence is also necessary if evidence-based policy is to inform health strategy. This is possibly the most important area of the stewardship role in relation to purchasing but also the most tricky and difficult to achieve. Countries such as the UK and the Netherlands have invested heavily in evidence-based medicine and evidence-based policy although the impact of this investment on practice is contested. The fact that much policy is not evidence-based raises issues about the nature of evidence and how it can best be deployed to influence policy (Black, 2001; Hunter, 2003b). For example, in respect of medicine and the interventions that are possible, a growing focus on evidence-based decision making has resulted in guidelines and protocols to govern clinical practice. In England, the National Institute for Clinical Excellence provides evidence to purchasers and providers on what constitute cost-effective interventions.

Many countries appear to have adopted, or are in the process of adopting, evidence-based clinical guidelines and protocols. In Italy, for instance, the National Health Plan envisages the development of a national programme on health care quality aimed at the continuous and systematic improvement, assessment and monitoring of all dimensions of quality. This aims to steer the behaviour of health care professionals towards appropriate and effective treatments and services. There is also the national programme for the elaboration, dissemination and evaluation of clinical guidelines. Its focus will be on implementation rather than on guideline development in order to encourage effective clinical practice.

In the Russian Federation, the Ministry of Health has announced the development and adoption of clinical standards and protocols as one of the major priorities in health policy. The intention is to make the clinical process more cost effective throughout the regions and medical organizations. In Estonia, the development of guidelines and protocols is also a major component of health policy but their impact on practice depends on the attitude and approach of providers.

In Spain, the approach to clinical governance has been variable. Most progress has been made in those health centres and services where there are enthusiastic clinicians. In Germany, too, progress is patchy. In some hospitals evidence-based clinical pathways are used although there is no legal obligation for them to do so. However, guidelines are an area of special policy emphasis. The introduction of disease management programmes, which are required to demonstrate they are evidence-based, is likely to accelerate the use of evidence and the adoption of a formal system of clinical governance.

Intelligence is crucial in terms of assessing the health needs of the population to informing health policy development and purchasing decisions. With few exceptions, though, the majority of countries surveyed are not in a position to undertake health needs assessment and to integrate its results into purchasing decisions. See Table 8.1 for some examples. Experience with health needs assessment and evidence-based protocols for purchasing is also dealt with in some depth in Chapter 7 on purchasing and public health.

Intelligence also informs the public about developments in health policy and the extent to which government targets and objectives are being met. In such a setting, the dissemination and manipulation of information to present policy and performance in the best possible light can be tempting for governments and local officials. In the United Kingdom, for instance, there have been a number of cases of 'gaming', where providers and purchasers colluded to fix waiting lists to show better results and demonstrate that government targets were being met. The point here is that intelligence is not value-free but is highly political and can be used for quite different purposes from that for which it was intended.

In most countries, information made available to consumers in making decisions about the purchasing of health services is limited. For example, in the Czech Republic, because the health care package is defined by law and is the same for all funds, little attempt is made to inform the public about their

Table 8.1 The integration of health needs assessment into purchasing decisions

Armenia	Estonia	Finland
Needs assessment lies within the responsibility of the MoH, but there is no information as to how this is informing purchasing decisions	Utilization statistics of the previous years are taken into account in contracting decisions. Public health programmes are reflected in the programme plan of the National Fund	Municipalities do not necessarily possess the capacity to undertake rigorous needs assessment

France	Germany	Hungary
So far limited	No	No

Italy	Latvia	Norway
Local health units are charged with public health monitoring and needs assessment but this is not necessarily linked to their purchasing function. The national and regional health plan sets out targets and priority interventions but is not linked to the purchasing function	Health status and care data are collected by district office of the regional funds. The extent to which these data are taken into account for purchasing decisions at the regional level differs	Regional committees have newly been set up to improve regional planning of health care services through the development of regional health plans. It is not clear how these relate to the purchasing decisions of primary care services

Russian Federation	Spain	Sweden
The prevailing view is that public health is the responsibility of public administration authorities rather than purchaser organizations. Needs assessment is becoming part of the purchasing process	Since 1999, regions have included needs assessment more systematically in the regional health plans. In Catalonia the health plan is used to set targets in contracts with providers	County councils undertake needs assessment for planning services

services. However, the influence of patient organizations in negotiations between funds and providers is growing. In Spain, only a low level of information is available to consumers in general. A key problem is that the current law on data protection prohibits the release of indicators showing the performance of individual hospitals and providers. In Estonia, the information available to consumers comprises a list of services, a list of contracted providers and statistics on average costs. No information is available on the quality of providers.

A similar situation prevails in the Russian Federation, where information about the cost and quality of services in the mandatory health insurance system is not generally available to citizens. In Italy, the availability of information to consumers is not considered an issue because all consumers must use the services provided by the local health unit (LHU) where they reside. Local health units and hospital trusts have begun to produce patient charters, which provide consumers with information on their rights and duties as patients and on the services they can expect to receive.

Overall, the availability and use of intelligence across Europe appears patchy although efforts are being made to improve both the quality of information collected and the use to which it is put. However, it is arguable how much attention is paid to evidence or intelligence by purchasers even when it is available. Neither may be a starting point for action to address health gain. Decisions often emerge from the national and/or local policy-making framework, planning processes, if any, in response to funding opportunities and the 'must dos' of national priorities and targets, where these exist. Often, problems in improving health and health care services are due not to a lack of quality intelligence but to shortfalls of other factors, including political will, clarity of purpose, the ability to manage change, and the flexibility to change direction.

Good stewardship

As we have argued, government may be deemed a good steward if purchasers ensure the delivery of health care according to public needs and in accordance with stated health policy where it exists. Such a redefinition of government's relationship with purchasers raises several fundamental questions, notably, what are the requirements for good stewardship? What barriers might stand in the way of achieving it? Earlier sections have addressed these questions to a degree. This final section attempts to pull together the arguments as well as expand on some of them.

The requirements for good stewardship

The power of government to affect the actions of purchasers is determined by the following factors:

- government's consistency in regulating purchasers according to its strategic vision;
- legislation and agreements to determine purchasers' actions;
- consistency of the reward system used for purchasers and their self-motivation;
- political will to apply sanctions when purchasers abuse their powers;
- government's strict observation of its own rules for financing health care services;
- government monitoring of purchasers.

The feasibility of monitoring purchasers' behaviour depends on at least three factors:

- the technical and economic wherewithal of health ministries;
- the administrative abilities and disciplines of government departments;
- the political feasibility and rationality of monitoring the purchasers' activities.

The barriers to good stewardship

There are many potential barriers to good stewardship – economic, political, social and cultural – which vary significantly among European countries.

Economic barriers

The two principal economic barriers are the gap between guarantees of public health care and available funding, and the high cost of formulating a strategic vision, introducing regulatory arrangements and institutions, and collecting and using intelligence.

Inadequate funding for state guarantees is a global issue but the gap is especially large in the CIS. The Soviet Union's constitutional guarantees of free health care were preserved or slightly reformulated in the constitution of the new states. Public health care expenditures decreased sharply during the transitional economies' decline in the 1990s, and although many of the countries have shown recent economic growth, GDPs are bound to be significantly lower in coming years than in 1991. Correspondingly, the resources for the public funding of health care will also be less than before the transition, meaning that state guarantees of free health care services are not covered. The shortfall of public funds is compensated by patients' out-of-pocket payments. Similar practices occur in other health care systems where funding does not keep pace with increasing expenditures, rising demand or exclusion of services from coverage.

The violation by government of its own obligations to finance health care services weakens its control over the purchasers (health authorities, public health insurance funds and private health insurance companies) and allows them greater scope for opportunistic behaviour as well as sanctioning the inefficient allocation of public funds, all amounting to an erosion of government's responsibility to the population for health protection. To avoid this situation, governments should carefully forecast health care needs, monitor and plan expenses for health care delivery in accordance with state guarantees, and revise the guaranteed health benefits package. If a gap already exists, government, and in particular the Ministry of Health, should ensure that politicians and society resolve the problem, publicizing the dire consequences accruing from inaction. The gap between guarantees and funding of health care can also be regional within a country. In this case, good stewardship means the reform of mechanisms for redistributing funds among regions.

Political barriers

Political barriers to good stewardship include the following:

- The high political cost of reviewing previous government obligations. This barrier is especially high for the CEE and CIS, where the potential for adjustment of guarantees according to available funding is limited by the significant political implications of changing the constitutional rights of the population. Overcoming this barrier is the task of the national government and parliament. Ministries of health could be more persistent in directing attention to the negative consequences of the status quo.
- The inability of government to force institutions to act in accordance with its wishes is one of the main causes of purchaser inefficiency. Such weakness is the key problem arising from the political and economic reforms in the CIS. The solution to this problem largely depends on the state, but health ministries, together with regional and local health care management bodies, could contribute to overcoming this barrier. Good stewardship might itself assist in the strengthening of government power and reinforcement of legal institutions.
- The divergence of fund allocation policies among different government bodies at the same level entails a high political cost of reaching concord among the various bodies. Overcoming this barrier depends on the capacity of health care management bodies to build and sustain coalitions by engaging the actors, using new tools and creating new forms of common activities.
- The divergence of policies and conflicts of interest among government bodies at different levels entail high political costs of achieving alignment of the various policies. Good stewardship presupposes the ability to monitor the policies of different actors at lower levels, to reveal the points of divergence in vision and policy implementation, to organize discussion of them, and to ensure compliance.

Social and cultural barriers

Social and cultural barriers to good stewardship include the following:

- rent-seeking behaviour of officials dealing with the regulation of purchasers but also the risk of purchasers 'capturing' the regulators in order to pursue the same rent-seeking behaviour;
- closed social networks and clannish links between government officials, purchasers and providers, which prevent the enforcement of legal agreements and the allocation of public funds according to efficiency criteria;
- double standards of government behaviour and the attitudes of officials, purchasers and providers towards the guiding vision;
- public mistrust of government;
- peculiarities of the social contract, such as governmental and public support in the CIS for partial substitution of public health care funding by informal payments by patients, along with refusal to accept revision of free health care guarantees;

- the former command-and-control management culture of officials expected to carry out the stewardship functions, which is widespread in the CIS;
- human capital barriers – the inability of officials to alter their behaviour and allocate funds according to efficiency criteria instead of spreading funds across all providers.

The need for large-scale management and organization development programmes, and the need to attract new people to carry out the new functions of government, constitute serious barriers to ensuring good stewardship.

Last word: some guidance for policy makers

As this chapter has sought to demonstrate, stewardship is the very essence of good purchasing and good government. Yet, many countries are falling short of realizing their full potential for good stewardship, especially of the purchasing function. Serious shortcomings in the performance of their health systems persist, causing unacceptable numbers of avoidable deaths or persistent poor quality and unresponsive services. For the most part, purchasers fail to realize or exploit the creative potential of purchasing. They remain, by and large, passive reimbursers of providers. In this regard, 'poorly structured, badly led, inefficiently organized and inadequately funded health systems may do more harm than good' (World Health Organization, 2000). The uses to which resources are put are a test of good stewardship in purchasing. Many resources continue to be misallocated to inappropriate or ineffective interventions.

No country has the perfect health system or is able to provide solutions to all the dilemmas posed by stewardship in purchasing. Few would disagree with the laudable aims of stewardship or with its centrality in the effective running of health systems but, as the preceding sections have sought to demonstrate, there are a number of delicate balances to be achieved in the realization of stewardship and these are offered to policy makers in the form of guidance as they ponder how to make stewardship more effective through better purchasing and more effective exploitation of the opportunities it affords. Policy makers might wish to take note of the following points:

- achieving a balance between central control and local autonomy to clarify their respective stewardship roles;
- acknowledging the widespread public distrust of government while striving for transparency in decision making and recognizing that the complexity of health care decisions may not always allow for the optimal level of transparency;
- getting the right balance between the means and ends of policy so that those charged with implementing policy are fully committed by virtue of having been involved in its creation;
- finding a better balance between 'upstream' and 'downstream' interventions since more might be achieved in improving population health if investment in prevention was given a higher priority;
- recognizing that the stewardship role includes setting the direction of health policy or providing a vision backed up by appropriate intelligence;

- ensuring that appropriate trust-building incentives and a regulatory framework are in place to create the conditions for good stewardship through effective purchasing;
- establishing a set of 'procedural rights' (Bynoe, 1998) including rights to be heard, to consistency and relevance in decision making, to unbiased decisions, to rationale for decisions, and to review;
- ensuring that managers and practitioners have the skills to undertake stewardship tasks and function as effective regulators and effective purchasers.

In addition, as we have sought to show in the preceding sections, a number of conditions need to be in place for good stewardship to occur. In particular, good stewardship is about:

- eradicating the double standards evident in government behaviour and fostering trust in government;
- making the regulation and distribution of funds more transparent;
- increasing the accountability of officials dealing with these matters;
- providing training and development programmes, monitoring health care purchasing and communicating best practice.

Addressing these concerns will require sustained commitment and constant vigilance on the part of policy makers. The matters raised are dynamic and ever shifting, and require regular monitoring and revision in line with changing mores and knowledge. Good stewardship entails being attentive to such concerns and responding to them sensitively but purposefully, with the public interest always to the fore.

References

Black, N. (2001) Evidence based policy: proceed with care, *BMJ*, **323**: 275–279.

Bynoe, I. (1998) Beyond the Citizen's Charter. *In*: Franklin, J., ed. *Social policy and social justice*. Cambridge, Polity Press.

Daniels, N. (1998) Accountability for reasonableness. *BMJ*, **321**: 1300–1301.

Day, P. and Klein, R. (1987) *Accountabilities*. London, Tavistock Publications.

Degeling, P., Hunter, D.J. and Dowdeswell, B. (2001) Changing health care systems. *Journal of integrated care pathways*, **5**(2): 64–69.

Department of Health (1998) *The health of the nation – a policy assessed*. London, The Stationery Office.

European Commission (2001) *The internal market and health services*. Report of the High Level Committee on Health. Luxembourg, Directorate G: Public Health.

European Health Management Association (2000) *The impact of market forces on health systems. A review of evidence in the 15 European Union Member States*. Dublin, European Health Management Association.

Figueras, J., Robinson, R. and Jakubowski, E., eds. (forthcoming) *Purchasing to improve health systems performance: Case studies in European countries*. Copenhagen, European Observatory on Health Systems and Policies. World Health Organization.

France, G. and Taroni, F. (2000) Starting down the road to targets in health: the case of Italy. *European journal of public health*, **10**: 25–29.

Ham, C. (1996) *Public, private or community: what next for the NHS?* London, Demos.

Hunter, D.J. (2002) A tale of two tribes: the tension between managerial and professional values. *In*: New, B. and Neuberger, J., eds. *Hidden assets*. London, King's Fund.

Hunter, D.J. (2003a) *Public health policy*. Cambridge, Polity Press.

Hunter, D.J. (2003b) Evidence-based policy and practice: riding for a fall? *Journal of the Royal Society of Medicine*, **96**: 194–196.

Hunter, D.J., Vienonen, M. and Wodarczyk, W.C. (1998) Optimal balance of centralized and decentralized management. *In*: Saltman, R.B., Figueras, J. and Sakellarides, C., eds. *Critical challenges for health care reform in Europe*. Buckingham, Open University Press.

Klein, R. (1995) *The new politics of the NHS*. London, Longman.

Lewis, S., Saulnier, M. and Renaud, M. (2000) Reconfiguring health policy: simple truths, complex solutions. *In*: Albrecht, G.L., Fitzpatrick, R. and Scrimshaw, S.C., eds. *The handbook of social studies in health and medicine*. London, Sage.

Moran, M. (2001) Not steering but drowning: policy catastrophes and the regulatory state. *The political quarterly*, **72**(4): 414–427.

O'Neill, O. (2002) *A question of trust*. BBC Reith Lectures 2002. London, BBC.

Osborne, D. and Gaebler, T. (1993) *Reinventing government*. New York, Plume.

Saltman, R.B., Busse, R. and Mossialos, E. (2002) *Regulating entrepreneurial behaviour in European health care systems*. Buckingham, Open University Press.

Selznick, P. (1985) Focusing organizational research on regulation. *In*: Noll, R., ed. *Regulatory policy and the social sciences*. Berkeley, University of California Press.

Travis, P. *et al.* (2002) *Towards better stewardship: concepts and critical issues*. Geneva, World Health Organization.

Van de Ven, W. and Ellis, R.P. (2000) Risk adjustment in competitive health plan markets. *In*: Culyer, A.J. and Newhouse, J.P., eds. *Handbook of health economics*. Volume 1A. Amsterdam, Elsevier.

Van de Ven, W. *et al.* (1994) Risk adjusted capitation: recent experiences in the Netherlands. *Health affairs*, **13**: 118–136.

Walshe, K. (2002) The rise of regulation in the NHS. *BMJ*, **324**: 967–970.

World Health Organization (2000) *World Health Report 2000*. Geneva, WHO.

chapter nine

Purchasers, providers and contracts

Antonio Duran, Igor Sheiman, Markus Schneider and John Øvretveit

Introduction

Contracts are the most visible and practical part of purchasing. They are a key tool that defines the relationship between principals (purchasers) and agents (providers). They can be used to reflect the purchaser's health objectives and the health needs of the population, and to make clear what services are to be provided and under which terms. They also have an important function in specifying the risk-sharing arrangements that apply to either the purchaser or provider in the event of unplanned events (see Box 9.1).

Box 9.1 Contracts in countries with separate purchaser and provider functions

In countries with separate purchaser and provider functions, contracts constitute the foundation for health care delivery by:

- linking financial resources to health services outputs and outcomes;
- clarifying the responsibilities of purchasers and providers and improving accountability;
- focusing health care delivery on what really matters to the purchasers and consumers;
- allowing periodical adjustments and renegotiations of health care delivery in line with supply and demand.

In recent years there have been major developments in contracting worldwide. In Europe, contracts are being widely introduced in Beveridge systems, in countries such as England, Italy, Portugal, Spain and Sweden among others. Contracts are also playing a pivotal role in the reform of former communist Semashko-type systems. Following the shift to Bismarck-type funding in countries of Eastern Europe, contracts are increasingly used as a new model for relationships between purchasers and providers. For instance social health insurance funds act as sole purchasers in the Baltic states, Bulgaria, Hungary, Kyrgyzstan and Slovenia and competing health insurers act as purchasers in the Czech Republic, Slovakia and the Russian Federation. In Kazakhstan the law requires government at all levels to contract providers through special units (*Densaolik*, the inheritors of the collapsed health insurance fund). In Armenia, contracting is implemented through the State Agency of Health, a governmental body acting as a third party purchaser.

This chapter analyses the role of contracts as purchasing tools. It describes the various types of contracts as well as their advantages and disadvantages; looks at output specification – a central element in contracting design; considers contracting under conditions of market competition, with an outline of selective contracting in the European Region; covers market and public governance of contracts, regulatory mechanisms and penalties and incentives; and focuses on implementation, first considering the contracting process in relation to the planning cycle, then analysing the obstacles to contract implementation.

Types of contracts

The actual content of a contract can vary considerably. The most frequent items covered are: type and volume of services, duration, price, invoicing, extra-contractual referrals, eligibility, organizational requirements, levels of human resources and facilities, monitoring, remuneration levels, confidentiality of information, sanctions and rewards. Quality standards are a crucial item, usually including waiting times, outcome, audit procedures and targets.

In our analysis of contracting, we distinguish between contractual arrangements to secure the safety net of health care delivery and those related to the actual health care to be delivered within a given timeframe. The first we call *market-entry contracts* and the second *process contracts* (among which a further distinction is made among input, performance and service contracts). Table 9.1 outlines the major differences among them. Another relevant distinction is between hard contracts and soft (also called 'relational') contracts. Roughly speaking the former are contracts in which participants are willing to use legal mechanisms in case of non-compliance. By contrast, soft contracts are less explicit and allow for different non-legal mechanisms to adjust deviations from the original terms of the contract (Dawson and Goddard, 1999).

Market-entry contracts

Licences for doctors or hospitals are market-entry contracts. In all European

Table 9.1 Generic classification of provider contracts in health systems

Purchaser objectives	Market entry contracts	Process contracts		
		Input	Performance	Service
Health objectives	Yes, explicitly formulated, or laid down in ethical codes	No	Yes, explicitly formulated in the contract	No
Health safeguards	Public review	Professional rules and supervision	Internal and external monitoring	Professional rules and supervision
Incentives	By regulation of property rights	Input oriented	Outcome oriented	Output oriented
Access to care	By certification of need	Subscription, obligation of acceptance	Social dimension of health; waiting times	Extra payment for remote areas
Quality	Licensing criteria, accreditation criteria	Disclosure of structure	Disclosure of outcome indicators	Disclosure of process indicators
Cost control	Limitation of contractors	Standards for skill mix, incentives for substitution	Pre-authorization	Budgets, pre-authorization

countries, licensing or accreditation procedures have been set up to secure a high quality safety net for health care delivery organizations, thus guaranteeing an acceptable standard of care. This is often done in combination with planning procedures. One problem with market-entry contracts is their necessary coordination with process contracts (see below).

Market-entry contracts are long-term contracts and are usually a prerequisite for process contracts. They do not link payments to services but only describe the obligations to be fulfilled in order to take part in the health care network. These obligations are usually conditional; licensed providers can be contracted by a public purchaser but the latter can deny them a contract due to, for example, overcapacity. Selective contracts, which combine market-entry and process contracting to a selected group of providers, are seen by many as a means to reorganize supply structures and to adapt them to health needs and policy objectives. Experiences in selective contracting are discussed further below.

Arguments for long-term contracting stress the benefits of securing more efficient investments. The precondition is that returns are clearly related to the contracting period, which may raise time–terms conflicts if the contracting period is too short, a point well illustrated in the recent English experience.

Process contracts

Three types of process contract are analysed, namely input contracts, performance contracts and service contracts.

Input contracts

Typically, input contracts are salary contracts: for example, nurses and doctors are paid for the time spent delivering services. These contracts do not usually have explicitly formulated performance goals, but jobs are usually described and major responsibilities are indicated with varying degrees of specificity (for example, catchment areas for GPs, or major services to be provided). Another example of an input contract is one covering ambulance service stations. The purchaser may contract for the provision of emergency care as needed 24 hours a day during the year.

Performance contracts

Unlike input contracts, performance contracts incorporate indicators for monitoring and evaluating health improvements, enabling purchasers to substantiate claims for better provider performance and to settle disputes. The definition of performance is usually much broader than health and would include other elements such as access to care, quality and cost control. Each of the objectives typically calls for special safeguards to reduce the individual hazards of inappropriate provider behaviour.

A performance contract with a GP may include targets for specific priority services (for example, immunization rate, first three months of pregnancy check-up rate, and so forth), expected health gains (for example, reduction in child mortality), requirements to follow clinical protocols and the like. Requirements for the GPs to organize medical and community care for the catchment area residents in a given way – as a gatekeeper, for example – are also regular performance provisions of this type of contract. Sometimes more detailed service delivery and cost containment gains are specified (targets for inpatient care and drug utilization, referral rates to specialists, and so forth). Reaching these targets is usually rewarded by bonuses. The timeframe for performance evaluation may also be specified, for example, quarterly for referral rates, annually for infant mortality. The recently introduced GP contract in England (2004) provides an ambitious example of a performance contract with payment-related quality 'points' awarded on the basis of 146 performance indicators.

More generally the scope of GP performance indicators varies according to the prevailing method of payment. In theory, salary payment is based on GPs being professionally motivated, but experience sometimes questions this assumption. In capitation schemes the role of performance indicators is high but it differs according to the precise capitation arrangement. In fundholding schemes, for example, the need for performance indicators is usually lower than in other capitation schemes, because GPs have incentives for health gains and cost containment. Performance indicators are harder to specify in fee-for-service systems, as a physician may not have a clear zone of responsibility.

Performance contracts will have legal provisions found in most types of contract, concerning, for example, their duration; rights, duties and obligations of contracting parties including rewards and penalties; and a monitoring mechanism and arrangements such as auditing and reporting. In addition, a health performance contract with a hospital may include explicit specification of such health, quality and satisfaction objectives as waiting list reduction targets, or a detailed description of the transactions, including such specific performance indicators for selected hospital units as planned volumes of specified quality of care, for example.

In contrast to input-related funding, a key aspect of performance contracts is that they offer an opportunity for purchasers to escape from provider domination. Purchasers can influence provider behaviour, ensuring that an appropriate mix of services is supplied on specified terms of cost, quantity and quality. These objectives critically depend, however, on information about consumers' health and the value of providers' activities. Performance contracts only achieve 'the combined advantages of greater flexibility and scope for innovation, while maintaining control over strategic objectives and financial protection' (England, 2000a) if very refined information tools are available. In fact, practical and timely performance measurement is a prerequisite for good performance contracting.

No country has yet developed an 'ideal' performance contract. In this connection, one area of considerable future interest concerns contracting and chronic disease management – how a purchaser can contract for complete episodes of care covering more than one provider for long-term or complex cases (diabetes, stroke and so forth).

Service contracts

Service contracts place the types of services to be delivered at the centre of the contractual arrangements, thus making a clear description of the services involved crucially important. In most cases, performance contracts are linked to service contracts.

The most common classification includes three types of service contracts – block contracts (simple or sophisticated), cost-and-volume contracts, and cost-per-case contracts (Savas et al., 1998)[1] – which are described below.

Block contracts

Block contracts are similar to giving a budget for a defined block of services, shifting all risks of volume changes to the provider. The provider agrees to a sum in exchange for a broadly defined block of services over a period of time, usually a year, but activity levels are not detailed. The payment (received periodically) is usually determined by reference to the previous year's provider costs or the level of provider inputs. To substantiate input funding, various normative rates are used, such as bed capacity or per-patient staffing ratios. Block contracts have some advantages:

- because they are based on previous experience, they provide certainty about the financial flows for both parties;
- they minimize the level of administrative and information costs;
- there is little incentive for providers to engage in some practices that are detrimental either to patient or purchaser interests (for example, increasing inappropriate admissions).

Block contracts are frequently favoured when a contracting system is first introduced because there is usually insufficient information for more sophisticated forms of contracting. Their main disadvantage is that there is little incentive to respond to patients' demands. In cases of overprovision, this type of contract also tends to preserve provider excessive capacity while limiting access because there is no incentive to increase workload and activity levels.

Block contracts may be altered to include 'indicative' targets for activity along with minimum and maximum activity thresholds. Activity levels can be specified in terms of numbers of inpatient cases/outpatient visits, numbers by specialty groupings, or particular clinical conditions. The purpose of target inclusion has been described as to allow both purchasers and providers to feel their way into contracting and to ensure the generation of data for performance review, negotiation and more focused contracting in subsequent years (Accounts Commission for Scotland, 1997). These more sophisticated block contracts offer an incentive for providers to increase their activity levels and earn additional income while purchasers control risks by setting thresholds appropriately.

Cost-and-volume contracts

Cost-and-volume contracts include payments for explicitly quantified services, which may be more or less broadly defined: number of outpatient attendances, patients to be treated in one specialty (usually with differentiation of high-, medium- and low-cost categories) and even numbers treated for a specific clinical condition. These contracts can be viewed as a combination of a sophisticated block contract and a cost-per-case contract (see below). As in block contracts, the purchaser agrees to pay a lump sum for a specified number of cases, and must make additional payments beyond that threshold level. Under this contract type, however, the additional payments are agreed on a cost-per-case basis and may set an upper limit on the number of cases that will be paid.

In contrast to block contracts, cost-and-volume contracts spread risk sharing between purchasers and providers. They usually set accepted deviations of actual and planned volumes of care for the same amount of money (risk corridors); if the planned activity is 100 cases and the risk corridor is 10%, then a hospital with 90 cases will get the same revenue as one with 100 or 110 cases. Volumes of care beyond these risk corridors are reimbursed at a lower rate. Thus, by choosing this type of contract the purchaser and the provider can share the financial risk for overprovision. Planning volumes of care and assuring the active role of the purchaser in determining the cost-effectiveness of interventions are necessary for making cost-and-volume contracts.

The main advantages of cost-and-volume contracts are:

- they permit the purchaser to be more specific about precisely what is expected from providers;
- the incentive for the provider to increase activity and reduce costs is higher, as there is greater assurance about the level of payments to be received for exceeding the block portion of the contract;
- the incentive for overprovision is much smaller than in cost-per-case contracts;
- planning and market-type negotiations between purchasers and providers are encouraged, with an incentive for collecting good managerial information.

The disadvantages of cost-and-volume contracts are:

- they require more detailed information on costing than block contracts, even with cases measured at specialty level, which results in higher transaction costs;
- volume is usually specified in broad terms (for example, the average number of cases by specialty), so hospitals have an opportunity for cost creeping by selecting relatively easy cases and allocating costs in a way that maximizes their income at the expense of purchasers;
- patient access may be limited, particularly if hospitals are close to the upper limit of the risk corridor;
- by providing incentives to increase volume and/or reduce costs, there is an inherent risk to quality, necessitating a high degree of quality monitoring.

Cost-per-case contracts

Cost-per-case contracts are based on a single cost set per episode of treatment, so are more precise in terms of output specification. These are usually measured in terms of the number of cases and services across diagnoses. The advantages are substantial: once the price is fixed, the provider has an incentive to provide at the lowest possible cost. For purchasers, paying only for the precise services they contract also offers the advantage of making total expenditure predictable. However, if the number of cases is not specified, all risks for overprovision are borne by purchasers, who have to pay for cases hospitals have chosen to take, including those that can be treated in outpatient settings or day care centres. The disadvantages also include the previously mentioned special costing requirements of cost-and-volume contracts, as the output specification across groups of diagnoses should be particularly precise. Transaction costs in this type of contract are usually much higher and may be particularly large if all clinical conditions in a hospital are included.

In many situations, cost-per-case contracts are used in addition to block or cost-and-volume contracts, for smaller numbers of services. In most European countries there is a general trend towards a higher level of care product specification in all types of contracts, reflecting a case mix. The main objective is to increase cost consciousness of providers and to avoid manipulation of the workload structure (Langenbrunner & Wiley, 2002). During the 1990s, prospective cost-per-case payments according to diagnostic groups (DRGs) became the dominant form of payment of inpatient services and they are increasingly used for outpatient services. It should be noted that the difference between prospective and retrospective payment is vital here for the sake of expenditure predictability and control. Clearly the types of service contracts and level of specification will be directly linked with the payment system. Chapter 11 provides a detailed analysis of different payment systems available and their use in contracting.

To summarize:

- Most developed countries have well established market-entry contracts in the form of licensing and accreditation.
- Most countries have performance contracts as an ideal in which much broader issues (access, quality, cost control and so forth) should be incorporated. In practice, however, performance contracts and service contracts can often be taken as rough equivalents.
- For different historical reasons, cost-per-case contracts are predominant in the United States and some of the postcommunist countries.
- Cost-per-case contracts are not very common in Western Europe, where cost-and-volume contracts are dominant. However, while Bismarckian systems have a long tradition of *hard* cost-and-volume contracts, NHS-type systems started with increasingly sophisticated block contracts and have been evolving towards more detailed but *soft* cost-and-volume contracts.

Output and quality specifications

As noted above, most service contracts are expected to identify the output and the quality of care required (see Box 9.2). In practice, output specification depends on the prevailing approach to provider payment methods. Volumes of inpatient care are usually defined in terms of the total number of cases, specialty cases, bed-days (total or by specialty) and, increasingly, 'finished' cases across diagnosis or groups of diagnoses.

In many countries with block and cost-and-volume contracts, the level of activity is specified in rather broad terms. For example, agreements between purchasers and hospitals in England set outputs and prices across the broad specialties and services. For each category the number of emergency, elective, day care cases and consultations is given (England, 2000b).

The output of primary care and specialized outpatient care is usually defined through reference to the prevailing method of payment. In fee-for-service schemes, reference is made to the number and cost of services. In per capita funding schemes, the size of the enrolment is usually defined in the contract; a list of activities subject to additional reimbursement is also sometimes included. A detailed discussion of alternative payment methods to contract ambulatory providers is given in Chapter 11.

While all contracts specify reimbursement arrangements, in some cases the volume is not always well specified. This was particularly the case in many countries in Eastern Europe where emerging health insurance models have been

Box 9.2   Elements in contract design

- Contract framework.
  - Objectives, contracting partners, relations, arbitration, committees
- Contract structure.
  - Type of contract
  - Output definition and size
  - Time
  - Subcontracts (by speciality, client group and so forth)
- Payment arrangements.
  - Incentives and sanctions, risk-sharing
- Detail (degree of specification of services, quality and so forth).
- Monitoring, verification and validation methods.

Source: Adapted from Øvretveit (1994).

based on market incentive principles – the money follows the patient. In contrast to those Western European countries with established traditions of contractual relationships, in many CEE countries there is little negotiation of contracted volumes of inpatient care based on data on efficacy and cost-effectiveness of care, as well as revealed inefficiency (Busse *et al.*, 2001). The result is a well documented tendency in these countries of increased hospital utilization with a high proportion of inappropriate cases (25%–35% of all hospital cases in the Russian Federation) (Busse *et al.*, 2001; Hollo & Orosz, 2001; Kozierkiewicz & Karski, 2001). Still, the admission rates in hospitals in many of these countries are lower than in some Western European countries.

In the Russian Federation, in particular, most contracts for inpatient care are of a cost-per-case type (cost-and-volume or block contracts are rare) and do not specify the volume of inpatient cases purchased. Health insurers do not negotiate utilization of care with providers but rather limit themselves to paying bills; although some control case appropriateness retrospectively. In addition, contracts do not specify risk sharing between purchasers and providers; financial risks of increased numbers of cases are borne by purchasers, at least in theory. In practice, health insurers are financially responsible only within the funds allocated to them by the Territorial Mandatory Health Insurance Fund; since these are usually not enough to cover all costs, risks are eventually shifted to patients in the form of informal payments for services (Sheiman, 2001).

Since cost-per-case payment creates incentives for overutilization of inpatient care, there has been an increasing trend for contracts to specify a cap on reimbursement, without contracted commitments to volumes of care. This is the case in the Czech Republic, Hungary and Kazakhstan.

A more detailed mix of services as the basis for provider payment is now seen in many countries as a tool for increasing efficiency. Various versions of DRG-type payment systems are either in place or in the process of elaboration (see Chapter 11). However, the existing evidence suggests that even very precise output measurement does not necessarily change adverse hospital incentives unless contracts explicitly specify volumes of care. This, in turn, requires significant changes in the contracting process including strengthening strategic and operational planning of both purchasers and providers, and making purchasing more selective.

Contractual specification of outputs should also be supplemented with risk-sharing arrangements, specifying possible deviations of volumes of care and the pattern of their reimbursement. For example, in some regions of the Russian Federation (Kemerovo, Samara, Murmansk, Kaluga, Tver oblasts) cost-per-case contracts in 1999 gave way to cost-and-volume contracts. Rather than paying retrospectively for actual volumes of care, insurers started to negotiate hospital utilization and defined admissible deviations from planned utilization targets (risk corridors) within which planned volumes are paid for. Polyclinics are also involved in planning volumes of inpatient care and have economic incentives to increase their workload. Furthermore an improved general planning framework and new contracting mechanisms have reduced structural distortions. In the Kemerovo oblast, the number of bed-days per 1000 residents fell from 2375 in 1998 to 1922 in 2000, the admission rate from 182 to 171 and the average length of stay from 13 to 11.2 days. The number of day care cases more than doubled, thus decreasing the need for hospital beds. With the growing use of cost-and-volume contracts similar evidence has also been accumulated in other regions (Sheiman, 2002).

German health funds contract for outpatient services with panel doctors associations and dentist associations, based on framework contracts organized at federal and *Länder* level including also volume corridors to avoid inappropriate expansion of services. There are no individual contracts between the practitioners and health insurance funds; however, the use of volume corridors allows benchmarking for each practitioner. Framework contracts have also been employed to improve the quality of care for certain diseases such as diabetes and breast cancer. These 'disease management' contracts clarify the rights and obligations of the various contracting parties, including the participating patients. Patient participation in these programmes is voluntary. In contrast, contracts for inpatient services are carried out individually for each hospital, though they are based on agreed framework contracts at federal and *Länder* level. Health funds control costs by negotiating budgets based on case mix and volumes. The medical review services of each health insurance control for the appropriateness of care.

In order to reduce waiting lists and thus increase access to care it is also important to specify separately contracted volumes of elective and emergency care. For instance, this is done in the United Kingdom to commit providers to reaching precise targets. It is also a good leverage for shifting the balance of power between the purchaser and the hospital, removing from the latter the opportunity to make inappropriate admissions under the traditional guise of 'emergency cases'.

The degree to which quality is defined in contracts closely depends on the available information. Also, some difficulties emanate from the very nature of medical services. Often outputs beyond traditional health services make it difficult for purchasers to identify what they pay for (see, for example, the difficulty with introducing preventive services such as 'health education' in primary health care contracts) but progress has also been achieved. In the context of introducing GP fundholding schemes in the UK during the 1990s, many battles were fought between GP practices and hospitals. GPs wanted quality targets in their contracts related not so much to professional medical issues in the narrow sense but to things that mattered to the GP and the patient, such as the content and speed of discharge letters, the length of wait before being seen by the hospital for an initial consultation and the possibility of being seen by the consultant on a certain minimum proportion of visits. In the end, most of the practices could review quality specifications of hospitals on a regular basis (Glennerster *et al.*, 1993). (See also Box 9.3.)

Box 9.3   Primary-care-based purchasing in the United Kingdom

In 1994, a three-year pilot programme was introduced in the United Kingdom that extended the scope of the existing GP fundholding scheme. This was known as total purchasing (TP). Through total purchasing, a set of pilot sites – covering average populations of around 30 000 people – were allocated budgets with which they could purchase potentially all of the community, secondary and tertiary care services of their registered patients.

The move from GP fundholding to total purchasing greatly increased the importance placed on the contracting process. The most common contract form used by the TP sites was the sophisticated block contract described in this chapter. Through the use of these contracts, GPs at the TP sites were able to influence the quality of services provided for their patients by hospitals. As one respondent commented: 'It's a springboard to open more doors. We spoke to [hospital] clinicians and addressed meetings to get their support for the changes we wanted to make. We wouldn't have been invited to such meetings if we were not going down the contracting road' (Robinson *et al.*, 1998).

With the election of the Labour government in 1997, the TP experiment was ended. However, the subsequent nationwide introduction of primary care trusts (PCTs) means that the focus on primary-care-based purchasing has been retained and extended. Each PCT now places contracts with providers (currently known as 'service agreements') as part of a service and financial framework process.

Quality might be specified in contracts by references to uniform requirements. National Service Frameworks (NSFs) have been issued recently in the United Kingdom in the areas of, *inter alia* coronary disease, cancer, mental care and services for elderly people. They are meant to serve as a device for implementing guidelines and protocols on best practice, and also as targets in relation to outcomes of services in specified areas. Hospitals make a contractual commitment to develop a quality development plan, including quality improvement targets, quality-focused job descriptions, auditing, reporting and monitoring arrangements, targets for consumer satisfaction, and so forth.

Specific requirements are set for emergency services (for example, that 90% of patients be clinically assessed within 10 minutes of arrival time and no patient wait more than 3 hours), for outpatient appointments (maximum time period from first referral), for waiting times for outpatient clinic and elective inpatient admissions, for consumer relations and information generation (England, 2000b).

In Andalusia, Spain, links between hospitals and the regional Ministry of Health adopt the form of a programme contract (in essence, a sophisticated block contract) defining criteria to achieve the objectives set out in the Andalusian Health Plan and a strategy defined by a Quality and Efficiency Framework Plan.

In many Eastern European countries, quality is incorporated into contracts through references to licensing and accreditation status of contracted providers. This has allowed adding requirements for equipment, skills of the staff and sanitary status of facilities. It also has limited the risk of certain services falling to providers with no capacity to deliver them. However, one-time procedures are usually not enough for ensuring quality. In Bulgaria, for example, the Ministry of Health has produced a national health map but contracts pay far more attention to bureaucratic specifications than to the definition of appropriate care.

With respect to quality of processes, contracts usually refer to clinical standards and protocols for each region and sometimes for the entire country. In the Russian Federation, for example, regional standards establish requirements for service delivery (including the average length of stay) and the expected outcome in terms of patients' health status after treatment. According to the standard contract, health insurers can check the performance of providers and penalize them for poor quality. Sometimes the requirement to match standards causes a defensive strategy by providers leading, for instance, to extended lengths of stay and overprescribing.

Chapter 10 on purchasing and quality widens the above discussion and provides a more detailed account of the main mechanisms to introduce quality specifications into contracts.

Competition and selective contracting

The potential for the contracting process to bring about change is higher when a purchaser can select among competing providers. In a growing number of countries the law now allows selective contracting to take place but in practice there are several obstacles to its implementation.

In the Netherlands since 1992 health funds have not been obliged to contract with all individual providers (Exter & Herman, forthcoming). However, their actual freedom to negotiate contracts is limited by rigidly defined entitlements and government price regulation. Health funds in the Netherlands are also concerned that by limiting contracts with some providers they risk that unhappy insured will switch to another insurer. The experience in the Netherlands also shows that selection is only possible when there is overcapacity; thus in practice it is not possible to refuse contracts for services when there is a waiting list. In a system of scarce resources selective contracting can help to tailor performance contracts with individual providers but cannot be used to refuse market entry.

In Germany, despite several reform proposals, health insurance funds are not allowed to contract selectively and cannot deviate from collective contracts. Selective contracts were proposed in 2003 for all ambulatory specialist care. However, these proposals experienced fierce opposition from the association of physicians practising under statutory health insurance conditions.

Many CEE countries with SHI models, at least formally declared the right of purchasers to select providers. There have been some striking examples of the denial of contracts to providers. In the Czech Republic, in 1997, the General Health Insurance Fund, which insures about 75% of the population, denied contracts with 176 new providers and terminated contracts with another 130 existing providers. This was done as an element of the government policy to limit the number and capacity of health care providers. However, another eight smaller companies have not followed this line (Busse *et al.*, 2001). In Slovenia, selective contracting is possible and health care providers engage in contract tenders and bidding. However, in practice, due to a relative shortage of health care providers the contracts are often not selective.

Despite these isolated examples of selective contracting, the prevailing picture in many countries is still non-selective contracting. This can be attributed to many factors. First of all there have been implementation problems. Regulation is needed enabling purchasers to contract selectively through a set of approved rules and procedures, but examples of this kind of regulation are rare. In England there is an expectation that primary care trusts will contract with local providers, although the concept of 'contestability' among providers is accepted in the cases of local failings.

Regulation in Kazakhstan means that all government agencies, including health authorities, are required to purchase services through a tendering process. The bidding procedures are specified as a uniform process for all public services with no or little account of specific characteristics of the health sector. The absence of requirements regarding costing procedures and quality targets has created a good environment for providers to win contracts by setting prices much below actual costs, while quality characteristics have not been adequately accounted. The tradeoff between cost and quality has not been regulated enough. Thus the problem is not only the existence of competitive regulation but also its quality.

A second obstacle to selective contracting is the opposition of the medical profession. For decades, the prevailing pattern of resource allocation has been either totally non-contractual or contractual with all physicians and hospitals. Collective contracting with physician associations is still strongly advocated by the medical profession. The laws allowing contracting with individual providers in many countries have not been supported by a mandate to select them according to obligatory procedures.

This opposition has been reinforced in some countries by the pluralistic model of health purchasing with many insurers competing for insurees. For example, in the Russian Federation around 400 health insurance companies tend to contract with all providers in the local area in order to attract more clients. The eight insurance companies involved in SHI in Moscow city have contracts with all the local hospitals and polyclinics. In the Czech Republic consumer organizations oppose selective contracting: there are examples of the organized collective change of membership of insurers who denied contracts with local hospitals (Hava & Dlouhy, 2002). Contrary to expectations, the pluralistic model of health purchasing in these cases has inhibited a selection process. The balance of power is still in favour of providers, particularly those of secondary and tertiary care.

Yet another obstacle is the lack of political will to close excess capacity and lay off staff of medical facilities that have not been awarded a contract. In the United Kingdom, even in the early, more competitive stages of health reform, the government strictly controlled competition between providers lest the efficiency consequence, such as hospital closures, threatened other goals such as equality of access to services, or embarrassed the government politically. The internal architecture of the NHS was substantially altered along the lines of a big corporation but it remained the direct responsibility of central government and, therefore, subject to political controversy. As noted in Mays *et al.* (2000),

> When the potential effects of competition threatened to cause chaos in central London, for instance, the government stepped in with a review of services designed to limit the play of market forces. Ironically, the conditions for extensive competition between acute hospitals existed to a greater degree in London than elsewhere.

In some countries of CEE/CIS there are also some historical institutional constraints to provider competition. In some countries even the strong financial pressure arising from health sector underfunding has not contributed to closures of hospitals. This is particularly so in big cities where the excessive capacity is obvious but the political resistance to such action is greatest and the opposition of the medical profession is strongest. Only small hospitals in remote areas of Albania, Armenia, Kazakhstan, Kyrgyzstan, Moldova and the Russian Federation have been closed – often with a very destructive outcome for the local population in terms of access to services. This is because the Semashko model is based on a hierarchy of providers in a segmented market with little overlapping of facilities (oblast, city, rayon, rural hospitals). Payment rates (tariffs) are the same for each specific type within the vertical hierarchy of medical facilities, so price competition can only exist between providers at different levels. In the Baltic states, Kazakhstan, Kyrgyzstan and the Russian Federation, selective contracting, if it exists, focuses on the choice of the level of care (for example, tertiary care facilities in many the Russian Federationn regions are losing contracts to city hospitals and some specialties are increasingly concentrated in inter-rayon hospitals). In the Baltic states, where big city polyclinics have been restructured to free-standing solo and group practices, the potential for selective contracting in outpatient care is increasing; providers in Estonia, for example, have competed for contracts through a formal tendering procedure since 2002 (Jesse, forthcoming).

Governance

Regulation

Health care contracts are usually incorporated within a legislative framework and governed by regulations. A perfect contract would describe all parties' obligations in all possible future states to the fullest extent possible. As a result, there would never be a need for the parties to revise or renegotiate the contract (Hart, 1995). However, the costs of making complete contracts are too high, and the purchaser will never be in a position to foresee all possible changes in the morbidity of a population and the implications for medical care. In reality, therefore, contracts are incomplete; they need to be revised and renegotiated all the time. That is why regulation is required to secure fulfilment.

Regulation is also needed to ensure compliance of contracts with health policy objectives. The government may want to make contracting more competitive and therefore sets tendering procedures while monitoring the process of placing contracts. Purchasers may in turn be more interested in contracting with providers that look more attractive to good risks, or for the same reason, to select more costly medical interventions with unclear clinical outcomes. They may also be reluctant to pay for additional costs of training primary care providers, or for experimental medical interventions designed to lower health costs in the long run. The government would then set restrictive legislation with specific safeguards to avoid the conflict between short-term purchasing decisions and long-term health policy objectives. Sometimes this legislation causes purchaser dissatisfaction and calls for deregulation. The true role of regulators is to find an optimum balance between contracting freedom and regulation (Sheiman & Wassem, 2002).

Regulatory targets

Purchasers and providers are required to follow certain targets reflecting general health policy objectives, such as health gains, utilization targets and a certain planned structure of health expenditures by health sectors. These targets may come from national and regional plans of service restructuring and quality improvement. Sometimes targets of accessibility are set, stating, for example, maximum waiting lists or criteria of physical access in terms of travel time. Both purchasers and providers are then supposed to transform these targets into the language of contract commitments – to adapt them to specific needs of the population they represent.

Rules and procedures

Costing and pricing requirements are inherent in any contracting system. In England, for example, the government has issued regulations for national tariffs designed to provide a common basis for contracting (Grant & Collini, 1996). In the Russian Federation a new draft law on health insurance sets the requirement on limit prices. Open information on provider prices is a requirement for competitive contracting.

Sometimes regulations stipulate government approval of contracts. In Germany at present, almost all negotiated contracts of health funds must be given to supervisory units of federal or state governments for informational approval or for agreement in substance. The major criterion for evaluating a contract is its impact on cost containment strategy. For example, the supervision unit can disapprove of any contract between an insurance fund and the local medical facility for development of some services if there is an excess capacity for similar services in the local area, on the grounds of 'conflict with cost containment'. Health funds are also given the freedom to cancel contracts with inefficient hospitals.

The need for a more restrictive regulations strategy may also arise when purchasers have to deal with providers as local monopolies. For instance, in a region with low population density it is rather likely that only one hospital can exist or that there are so few physicians available that it is unrealistic not to contract with any of them.

Contract monitoring and evaluation requirements are central to regulation. Purchasers are supposed to formally assess contract implementation and sometimes to report to an independent governmental agency. Evidence regarding such assessment varies across countries. In countries where contracting is at the initial stage and contracting culture is still low, the focus tends to be on contracts as such rather than on contract implementation.

There are, however, attempts to regulate the content of contracts by introducing a model contract including all government requirements. In some emerging SHI systems in the CIS (the Russian Federation, Kazakhstan, Kyrgyzstan) a model contract was used during the initial stages of health finance reform. It was designed to describe all parties' obligations in all possible future states to the fullest extent possible. This type of contract is doomed to be very general and does not leave room for negotiating and renegotiating according to actual health needs. As also seen in the United Kingdom, contracts are becoming increasingly flexible. Regulation does not need to set strict limits on the contract scope, apart from general provisions (contracting parties, timeframe, conditions of termination and so forth).

Collective contracting

Collective contracts may regulate purchaser–provider relationships between physicians' associations and insurers. Agreements between third-party payers and associations of providers serve as the basis for individual contracts, with more or less intervention from the state, as is the case in all social insurance systems with framework contracts. Framework contracts are part of the governance tools that safeguard contractual relations while reducing transaction costs of repeated contracting. The tradeoff is that the hazards of a bilateral monopoly might increase.

In some countries, mostly outside of Europe, there are also restrictions on offering insurees a choice of insurance contracts, including managed care alternatives that would control utilization by restricting the choice of provider in return for lower premiums.

Other areas amenable to regulatory action include the approaches to the link between contracts and the broader planning process, the specification of service outputs, provider payment methods, conditions for selective contracting, and incentives and penalties.

Incentives and penalties

In theory, whenever a contract is signed, incentives and penalties are either implicit (soft contracts) or explicit (hard contracts) for stakeholders to perceive, as are the guarantees in case of failure to deliver; but is this so in practice?

In the United Kingdom the first contracts introduced in the 1990s did little more than conserve the existing volumes of activities and costs. Hospital trusts were tempted to fulfil and even exceed the contractual volume of activities in the middle of the year and then require more money. Unclear specification of workload structure created incentives for inflating activities by, for example, counting outpatient minor procedures as day surgery cases. It took some time to refine contracting mechanisms and incentives to better specify contractual commitments regarding volumes of activity and cost control.

Another example from the English NHS illustrates the power of financial incentives in contracts. In the past, despite universal acknowledgement of its benefits, many GP practices achieved only a 40%–60% uptake of cervical screening. With the introduction of a financial incentive in the contracts, linking GP income to the level of uptake, most practices managed to go above 90%. However, it was also recognized that the increase was at least in part due to a previous growth in the number of nurses and other PHC staff in GP practices, who took over much of the responsibility for the programme (Steve Engleman, personal communication). In addition, the workload and characteristics of a practice's patient population are likely to influence uptake levels. Lynch (1994) has pointed out that the exclusion from the payment calculations of immunizations in excess of the set minimum values – 90% and 70% – penalizes GPs who miss the target by a small margin. A payment system based on a smoother sliding scale, with an intermediate target of 80% accruing payments equivalent to two-thirds of the high target fee, would more equitably reward GPs for the provision of this service. Careful thought is required to ensure a choice of incentive (or constraint) so that the means by which the outcome is achieved is consistent with the ultimate objective.

In most of the CEE, contracts are increasingly explicit about protecting insureds' rights and imposing financial penalties in case of inappropriate care. Compared with the previous command-and-control methods, these new commitments have created some incentives for increasing the workload of providers, collecting new management information and enhancing the interest of providers in cost level and structure. Third-party control activities as well as protection of the insureds' rights have brought higher clinical discipline and accountability. The example of the Russian Federation is given in Box 9.4.

However, only the first steps have been made in developing a culture of contractual relationships with mechanisms for monitoring and evaluating the

Box 9.4 Contractual mechanisms for influencing providers in the Russian Federation under SHI

Performance-related methods of payment. Around 90% of providers contracted by SHI insurers are reimbursed for the actual outputs measured through various units of volumes of care. This allows purchasers to encourage an increase in providers activity and sometimes to improve the structure of health care provision. But the fact that performance-related payment is used only under SHI contracts while the government traditionally allocates resources directly for inputs of providers attenuates to a great degree the positive impact of SHI contracts. The government is also looking for ways to allocate resources according to actual provider performance.

Control of volumes and quality of care. Medical and economic expertise is required here. Insurers may either have special medical quality control units or hire experts. They selectively check cases (including medical records) against proper treatment standards, which are developed regionally with requirements for the process and outcome of the medical interventions for most diagnoses. According to the World Bank survey of health insurers, 85% of the latter conduct medical reviews. Economic assessment is conducted to discover inappropriate hospital admissions and to monitor particular services. Sixty-six per cent of all insurance companies and 72% of fund branches report pre-admission controls, although the survey of health insurers does not demonstrate their actual scale. There is some evidence, particularly in big cities, that a high percentage of admission cases are not referred by primary care providers. In 2000, Moscow polyclinics had not referred 67% of SHI-insured admissions of the biggest Russian Federationn insurance company, RosnoMed; 31% of inpatient cases had not received outpatient care three weeks prior to admission and 19% of admissions were rated by company experts as inappropriate. Thus, the incidence and actual impact of pre-admission controls is not clear and likely to be insignificant in most of the Russian Federation regions. Most admission decisions are made by hospitals themselves. Around 85% of health insurers control average lengths of stay of admissions, and even a higher percentage control appropriateness of the diagnostic procedures in hospitals, as well as drug use. There are reasons to believe that the control of average lengths of stay (LOS) really influences hospital performance. Usually this control is aimed at identifying cases with LOS lower than approved standards (in an attempt to neutralize economic incentives to discharge patients prematurely). The insurer can impose financial penalties on hospitals for such behaviour, so hospitals tend to stick to the average lengths of stay standards. The negative side of this is that this type of control leads to a defensive strategy by doctors, who tend to keep patients the standard number of days whether necessary or not.

Protection of the insureds' rights. Patients can complain to health insurers regarding negligence of medical staff, inappropriate outcome of interventions, premature discharges, denial of services, and so forth. According to the legislation, these cases are subject to the expertise of health insurers, which have the right to impose financial penalties on providers and reimburse the damage to the insured. There were 1 203 152 complaints in 1999, of which 25% proved to be appropriate – most due to limitation of provider choice and unavailability of drugs for the groups entitled to free or partially paid drug benefits. Health insurers found that 33% of approved complaints were attributable to poor performance of medical facilities, 10% to poor decisions of health authorities, 9% to SHI funds, 8% to the insurers themselves and the rest to other organizations. However, because of underfunding, only 5% to 6% of the total number of complaints deemed appropriate by health insurers triggered financial penalties to providers.

performance of contractual commitments. The main emphasis is still on relatively simple incentives for providers, who are driven by their own interests, rather than broader objectives of a purchasing strategy. Data are lacking on clinical effectiveness of medical interventions and there are no strong incentives to collect it (and some countries also lack the equipment and skills to do so). Performance evaluation is seen mostly in control measures with penalties imposed for poor quality and inappropriate volumes of care rather than the analysis of 'zones of inefficiency' and quality assurance. Planning of rational 'routes' of patients and the choice of cost-effective medical interventions is still at the very first stage.

Even controls and penalties are not easy to implement due to underfunding and lack of modern control capacity in some countries. Action does not always ensue if the provider organization deviates from the agreed contract. For example, sanctions in Bulgaria after two years of SHI functioning mostly cover administrative misdemeanours. In 2001, of the 13 840 contracts signed with providers, 8274 (59.75%) were audited. Auditors found 10 020 infractions and the sanctions imposed amounted to a total BGN 959 757; but only two-thirds of the sanctions (73%, BGN 703 917, a very small fraction of the approximate BGN 400 million paid by the fund to health providers during the year) were actually paid (Bulgarian National Health Insurance Fund, 2002).

In the Czech Republic the modification of contractual incentives has taken place following the failures of the first stage of SHI model implementation. Open-ended health funding coupled with unregulated fee-for-service provider payment inflated health care expenditures and bankrupted some insurance companies, leaving CZK 2 billion in unpaid debts, mostly to hospitals (Langenbrunner & Wiley, 2002). Proving that the contracting system has learned its lessons, in the new contractual arrangements health insurers set a ceiling on the volume of services and penalties for above-average costs and monitor contracts financially. They also hire external reviewers for checking clinical aspects and appropriateness of care; the volume of services above the negotiated and above-average costs of providers may not be reimbursed (Hava & Dlouhy, 2002).

The experience of many countries demonstrates that contracting is not a magic tool. Its potential is better realized if mistakes of the previous stages are analysed and a system of incentives and penalties is adapted to new objectives. There is now a tendency to specify mechanisms that would come into play if either party fails to meet its contractual commitments rather than to specify every detail. There is a shift to 'soft' service agreements with contracting parties depending more on cooperation and a continuity of relations, as opposed to competition. Many commentators consider this a sign of maturing contracting (Sheiman & Wassem; Robinson, forthcoming, 2002).

Implementation

The contracting process

The details of the contracting process vary substantially across countries. However, there seem to be some common features in contracting as an integral part of health policy implementation. In many instances, contracts are increasingly incorporated into the broad planning process. Figure 9.1 shows how the contracting cycle can be linked to the planning cycle.

The planning process begins with an assessment of the population health needs and the establishment of a set of health priorities (see Chapter 7 on purchasing and public health). This forms the basis for developing a purchasing strategy and is followed by the establishment of a set of service requirements and targets to be achieved through contracting.

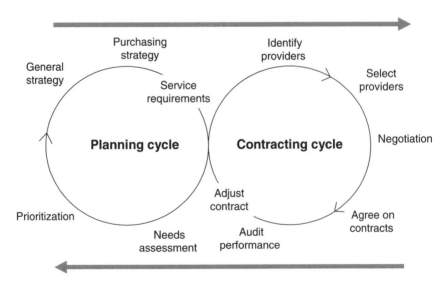

Figure 9.1 Planning and contracting cycles.
Source: Øvretveit (1994: 135).

The contracting cycle starts with identifying and selecting providers. As noted earlier, some purchasers may have little choice of provider whereas others may have a choice or wish to create a choice by encouraging providers to come forward. Key issues are finding out provider costs and likely reliability in meeting contract requirements. The second step is negotiating and agreeing a contract. Key issues at this stage are which type of contract to use, what measure of output and how to pay for it – see above. The third stage of contracting is managing the contract, a central part of which is monitoring. Often, purchasers do not have sufficient personnel for carrying out the many purchasing tasks and nowhere are the personnel constraints more apparent than when it comes to considering how to get and use information for monitoring contracts.

The case of the English NHS provides a useful lesson about the process of contracting and its linkage with planning. Contracts here are a final point of a planning cycle. This is particularly true for the recent stage of the reform with a new strategy of more cooperation between purchasers and providers, and their joint planning in contracting. Government guidance has required purchasers to draw up strategic purchasing plans that demonstrate to providers their purchasing intentions for the next three to five years. They cover an estimate of health care needs and priorities, plans of reorganization of service delivery to meet these needs, expected significant budgetary allocations, guidance on information requirements, quality standards and quality assurance procedures (England, 2000b). Operational purchasing plans for the following year are also part of a contracting process, covering the services a purchaser plans to contract for and the budget constraints.

Operational plans are also developed in some SHI countries. For example, before entering into contractual aspects such as volumes of inpatient care and substitution strategies, health insurers in the Netherlands and Germany must submit to the government operational plans not only reflecting expected internal operations (staffing, equipment and so forth) but also demonstrating their managerial capacity and purchasing intentions.

Knowing the plans of purchasers, providers then produce their annual business plans with details on specific targets and services to be provided, capital investment, bed capacity, sources of funding, and so forth. In the course of contract negotiations these plans are linked to purchasing plans. The signed contract later becomes the basis for performance evaluation, a critical part of the contracting process and sometimes even more important than the contract itself. Actual performance indicators are compared with those contracted, the causes of deviations are examined and financial sanctions are imposed if appropriate.

The structure of health care provision in many of the CEE/CIS countries is not improving as much as expected in the course of the reforms, so the need for modifying the contracting process is seen as urgent. Emphasis is being placed on enhancing the planning function of contracting by incorporating contracts into a general planning process; ensuring joint planning by purchasers and providers; and on increasing the use of sophisticated block and cost-and-volume contracts with volume of care specifications and risk-sharing arrangements.

In the Russian Federation, contracting started changing in 1998 when the federal government set annual Territorial Programmes of State Guarantees and an SHI package of medical benefits. The programme, a combination of top-down and bottom-up planning, stipulates target volumes of care across specialties, types of medical facilities and population groups. The benchmarks are the Federal Programme of State Guarantees' restructuring targets (decrease hospital bed-days from 3.6 per resident to 2.8, increase rates for day care centres, outpatient surgery and so forth). Regional health authorities and the SHI fund develop targets negotiated with local health systems and medical facility managers. The approved programme operates as an umbrella contract, with local insurers expected to base their contracting decisions on cost and utilization targets.

There is early evidence of more coordinated action resulting in lower admission rates and average lengths of stay, and the establishment of new day care centres, plus the intangible outcomes of new planning and managing skills for both purchasers and providers. However, this can be attributed mostly to the government being tougher on planning targets rather than to the contracting process. Contracts remain poorly linked to planning for many reasons. First, health insurance companies are not much involved as a contracting party in the planning process (sometimes they do not even know about planned targets). Second, prevailing cost-per-case contracts and retrospective methods of payment for actual rather than planned volumes of care (that is, without risk sharing) place serious limitations on reaching utilization targets; providers tend to increase their workload and usually exceed utilization targets. Third, the requirement of accountability for efficiency gain does not exist in many countries; insurers are not accountable to the government at that level and therefore have no incentives to look for more cost-effective options of service delivery.

Hungary may serve as an example of a formal purchaser and provider contracting process with practically no role for the contracting parties because major parameters of the contracts are predetermined. The National Health Insurance Fund has to contract with the providers determined by the Ministry of Health and local governments. Decisions on provider capacity and payment methods are made by Parliament, those on price, volume and quality of care by the Ministry. The discretionary power of the Fund is very limited, thus making contracts a formal exercise (Gaal & Eletovits, 2002).

Another mechanism may also operate so that regulatory capture by professional organizations leaves no room for service planning by the National Health Insurance Fund. In Bulgaria, for example, the cornerstone of the contracting and payment systems is the annual National Framework Contract (NFC) between the National Health Insurance Fund and the Bulgarian Medical Association (BMA) and the Bulgarian Dentists Union (BDU). However, the NFC is negotiated through an extremely rigid process, whose complexity and procedural detail results in a mechanistic, non-responsive financing system that cannot be managed in the regions or indeed in the hospitals. As a result, the allocation of funds (and hence access to services by the community) remains essentially as it was before the Fund was set up (Duran *et al.*, 2003).

Obstacles to implementation

Low operational autonomy of providers

To act as contracting parties, providers must have flexibility to respond to purchasers' demands and, in particular, be able to increase or decrease capacity, borrow money within limits, take financial responsibility for performance, and so forth. That is why hospitals' operational autonomy is an issue for many Western countries such as Italy, Norway, Spain, Sweden and England that want to give hospitals more rights and responsibilities, making contracts a mode of interaction with the payer. However, political factors have sometimes prevented this from happening. In Spain, for example, many regional health services have consolidated the bureaucratic integrated model, with indicative shadow contracts. A number of regions, however, have tried something different. They have started using contractual arrangements with new QUANGO provider organizations while maintaining the system's public nature under Spanish law. Three main variants are being used: public law ruled organizations, consortia and public foundations (Martin, 2003). In general, it is understood that all three forms of 'reformed' ownership and management should make a more effective use of contracts and promote more efficient resource allocation. However, the increased real importance of these new provider organizations in the Spanish health sector stems from their use by most political forces to promote their own strategic objectives.

In many Eastern European countries, legislation explicitly precludes or limits contracting since providers are entities directly managed by the government. In the Russian Federation the new budgetary code considers medical facilities 'budgetary institutions' run by government at different levels on a non-contractual basis and funded from general budget revenue according to items of expenditure (inputs); the scope for contracting is left only for SHI funds. The operational inflexibility of budgets imposes further limits; providers cannot adapt their capacity in response to actual needs and contracting requirements. Similar legal limitations exist in many countries of the CIS. The rights and responsibilities of providers as prudent sellers of their services do not match with the new financial arrangements.

To make contracting viable, many of these countries had given a new legal status to health providers. The Baltic states have restructured state-owned polyclinics into free-standing practices and independent contractors. State-owned hospitals gained the status of public non-profit organizations with new contracting rights and responsibilities in Bulgaria, the Czech Republic, Estonia, Latvia and Lithuania. In Kazakhstan most health providers are now state enterprises able to contract with the government. In the Russian Federation a draft law on public non-profit organizations is being discussed.

Poor managerial skills

Poor managerial skills has proved a particular problem in parts of Eastern Europe and has meant that contracting has by no means become the prevailing pattern of relationships between purchasers and providers. For a start, there is little real experience with modern insurance schemes and contracting. Contract handling requires particular skills (among them identifying cost-effective medical interventions, negotiating and monitoring providers' performance, and communication strategy) that are not needed under direct public service provision. Furthermore, contracting implies decentralized resource allocation because bids are likely to involve locally based providers who are too numerous to be dealt with at a central level and are better known to locally based purchasers. Effective contract management skills are thus required at the middle and bottom levels, where capacity may be particularly weak. An additional difficulty is that some reform teams have shown a preference for technical approaches that are sometimes even more complex than those in many Western countries. Furthermore, the corresponding capacity building exercise has been patchy and discontinuous. Capacity building is in many countries being achieved through 'learning by doing' and unfortunately these processes sometimes focus on collecting revenue rather than improving efficiency.

Inadequacy of health funding

Since contracts express a clear-cut commitment on the part of a purchaser to reimburse the cost of provided services, attempts to start contracting require a realistic assessment of its feasibility and of the readiness to make politically loaded decisions about the public/private mix in funding. Experience in the Russian Federation and Kazakhstan suggests that with public funding at 3% to 3.3% of GDP, contracting is not fully viable. Insurers simply cannot pay all providers' bills. Thus the debt is growing, payment rates are adjusted downwards, and providers lose interest in volume and quality contractual provisions. Providers in general seem to be jumping over contracted budgets and governments usually bail out debts, as has been the case in Albania with pharmaceutical companies, in Croatia with different providers and in Georgia and Bosnia and Herzegovina with payments to physicians. Nonetheless, some of the CIS countries are currently considering launching SHI and contracting schemes without first ensuring adequate funding. For example, in Armenia, Moldova and Azerbaijan, work has started on establishing SHI with public funding ranging from 1.3% to 1.7% of GDP and practically no formal copayments of patients. Kyrgyzstan is a special case: public underfunding has been partly compensated for by formal user charges, thus increasing the viability of contracting (Kutzin et al., 2001). The Baltic states, the Czech Republic, Slovenia and Slovakia have much stronger funding bases.

A disintegrated purchasing function

The scope for contracting is further limited by the disintegration of health finance in some Eastern European countries. Newly emerging SHI systems co-exist with the old financing mechanisms through direct (non-contractual) allocation of government resources to providers. There are too many actors in health finance (SHI funds, central and local treasuries and health authorities, sometimes commercial insurers), each trying to control large portions of funding.

In the Russian Federation the bulk of funding is not allocated by health insurers but mostly by local governments with little coordination among them. Contracts cover only one-third of public health expenditures. Thus providers receive most of their money on input bases. Similar disintegrated purchasing is considered now in Kazakhstan, Moldova and Armenia. The low incidence of contracting can partly be attributed to an inability to collect enough insurance contributions, but the unwillingness of traditional payers (health authorities and local governments) to lose control over money also plays its part.

By contrast, in the Baltic states, the Czech Republic, Hungary, Slovakia and Slovenia, SHI actors control most of public money (the role of health and finance authorities in funding is limited to major investment and some legislation-delimited marginal areas). Purchasing is increasingly integrated, which facilitates financial and medical services delivery planning, with the focus on efficiency gain. The recent positive example is Kyrgyzstan, which has started the shift to a single purchaser model through integrating general budget revenue and SHI contributions (Kutzin *et al.*, 2001).

Overall and in spite of the implementation difficulties, progress is being made. Contracting in many of the countries under discussion is proving a useful exercise, with promising preliminary results: advocacy of performance-related provider payment methods, collection of management information, growing cost consciousness, new managerial skills and sometimes modest efficiency gains.

Summary and conclusions

The main lessons learned from experience with contracts can be summarized as follows.

There is not, as yet, a comprehensive body of evidence that contracts have a decisive influence in improving results in the health sector where, although many of the contractual caveats apply, uncertainty and doctor–patient asymmetry of information (the source of the agency relationship between them) reign. Conspiracy, corporatism, risk selection, market domination, segmentation, bounded rationality, and so forth, are also mentioned as limits to fair contracting.

Despite the undeniable complexity of purchasing in the health sector, European policy makers seem committed to using contracts extensively as a way to set up clearer relationships between purchasers and providers, increase cost-effectiveness, quality and responsiveness, as well as achieving equitable financing of their health systems. This is done in an environment of health system functions separation.

While all countries, both in Western and in Eastern Europe, have market entry contracts to allow health care facilities to get licensed, the use of process contracts is very much conditioned by the political context and the availability of regulatory and managerial tools.

For historical and system-related reasons, some European countries are using some contract modalities more than others. Cost-per-case contracts, the most frequent form in the United States, are also extensively used in CEE and CIS after the fall of communism. Countries with established Bismarckian systems in Western Europe are mostly refining their cost-and-volume contracts. Beveridge-system countries have started with increasingly sophisticated block contracts and are moving to cost-and-volume contracts.

Hard (fully legally binding) contracts in a competitive environment are not common in Europe. In many European countries, there is a shift to 'soft' service agreements with contracting parties depending more on cooperation and continuity of relations (relational agreements), as opposed to competition, while trying to improve the information on population health gains and on the cost function of health care services provision. Many commentators consider this a sign of 'maturing' contracting in the health care field.

In general, countries are learning to specify outputs related to health needs as circumstances and information permit. There is a certain trend to move from contracting with few provisions, mostly on costs and volume, to more sophisticated specifications such as provisions on expected health gain, quality assurance, access, and cost containment and utilization targets.

Volumes of inpatient care are usually defined in terms of total number of cases, specialty cases, bed-days (total or by specialty) and, increasingly, 'finished' cases across diagnoses or groups of diagnoses whereas in PHC they are related to patient consultations and procedures, depending on method of payment. Adaptations are usually made within self-governed or public arbitration boards. However, no health feedback, population-based monitoring is usually made when contracts are updated.

Further research is needed into improving performance contracts. An area of particular interest, given the age structure of the European population, is relational contracting and disease management – how a purchaser can contract for complete episodes of care covering more than one provider for long-term or complex cases.

The attractiveness of selective contracting is growing in many countries and few decision makers question its strategic imperative, particularly in countries with overcapacities. However, the advocacy of selective contracting is currently still weak and the opposition powerful. In some countries, removing barriers against selective contracting will probably take time.

Regarding the process of contracting, two main lessons have been learned. Contracting parties should be involved in a planning process and have an input on expected contractual outputs; in doing this they will be made accountable for reaching the targets. But contracts should not be linked to planning targets to a degree that stakeholders are expected just to endorse planning decisions of one or more of the parties, with little or no participation from the others.

The development of sound incentives and penalties as well as the entire regulation of contracts should not be seen as a one-time decision. It rather requires ongoing contract monitoring and evaluation. Contractual aspects cannot be left to the discretion of contracting parties: the role of government is critical for reaching health policy objectives.

Low operational autonomy of providers and insufficient managerial skills are key obstacles to implementation of contracting throughout the European Region, albeit in different degrees. In addition, some CIS countries face inadequate and rather unpredictable health funding as well as a disintegrated purchasing function.

Capacity building in many countries, in both East and West Europe, is mostly being achieved through 'learning by doing'. In some Eastern European countries this is true to such an extent that new managerial capacity is probably the major output of introducing SHI funds.

Notes

1   A similar but rather more detailed classification has service contracts divided into six types, namely: block contracts; block, indicative cost and volume; block indicative specialty cost and volume; stand-alone specialty cost and volume; case-mix standalone specialty cost and volume; and single item (Øvretveit, 1994).
2   'New entry and potential entry is coming not from hospitals but new kinds of suppliers encouraged by GP Fund-holders and District Health Authority purchasers and competing for only some of a hospital's activity-day surgery, specialist outpatient clinics and diagnostic testing (. . .) Even in areas that appeared secure monopolies, accident and emergency services, primary care centres as partial substitutes for hospital provision are receiving attention from purchasers. The cumulative effect of these trends is that existing secondary units must cut costs and reduce the scale and type of work they do unless they can attract new contracts and discourage any existing purchasers from switching contracts' (Dawson, 1994).

References

Accounts Commission for Scotland (1997) *Expanding on contracting*, Bulletin 1, August.
Bulgarian National Health Insurance Fund (2002) *Report on the NHIF activities in 2001*. Sofia, Bulgarian National Health Insurance Fund.
Busse, R., Prymula, R. and Petrakova, E. (2001) Implementing hospital reform in the Czech Republic. *Eurohealth*, **7**(3): 31.
Contracts for Health Services. (1990) *Operating contracts*. London, Working for Patients.
Dawson, D. (1994) *Costs and prices in the internal market*. Discussion Paper 115. York, University of York, Centre for Health Economics.
Dawson, D. and Goddard, M. (1999) Long term contracts in the NHS: a solution in search of a problem? *Health Economics* **8**: 709–720.
Duran, A. *et al.* (2003) International consultant in contracting/payment methods to health care providers and quality assurance/medical audit. Project final report by Tecnicas de Salud. Republic of Bulgaria, Health Sector Reform Project, World Bank Loan No. 4565BUL.
England, R. (2000a) *Contracting and performance in the health sector, a guide for lower and middle income countries*. London, Institute for Health Systems Development (IHSD).
England, R. (2000b) *Contracting and performance management in the health sector. Some points on how to do it*. London, Institute for Health Sector Development.
Exter, A. and Hermans, H. (forthcoming) *Case study on the Netherlands*. In Figueras, J., Robinson, R. and Jakubowski, E., eds. *Purchasing to improve health systems performance: country case studies*. Copenhagen, European Observatory on Health Systems and Policies. World Health Organization.
Gaal, P. and Eletovits, T. (2002) *The purchasing function in the Hungarian health care system*. Copenhagen, European Observatory on Health Care Systems.
Glennerster, H. *et al.* (1993) GP fund-holding: wild card or winning hand? *In*: Robinson, R. and LeGrand, J., eds. *Evaluating the NHS reforms*. London, King's Fund Institute.
Grant, K. and Collin, E. (1996) *The evolution of management in the UK National Health Service, 1948–1995*. London, Institute for Health Sector Development.

Hart, O. (1995) *Firms, contracts and financial structure*. Oxford, Oxford University Press.

Hava, P. and Dlouhy, M. (2002) *European purchasers questionnaire for the Czech Republic*. Copenhagen, European Observatory on Health Systems and Policies.

Hollo, I. and Orosz, E. (2001) Hospitals in Hungary: the story of stalled reforms. *Eurohealth*, **7**(3): 22–35.

Jesse, M. (forthcoming) Case study on Estonia. In Figueras, J., Robinson, R. and Jakubowski, E., eds. *Purchasing to improve health systems performance: country case studies*. Copenhagen, European Observatory on Health Systems and Policies. World Health Organization.

Kozierkiewicz, J. and Karski, J. (2001) Hospital sector reform in Poland. *Eurohealth*, **7**(3): 32–35.

Kutzin, J. *et al.* (2001) *Innovations in resource allocation, pooling and purchasing in the Kyrgyz health care system*. London, DFID/World Bank Conference.

Langenbrunner, J. and Wiley, M. (2002) Hospital payment mechanisms; theory and practice in transition countries. *In*: McKee, M. and Healy, J., eds. *Hospitals in a changing Europe*. Copenhagen, European Observatory on Health Care Systems.

Lynch, M. (1994) The uptake of childhood immunization and financial incentives to general practitioners. *Health economics*, **3**(2): 117–125.

Martin, J.J. (2003) Nuevas fórmulas de gestión en las organizaciones sanitarias, Documento de trabajo 14. (New management formulas in health organizations.) Madrid, Founción Alternativas.

Mays, N., Mulligan, J. and Goodwin, N. (2000) The British quasi-market in health care: a balance sheet of the evidence. *Journal of health service research and policy*, R, 1, January.

Øvretveit, J. (1994) *Purchasing for health*. Buckingham, Open University Press.

Robinson, R., Robinson, J. and Raftery, J. (1998) *Contracting by total purchasing sites*. Working paper, Total Purchasing National Evaluation Team. London, King's Fund.

Robinson, R. and Steiner, A. (1998) *Managed health care, US evidence and lessons for the NHS*. Buckingham, Open University Press.

Robinson, R. (forthcoming) *Case study on England*. In Figueras, J., Robinson, R. and Jakubowski, E., eds. *Purchasing to improve health systems performance: country case studies*. Copenhagen, European Observatory on Health Systems and Policies. World Health Organization.

Savas, S. *et al.* (1998) *Contracting models and provider competition*. Buckingham, Open University Press.

Sheiman, I. (2001) Paying hospitals in the Russian Federation. *Eurohealth*, **7**(3): 79–82.

Sheiman, I. (2002) Shall we improve structural inefficiency? *Meditsinski vestnic* 2 (in Russian).

Sheiman, I. and Wassem, J. (2002) Regulating the entrepreneurial behaviour of third-party payers. *In*: Saltman, R., Busse, R. and Mossialos, E., eds. *Regulating entrepreneurial behaviour in European health care systems*. Buckingham, Open University Press.

United Kingdom Department of Health (2002) *Reforming NHS financial flows*. London, DoH.

Williamson, O.E. (1996) *The mechanisms of governance*. Oxford, Oxford University Press.

chapter ten

Purchasing for quality of care

Marcial Velasco-Garrido, Michael Borowitz, John Øvretveit and Reinhard Busse

Introduction

This chapter adds the critical dimension of quality to the theoretical framework on health purchasing. Previous chapters have discussed at length the theoretical underpinnings for separating the purchaser from the provider and the introduction of contracting. The objectives behind these reforms are primarily economic: to increase the efficiency of the health care system and eliminate administrative rigidities.

There is a need to develop a conceptual framework for quality in health purchasing – improving the aggregate level of health in the population. It should not be forgotten that quality is an integral component of efficiency. One cannot measure efficiency without linking it to quality of care. If the goal of contracting is to improve health systems performance, it should improve the quality of care, which should lead to better outcomes. Quality of care is one of the key intermediate indicators that link inputs with outcomes. To achieve improved health outcomes, purchasing must focus on improving the quality of health services.

The growing concerns about the quality of health care have led many countries in the European region to implement national quality strategies that include a diversity of interrelated interventions and programmes such as accreditation systems, hospital quality management (for example total quality management, European Foundation for Quality Management) or other forms of external assessment of quality, such as providers' league tables or auditing (see Federal Ministry of Labour, Health and Social Affairs, 1998; Federal Ministry of Social Security and Generations, 2001).

The central question is: how can purchasing be used to enhance the quality of health care delivery? This question concerns the issue of intentionally promoting quality through purchasing, especially through contracts (Chapter 9). Obviously, an essential first step is to define and specify 'quality'. In the first section of the chapter we will briefly discuss the aspects of quality that purchasers need to consider and present the most relevant concepts related to its measurement. In the second section we will explore the mechanisms available to link purchasing with quality improvement, whereby our aim is to attempt a systematic analysis of the options used in Europe to promote quality through contracts. This overview does not attempt to cover all European countries exhaustively. In the boxes, examples are presented with some level of detail to illustrate some of the options described. When possible, examples were taken from original contracts; other sources used have been published literature and the material from the case studies produced for this study (Figueras *et al.*, forthcoming). In the third section we will discuss the options described and draw some conclusions.

Framework for quality

Aspects of quality relevant to purchasing

Quality of care is the degree to which health services for individuals and populations increase the likelihood of desired health outcomes and are consistent with current professional knowledge (Campbell, 1975). Quality of health care is a matter of achieving better health outcomes. The definition underlines a very important aspect of quality: its relationship to scientific knowledge about effective interventions. High quality care can be achieved when interventions that work are applied to the right patients at the right moment and at the right place. Improving quality in health can thus be seen as a matter of finding out and defining what is the best clinical practice and of promoting evidence-based everyday practice following such defined 'best practice'. Best practice can be defined in the form of evidence-based clinical practice guidelines or evidence-based recommendations. Systematic reviews of the evidence on effectiveness and health technology assessments – which have a broader scope than traditionally systematic reviews as they include the assessment of organizational, societal, ethical and economical aspects of the interventions (Busse *et al.*, 2002) – represent ideal underpinnings for the development of clinical practice guidelines and quality standards, because they help to identify which interventions are effective and which factors determine their success.

Quality of health care can be improved by translating evidence from research into practice. This approach should lead to reduction of practice variations and should promote appropriateness (that is reducing overuse, underuse and misuse). The efforts made to obtain results from technology assessments and from systematic reviews, and to produce high quality evidence-based clinical practice guidelines may, however, be a waste of resources if no attention is given to their adoption. For example, the actual management of asthma does not satisfactorily meet the recommendations from evidence-based guidelines in Europe, leading to poor control of the illness and poor outcomes (Vermeire *et al.*, 2002). Once the evidence has been systematically reviewed it must be turned into recommendations that, in turn, must be enforced. This is where one shifts from defining quality to purchasing, and finally monitoring quality.

Nevertheless, quality of health care delivery is not only a matter of transferring evidence to everyday practice. Even if the providers are aware of, and act following, sound scientific evidence, other aspects of the process of health care, such as organization and system design, may impair performance and lead to poorer outcomes than desired. For example, medical errors are often attributable more to structural problems and system design than to mistakes by individual professionals (Cubanski & Kline, 2002). The application of quality improvement methodology to health care, known as total quality management or continuous quality improvement, has resulted in dramatic improvements such as reducing errors in anaesthesia (Berwick, 2001).

The fragmentation of a health care system is also an important threat to the quality of health care. A lack of continuity in care leads to delays in recognition of potentially avoidable complications from chronic illnesses, duplication of services provided (for example diagnostic tests) and uncoordinated, even contradictory, interventions. Waiting lists are another system-related threat to quality. Apart from the potential to lead to poor health outcomes or even cause harm, the structural quality problems lead to dissatisfaction, even frustration, among the public, the professionals and the politicians. The dissatisfaction of those groups with the quality of health care delivery in European countries is clearly related to the above-mentioned problems (Shaw & Kalo, 2002). This introduces a further aspect of quality: public satisfaction.

In conclusion, quality of health care is a broad, multidimensional concept, with a bewildering array of definitions, frameworks and approaches. It is problematic when purchasers do not clarify for providers what they mean by quality and what they want providers to achieve.

Specifying and measuring quality

The quality of health care can be assessed and monitored by three categories of indicators: input, process and outcome (Donabedian, 1988). Within this framework, quality assessment has moved away from the classical quality assurance, based on input standards, towards a systematic understanding of the processes of care that lead to improved outcomes. Current quality assessment approaches and frameworks characterize and monitor quality by using a mix of all three types of indicators. The underlying rationale is that structural and process quality are preconditions for outcome quality. This is not to say that high quality structures and processes are a guarantee for improving outcomes, because the outcomes of an intervention are also determined by the starting situation (for example the extent to which the patients are at risk at the outset).

The primary goal of health interventions is to decrease mortality and extend life, so at first glance the desired outcome of health care should be obvious: survival. Unfortunately, mortality is an incomplete measure of desired outcomes. First, differences in outcome take time to become apparent. Second, because deaths following many interventions are uncommon, differences may simply reflect random variations. Third, it neglects quality of life. Many interventions are not intended to decrease mortality but to enhance quality of life. For such interventions, other outcomes are relevant. Because of the limitations of mortality as an outcome indicator, alternative outcomes have to be measured. The first possibility is to measure control of disease by means of physiological parameters such as blood pressure or cholesterol levels. The link between such so-called surrogate parameters and the desired outcome (for example improving survival, improving health), however, needs to be well established, on sound scientific evidence. Another possibility is to measure other patient-relevant health-related outcomes such as hospital admissions, freedom from pain, complication rates, relapse rates, functional status, and so forth.

The choice of the outcome indicators depends on the specific disease, or type of care being assessed. For example, for mental health services, the number of hospital admissions can be a good outcome indicator. Elective surgical procedures can be assessed using rates of avoidable complications. Nevertheless the measurement of outcome indicators faces an important difficulty, namely, the fact that outcomes are related not only to the quality of care, but also to other factors beyond the influence of providers, such as severity of the condition, age of patients, co-morbidity and chance. Therefore, when these measures are used to assess performance, especially if the purpose is to compare performance of providers, some kind of risk adjustment is necessary. This requires sophisticated systems for collecting the necessary data. Drawing conclusions about performance based on outcome measures in routine quality monitoring can thus be difficult if the system is not comprehensive. However, this does not mean that outcome measurement should be abandoned but that it should only be used as a tool to identify problems to be analysed in much greater detail with data not available from routine health information systems.

The difficulties in using outcome indicators mean that routine monitoring of health quality must rely on valid process indicators. Process indicators describe adherence to practices more likely to result in desired outcomes. The interest here is not the power of health care to change outcomes generally but whether providers are doing what is known to be most effective, acting on current best evidence (Donabedian, 1988). Typical process indicators are the percentages of patients treated with a therapy known to be effective for a given condition. The causal link between the action promoted by the indicator and the desired outcome needs to be well established, ideally from evidence-based clinical protocols or guidelines. These kinds of indicators are useful to assess the extent to which health care is delivered according to best evidence. An example of a process indicator is the use of aspirin/anti-platelet agents in patients with a history of non-haemorrhagic stroke or of transitory ischaemic attack (TIA) when no contraindications are present. Key process indicators together with outcomes indicators can give a good picture of the performance of a provider.

Lastly, structural indicators refer to the inputs of the health care system – qualification, technical equipment, availability of information systems, and so forth – that reflect its ability to deliver good care. The assessment of structural quality also includes the administrative structure and processes that support the provision of care (Donabedian, 1988). The underlying assumption is that high quality structures will contribute to better outcomes. Structural quality might be a necessary condition but it is not sufficient for achieving high quality performance. These kinds of indicators are commonly used in the process of licensing and certification.

Measurement of quality, on the basis of well designed, evidence-based indicators, can provide purchasers with the information they need to track performance of providers. Behind any kind of indicator-based quality assessment or monitoring, a comprehensive and reliable system of data collection and analysis is needed.

How can purchasing promote quality?

Purchasers have an intermediary function between the public and the providers. They have responsibility for allocating the resources that the public has entrusted to them in a way that leads to better health. Thus, together with providers, they share the responsibility for the quality of health services. Purchasers' responsibilities for the providers' quality are exercised via the contract and its use as a tool to enforce quality. The purchasers' responsibilities include

- negotiating and agreeing the contract:
  - specifying appropriate quality requirements, including access and availability;
  - agreeing with the provider on responsibilities for collecting quality information;
- monitoring the contract:
  - receiving providers' quality reports, and checking their validity;
  - taking action on poor quality;
  - receiving complaints directly from the public;
  - obtaining feedback from the public about satisfaction with the service;
- reviewing the contract:
  - reviewing quality performance;
  - agreeing on changes to improve quality;
  - proposing to change contracts if quality performance is unacceptable and there are alternative services.

An attempt at systematizing the options available to purchasers to promote quality in purchasing follows, focusing on the issue of specifying quality requirements, as this is the precondition for the exercise of both monitoring and reviewing. For analytical purposes, we distinguish between quality specifications that have to be fulfilled prior to negotiating the contract and those that can be included in the contracts. Later we briefly discuss some mechanisms to reinforce quality specifications.

Quality requirements prior to contracting

Certain requirements have to be fulfilled by providers in order to become eligible for obtaining and retaining contracts. A quality threshold is the condition for the provider to be able to offer its services in the marketplace. Whereas licensing, certification and accreditation (Table 10.1) are independent from purchasing and exist already in many countries, purchasers can make use of them in order to promote quality by preselecting only those providers that meet minimum quality requirements. The purchaser might sign contracts with all licensed providers, accepting the standards set in licensing, (usually) by the legislature and controlled by government stewardship. However, it might set higher standards and only sign contracts with certified or accredited providers. The terminology, however, is often not applied as stringently as Table 10.1 suggests, and in reality overlaps exist.

Licensing limits or regulates the access to the marketplace of providers (health personnel and health care facilities), stating the minimum quality requirements for receiving contracts. This approach reflects the stewardship function of the state and focuses on structural issues (minimum equipment and qualifications).

Table 10.1 Types of requirements prior to contracts

	Licensing	*Certification*	*Accreditation*
Applied to	health care facilities, health care personnel	health care personnel	health care facilities
Required for	entry into practice	professional status and possibly reimbursement	status and possibly reimbursement
Purpose	restricts entry into marketplace to providers	limits entry into and duration in marketplace to providers for special purposes	public assurance of desired level of quality of care
Duration	permanent	limited	limited
Renewal	mostly unnecessary	required recertification	required re-inspection
Standards	minimum quality of structure	minimum quality of structure and process	optimal achievable quality of structure, process and often outcome
Performance based	no	sometimes	yes
Indicator of high quality	no	limited	yes

Source: Adapted from Hafez Afifi *et al.* (2003).

Licensing does not imply any monitoring system and once a licence is given renewal is usually not required.[1] In addition, having a licence is not an indicator of quality. Licensing is usually a legal requirement to practise.

Certification is legally voluntary and is only needed as prerequisite for a contract if the provider wants to offer care at a specialty level or use special techniques. It is based on a set of educational or training standards (structure and process). Duration is limited and recertification is thus needed. Certification and recertification usually focus on minimal technical requirements and a minimal number of cases.

Accreditation represents a further step in which, besides structural standards, performance is also considered. The purpose of accreditation is to make health care organizations focus on performance improvement (Scrivens, 2002). In accreditation, processes and outcomes are assessed according to standards reflecting an optimum achievable with existing resources (Hafez Afifi *et al.*, 2003). Accreditation programmes emphasize what can be improved, and assess the providers' approach to continuous improvement. Accreditation programmes have been started in several European countries, including Belgium, Finland, France, Germany, Ireland, Italy, Kyrgyzstan, Lithuania, the Netherlands, Poland, Portugal, Spain, Sweden and the United Kingdom (Heaton, 2000; Shaw & Kalo, 2002). Originally accreditation was run by independent organizations and participation was voluntary. Being awarded an accreditation could be seen as a kind of honour for achieving an optimal level of quality and a recognition of institutional competency (Hafez Afifi *et al.*, 2003). The tendency in Europe, however, is towards governmental accreditation programmes and mandatory participation if providers are to deliver services under contract with public purchasers. In Belgium, France, Italy and Kyrgyzstan, accreditation has become a legal requirement to enter (or to remain in) the publicly funded marketplace, which actually conflicts with the original formal definition of accreditation. In Lithuania, the assessment methods and standards of an accreditation system have been kept, including an internal system of quality assurance, but the system is called 'licensing' because it is a mandatory condition for a contract with the public purchaser (Cerniauskas & Marauskiene, 2000). In Europe, accreditation seems to be taking characteristics from licensing and could become a kind of 'extra licensing' for eligibility for the delivery of care funded by public purchasers.

Accreditation programmes require considerable investment and evidence indicates that providers improve their compliance with published standards and enhance their organizational processes in the months prior to external assessment, but there is little evidence of the long-term effect of these improvements on the quality of health care or on care outcomes (Shaw, 2003). Whereas licensing is undoubtedly a precontract condition, certification and accreditation, due to their dynamic nature, can be considered both precontract conditions and contract items, since the continuation of the contract depends on the renewal of accreditation or certification. In France, for example, if accreditation still has not been achieved at the time of negotiating the contract, a deadline for achieving it can be put into the contract.

Quality specifications in the contract

Irrespective of the requirements prior to contracting, purchasers can also include quality specifications in the contract as objectives the providers commit themselves to achieving. Ideally, the contract also specifies the indicators used to measure achievement of the objectives. Following the quality framework presented in the first section, quality requirements and objectives in contracts can refer to the structure, the process and the outcomes (Table 10.2).

Structural quality

The first option is to build mechanisms into the contracts that oblige the providers to involve themselves in appropriate and comprehensive quality assurance systems or initiatives (total quality management). The Council of Europe (1997) has recommended that purchasers should contribute to quality by requiring the establishment of a quality improvement system in their contracts with providers. Some total quality management approaches ensure that attention is paid to attitudes and cultural change as well as to systems and processes. Little is known, however, about the effectiveness and cost-effectiveness of these kinds of quality programmes (Øvretveit & Gustafson, 2003). There are examples of purchasers and regulators requiring providers to use inappropriate quality systems that only add costs and bureaucracy (Shaw, 2003). It seems more appropriate to leave the decision of which system to adopt to the providers, which can then choose according to their own circumstances. Purchasers will need to develop their knowledge about quality systems in order to be able to judge between the image and the reality of providers' total quality management programmes, and to be able to judge which systems are both appropriate to a particular provider and produce data which can be used for comparisons and benchmarking.

The difference between in-house quality initiatives and requiring accreditation is that the former are not necessarily monitored and measured against standards as would be done by an accreditation agency. However, quality management

Table 10.2 Types of quality specifications in contracts

	Requirements, specifications
Structural	implementation of systems of inhouse quality management detailed structural requirements implementation of systems of data collection
Process	mandating of evidence-based standards (clinical practice guidelines) targets for indicators (for example, proportions of patients treated with . . .) minimum volume of service agreements
Outcome	targets for health outcomes (for example, proportion of patients with outcome . . .) targets for patient satisfaction

systems frequently involve some external support or supervision, so the borders with accreditation might be blurred.

Another possibility is to specify more detailed lists of structural requirements that providers should meet. The specification of structural standards is being used in several European countries, with variable levels of detail. The specification is usually accompanied by a deadline for implementation. Mostly, specifications refer to organizational issues related to accessibility, delivery of care in a timely manner, safety and continuity of care. Table 10.3 gives some examples of specifications taken from existing contracts.

A particular type of structural requirement is the establishment of systems of documentation and data collection for purposes of performance monitoring. The implementation of disease-specific or intervention-specific registers is required in the master contracts between German sickness funds and hospitals. Similarly, the British general practitioner (GP) contract includes the implementation of patient documentation systems. Since 2004, 2% of the DRG reimbursement in Stockholm County is subject to the fulfilment of required quality reporting (Dr Gunnar Németh, personal communication).

Table 10.3 Selected examples of detailed structural requirements in contracts

Specification	Area	Source
implementation of pharmacological adverse effects reporting form	safety	French hospitals
appointment of a person in charged of anaesthesia	safety	French hospitals
development of cooperation with centres for specialized care (for example oncology)	continuity of care	French hospitals
availability of a receptionist via telephone or in person in the practice for at least 45 hours over 5 days, Monday to Friday	access	United Kingdom GP contract
10-minute minimum length of routine booked appointments with doctors	other	United Kingdom GP contract
a protocol for identification of carers and a mechanism for referral of carers for social services assessment	continuity of care	United Kingdom GP contract
at least 90% of patients to be clinically assessed within 10 minutes of arrival and no patient is to wait more than 3 hours	timely delivery	United Kingdom hospitals
maximum waiting times (service specific)	timely delivery	Estonian hospitals

Process quality

From the standpoint of quality, one method is to buy clinical protocols. In theory a purchaser could purchase protocols. This means that the purchaser could mandate that the care it pays for is provided in a certain way. This approach could be used to decrease overuse and misuse of health services. The idea is to support practices that, based on best available evidence, are expected to improve outcomes. Much effort is undertaken to develop evidence-based clinical practice guidelines (CPGs) in most of the countries of the European region (Council of Europe, 2001; Burgers et al., 2003). Such guidelines, properly adapted to local necessities and peculiarities, could theoretically be made objects of contracts. In the Russian Federation, purchasers are increasingly requiring providers to adhere to clinical practice guidelines. The problem of mandating clinical protocols or guidelines is that providers may see a limitation of their professional autonomy, leading to opposition and difficult implementation.

Adherence to protocols of care can be measured with process indicators, usually expressed in rates of patients being given effective interventions. Examples are vaccination rates, screening rates, rates of eligible patients treated with effective drugs, and so forth. Even if the contract does not include explicit clinical guidelines, a set of process indicators and targets to be achieved can be specified. Targets can be formulated as increments or as absolute rates to be achieved (Table 10.4). The former requires collection of data concerning the situation previous to the contract.

Volumes of services (activity levels)

Targets for volumes of service can be agreed for elective surgical procedures such as hip replacement or cataract surgery. Agreements on activity levels (or service volumes) promote quality indirectly in several ways. First, minimum volumes can be specified in order to promote reduction of waiting lists, which are one of the public's major quality concerns (Shaw & Kalo, 2002). Concerning volumes, there is ample evidence of the relationship of service volumes and health care outcomes, especially from surgical and medical-interventionist procedures

Table 10.4 Two selected examples of detailed process quality specifications

French hospital contract (details in Box 10.1)	GP contract (details in Box 10.4)
Indicator: prescription rate of morphine or derivates for pain control	Indicator: rate of patients with coronary heart disease currently treated with beta-blocker (unless contraindicated)
Target: increase of 10% per year	Target: 25% to 50%
Indicator: length (in days) of use of morphine pumps	Indicator: percentage of women aged 25 to 64 years who have received a cervical smear in the last three to five years
Target: increase of 10% per year	Target: 25% to 80%

(Sowden *et al.*, 1997; Tiesberg *et al.*, 2001; Halm *et al.*, 2002). Agreements on minimal service volumes thus can be seen as warrants of minimal quality levels. In Germany, minimum service volumes are one of the requirements for certification and recertification in order to be eligible to contract for delivering special services in the ambulatory care sector, and Social Code Book V requires such regulations for selected procedures in the hospital care sector as well (see Box 10.2). In the countries of CEE there are major concerns about appropriateness (especially about overuse). In contracts in Estonia or the Russian Federation, for example, maximum volumes of services are specified and reinforced with penalties, in order to reduce overuse and thus to improve appropriateness.

Outcome quality

As explained in the first section, the goal of health care is to achieve desirable outcomes and, complementarily, to avoid undesirable outcomes, to the maximum extent possible. Contracts can reflect these goals by specifying outcome targets. Like process targets, outcome targets can be set as proportions of patients achieving desired outcomes or as increments (conversely as decrements for undesirable outcomes). This is being done in, for example, the United Kingdom and France, and is expected to be done in Italy (see Boxes 10.1, 10.3 and 10.4). Health care outcomes can be measured relying on validated surrogate parameters, which are known to be directly linked to health outcomes. The new GP contract in the United Kingdom (see Box 10.2) specifies targets on validated surrogate outcomes, such as blood pressure targets, cholesterol levels and HbA1c levels for hypertension, cardiovascular diseases and diabetes mellitus.

Targets for hard health outcomes are also being included in contracts. For example, a French hospital contract stipulates that the rate of nosocomial infections should be reduced by 30% within two years. The above mentioned GP contract includes the percentage of patients on drug treatment for epilepsy who have been convulsion free for the last 12 months.

Additional measures to reinforce quality

If selective contracting is practised, it is expected that providers will do their best to meet the quality requirements agreed in the contract. The possibility of losing the contract if targets are not achieved would act as an important incentive leading to change. Similarly, the precontract requirement of minimal quality levels should also promote improvement among providers wishing to survive in the market. As we discuss further below, these expectations are difficult to fulfil in reality, because decontracting or selective contracting *de facto* does not exist on a large scale in many European countries.

Contracts can, however, include explicit incentives or penalties in relation to the achievement of quality targets. Financial rewards have been shown to be effective in the case of British GPs for increasing delivery rates of specific services such as vaccinations and cervical cancer screening (Hughes, 1993). An important limitation of linking payments to achievement of single targets is their potential unintended negative effects on overall quality of care. Concerns have

Box 10.1 Contracts with public and private hospitals in France

The French regional hospital agencies (*Agence Régionale de l'Hospitalisation*, ARH) are mixed institutions with participation by both the state and the health funds. The agencies are in charge of assuring the delivery of hospital care. They have the responsibility for purchasing hospital care within an administrative region. Both publicly owned and private hospitals can be contracted. The agencies negotiate and monitor the contract. Two different types of contracts are being used: one for public hospitals and one for private hospitals.

Contracts for public hospitals

Contracts for public hospitals are tailored to the single provider. The contract includes objectives related to quality of care, which vary depending on the needs for improvement previously identified. For each objective the contract provides detailed actions to be taken, indicators for monitoring quality and targets to be achieved. Further, persons responsible for each objective are specified in the contract, together with alternative actions. Depending on the objectives, indicators to measure achievement of the targets include implementation of structures for quality, process indicators (the rate of patients treated with 'X' and/or outcome indicators, for example, the rate of nosocomial infections).

Contracts for private hospitals

These are uniform for all hospitals. In the contract, providers commit themselves to achieving accreditation within a deadline. Additionally, the contract includes a list of more than 50 specifications of targets to be achieved within an agreed deadline. The specifications refer to structural standards, mainly concerning safety. Targets to be met include, among others, appointment of persons responsible for safety and quality in different areas, establishment of action protocols, or the establishment of documentation systems. The specifications refer to the following areas: waste management, internal emergency management, pharmacovigilance, nosocomial infections, patient satisfaction, safety of anaesthesia, haemovigilance, pain management and nursing.

Sources: (Polton, forthcoming), Contracts (www.arhmip.fr).

been raised about the possibility that providers might focus on the aspects of care being measured and rewarded, which could leave other important areas of care unattended (Casalino, 1999). Rotation of quality measures, or the use of broad sets of quality measures, while rewarding only for certain measures not announced in advance, have been postulated to minimize unintended effects (Casalino, 1999). The approach taken in the new GP contract in the UK seems to

Box 10.2   Quality requirements of contracts in Germany

1. Hospital care sector

1.1 Precontract
Licensing: Purchasers are allowed to make contracts only with hospitals that fulfil minimum requirements, which are not, however, indicators of high quality (German Social Code Book V [SGB V]).

Certification: Contract partners are required to develop a list of services that can be planned (mainly elective surgery) and for which there is a 'relationship between quality and volume'. For those services, delivery of a predefined minimum volume is the condition of remaining eligible for contracts, making them a mixture of precontract certification and of target volume agreement. As of 2004, North-Rhine-Westphalia, a German Länd, has fixed yearly minimum numbers of operation volumes for breast cancer centres allowed to be contracted for breast cancer treatment in 150. At the national level minimum volumes have been established for oesophagus and pancreas cancer surgery (each 10 procedures/year) and for transplantation (kidney 20/year, liver 10/year and bone marrow 12/year). Minimum volumes for PTCA and coronary by-pass surgery are currently under discussion. However, whether volume alone can be used as a quality indicator is still controversial (Velasco-Garrido & Busse, 2004).

1.2 In contract
Obligation to participate in QA: The SGB V provides that quality has to become an object of the contracts between purchasers and providers (§137). In the contract, providers are committed to participating in quality assurance measures that put special emphasis on the documentation of quality indicators in a standard way allowing for comparative analysis. An independent institute has been established (*Bundesgeschäftstelle Qualitätssicherung* – BQS) to assist the contract partners in choosing and developing the quality indicators to be monitored. It is also charged with collecting the data and presenting them in a comparable way. As of now, the contracts oblige the providers to document the quality of a set of surgical procedures (hip, hernia and cataract) and invasive medical procedures (PTCA, pacemaker implantation). The contract partners are charged by the legislation to further develop the list of areas for which quality documentation should be provided. The contract lists sanctions in case the documentation is not completed, that is for discrepancies between the number of cases claimed for reimbursement and the number of cases documented for quality assurance.

2. Ambulatory care sector

2.1 Precontract
Certification: In order to offer special services, mostly invasive procedures or medical imaging procedures, providers need to fulfil certification

requirements in addition to being licensed as specialists. This is the case for about 30% of the catalogue of ambulatory services. Certification is obtained when the facilities fulfil minimum technical requirements and the providers have undergone additional training, defined as a minimum number of cases done under supervision. Organizational requirements are also considered for certification. For example, a binding cooperation agreement with a heart surgery unit within a determined area (measured on time to access) is required to obtain certification for ambulatory PTCA.

2.2 In contract

Recertification is needed in order to retain the ability to offer special services within the contracts. Requirements for recertification are fixed in the contracts and vary depending on the service in question. The different approaches include minimum volumes of procedures done within a year (for example, 200 coloscopies within one year), or case verification and evaluation of skills of the physician (with thresholds for sensitivity, for example). The contracts also include agreements that physicians involve themselves in quality improvement interventions such as auditing or supervision with significant event reviews. These requirements are defined by the Federal Association of SHI-Physicians (KBV), the monopolistic providers' association. In fact, the KBV acts as a 'subpurchaser' between the payers (sickness funds, which contract the KBV) and the individual providers. The KBV as a subpurchaser has the ability to link quality of care to the contracts.

2.3 Examples of ambulatory services for which certification/recertification is required

Service	Certification	Recertification
arthroscopy	+	−
dialysis	+	−
pacemaker surveillance	+	−
PTCA	+	volume (150 procedures/year)
magnetic resonance imaging	+	volume
colonoscopy	+	volume (200 procedures/year)
mammography	+	evaluation /case-verification
lab. testing	+	−
photodynamic therapy	+	case-verification
ultrasound	+	−
cytology	+	evaluation /case-verification
ambulatory surgery	+	quality data collection and audit

Sources: Contracts (www.kbv.de); Dr. Bernhard Gibis: personal communication.

Box 10.3 Authorization, accreditation and contracting in Italy

---

1. Precontract

In Italy a three-step system of authorization and accreditation constitutes the precontract requirements:

- The establishment of new health care facilities and the modification of existing ones require an authorization from the municipality, which must reach an agreement with the regional health authorities.
- The authorization for delivering health care services is granted by the regional health authorities and can only be obtained after a minimum set of structural (including technological and organizational) requirements are fulfilled. Following the conceptual framework presented in Table 10.1, this approach could be considered as a kind of two-stage licensing.
- Accreditation is mandatory for ambulatory health care facilities, hospitals and long-term care estates, whether public or private, to become contractual partners of the Italian NHS. Accreditation is granted by the regional health authorities, which develop their own standards according to general guidelines provided by the Ministry of Health. Compliance with accreditation standards is periodically assessed by independent external surveyors. The standards are mostly related to structural and organizational characteristics such as safety regulations, administrative procedures, staffing requirements and health care delivery policies (guidelines). Additional criteria are implementation of inhouse quality management systems and participation in regular external quality assessment. A peculiarity of the Italian system is that the health needs defined within the regional health plans are to be considered when awarding accreditation.

Accredited providers are the subgroup of authorized providers from among which the local health authorities can choose. It is expected that the local authorities, in cooperation with the regional authorities, will base their decisions on comparisons among accredited providers.

2. In contract

The fourth step is the negotiation of the contract. Current legislation requires that the contracts include agreements on the quality of services, including maximum waiting times and health outcomes targets.

Sources: Donatini *et al.* (2001); Pellegrini (2002); Donatini (forthcoming).

Box 10.4 The new GP contract in the United Kingdom (2003)

The new contract between the NHS and the GPs is now in the process of implementation after it was approved by the GPs. One of the innovations is that practices (not individual GPs) will be rewarded for delivering clinical and organizational quality. The new contract addresses quality mainly in two ways. First, it states a set of quality-related contractual statutory requirements that have to be fulfilled by providers as a precondition. Practices are required to have leaflets for patients, a system to handle patient complaints, safety policies and a system of quality assurance. Second, a system of financial incentives for clinical and organizational quality has been designed. Traditionally, funding of GPs has been made (with the exceptions of target-oriented payments for cervical cancer screening and child immunizations) solely on the basis of the number of patients registered with a practice. In the new contract, quality rewards will comprise a substantial part of the funding for the practices. Performance will be measured using an outcomes and quality framework especially developed for this purpose. The contract's quality framework focuses on four main components:

- *clinical standards* linked to the care of people with chronic conditions: coronary heart disease (CHD), stroke or transient ischaemic attacks, hypertension, diabetes, chronic obstructive pulmonary disease (COPD), epilepsy, cancer, mental health, hypothyroidism and asthma;
- *organizational standards* covering records and information about patients, information for patients' education and training of staff, practice management and medicines management;
- *experience of patients*, covering the services provided, how they are provided and patients' involvement in service development plans;
- *additional services*.

These components have been operationalized in a comprehensive list of 146 indicators including structural, process and outcome indicators, which describe performance.

Examples of indicators, targets and points values of the new GP contract

Type	Indicator	Points	Target range
Structural	access to a receptionist via telephone and face to face in the practice, for at least 45 hours over 5 days, Monday to Friday	1.5	yes/no
Structural	practice establishes a register for patients with stroke or TIA	4	yes/no

Process	percentage of patients with a history of myocardial infarction currently treated with an ACE inhibitor	7	25% to 70%
Process	practice will undertake an approved patient survey each year	40	yes/no
Outcome	percentage of diabetic patients with blood pressure of 145/85 or less	17	25% to 55%
Outcome	percentage of patients 16 and over on drug treatment for epilepsy who have been convulsion free for last 12 months recorded in last 15 months	6	25% to 70%

The clinical standards have been developed on the basis of the currently best available evidence. To link payments to achievement of quality standards, a system of points has been developed. The maximum number of points achievable for each indicator is related to the workload associated with it. For clinical indicators, points will be awarded for achievement between a minimum and a maximum (which can be considered a kind of simple method for risk adjustment). Alternatively, they are based on a yes/no determination (for organizational or patient-experience indicators). For example, for controlling blood pressure in diabetic patients (that is BP 145/85 mmHg or less) a maximum of 17 points can be achieved. The threshold to obtain a score is 25% of patients; the maximum practically achievable has been set at 55%. If a practice achieves this target blood pressure in 55% of its diabetic patients it will obtain the full score for this indicator. If the target is achieved only in 30% of the diabetic patients, the practice will get a score for this indicator of only 5/30, that is 2.8 points. For conducting an approved patient survey annually, a practice can get 70 points. If the survey is conducted, the full score will be awarded; if not, zero points will be given.

The approach is not prescriptive: it is left to each practice to decide which domains and targets to concentrate its efforts on. However, the contract includes a bonus mechanism to reward 'broadness' of the quality improvement, in addition to the ones stated above, which reward 'depth' of the improvements. This new contract is thus to be seen as a tool to promote quality improvements in primary care, representing a mixture of precontract requirements, and linkage of payments to achievement of clinical and organizational targets and to quality assurance implementation. The initiative of the new GP contract 2003 seems to be unique in its scope on quality (Shekelle, 2003).

Source: GP contract (2003) (http://www.nhsconfed.webhoster.co.uk/gmscontract/).

address these limitations. Payments will be in part linked to the achievement of performance targets through a point system. Points will be awarded for depth of quality in particular areas and breadth of achievement across the framework, leaving providers the choice of indicators they will focus their efforts on (see Box 10.4). The effects of this approach, intended and unintended, remain to be seen.

In Germany, sanctions have been made explicit in the contracts in order to enforce the completeness of quality documentation. The hospitals are committed to building disease-specific patient registers for selected conditions. Discrepancies between reimbursement claims and the number of cases registered in quality documentation will be penalized. Excess cases will be reimbursed at a lower tariff. Financial penalties are being used in some CEE countries when agreed service volumes are exceeded. In Estonia and in the Russian Federation excess claims might simply not be reimbursed at all.

A deeper analysis of systems for paying providers goes beyond the scope of this chapter. Rewards and penalties, however, seem to be the option most used across Europe to reinforce compliance with quality agreements in the contracts.

Discussion and conclusions

In this overview we have attempted to provide a systematic review of the options available to link quality with the purchasing process. We have presented detailed selected examples of the developments and efforts being made in France, Germany, Italy and the United Kingdom to make quality of care an issue in contracts. These cases may serve as illustrations of the mix of options available to purchasers to make quality a central component of purchasing.

A mixture of the mechanisms described above is being implemented across Europe with the intention of promoting quality of health care. This seems appropriate because the different options have advantages and limitations. A combination of several strategies thus could have synergistic effects and help to overcome the problems of each single strategy. Probably the single most important thing that purchasers can do to improve quality is to require that providers have appropriate, documented quality systems. This approach requires providers to define responsibilities and processes for assessing quality, documenting deviations and making corrections. It leaves it to the provider to decide the detailed standards to use, as opposed to the purchaser specifying its own medical standards and protocols. This is not to suggest that purchasers should not set a few key standards but rather that an appropriate provider quality system would ensure that providers formulate the critical standards, which include those of concern to the purchasers, who then only need to ensure that the system is working.

Purchasers need to decide what they will include and exclude in their definition of provider quality. Such definitions should not be so prescriptive that they make it impossible for the provider to choose a quality system appropriate for its particular circumstances. The broad definition should form part of all specifications of services to be contracted, and each individual specification should then add any details of quality the purchaser views as necessary.

A purchaser's quality definition and policy then provide the context within which it conducts relations with a provider, and within which it specifies quality standards. These are complex tasks, which will require that purchasers themselves develop skills and expertise in the field of health care quality management. Purchaser organizations, whether they are allocating public or private resources, will need to engage specialized staff if they are to fulfil their part of the responsibility for the quality of health care services.

Within the free market logic, the ideal purchasing situation would be one where several providers would compete for contracts with several purchasers. Purchasers would have the choice among providers with different levels of quality. In this ideal situation, precontract quality requirements would be used to select preferred providers and quality specifications in the contracts would regulate the relations between purchasers and providers. Theoretically, not fulfilling the quality terms of reference should lead to revision of the contract and in the worst case to decontracting. In this situation purchasing could contribute to quality improvements because providers would have an incentive to improve. The highest potential is thus seen in selective contracting.

In the real world, selective contracting based on quality faces some obstacles. In Europe, purchasers mostly spend public money and are part of the state or exercise quasi-state functions. This means that they may have to fulfil several mandates, such as covering the health needs of the population or ensuring equal access, besides looking after high quality health care. In some situations these mandates may limit the power of purchasing to enhance quality. For example, accreditation in Italy takes into account health needs stated in the regional health plans. At least theoretically, it is possible that a regional health authority might award accreditation to health care facilities that may not achieve optimal quality standards in order to meet needs (for example to maintain bed capacity). This can also be the case when only one provider is acting in an area and purchasers may be forced to contract with it in order to guarantee equal access (for example in remote regions). In such conflict between quality and capacity or access, quality issues might be put behind. In Germany, inclusion in the so-called Hospital Plan of the *Länder* (which only requires licensing and is based on an assessment of capacity needs) guarantees the provider a contract with statutory health insurance, independently of its performance. This fact may limit the purchaser's ability to promote quality not only by avoiding preselection of high quality purchasers but also by downplaying the relevance of quality specifications in the contracts as long as decontracting is *de facto* not possible.

The entanglement between state and purchasers, which is to some extent present in all European countries, may be problematic when the latter fix precontract conditions that differ from general market entry conditions. The quality requirements to deliver care for public money are becoming higher as are the requirements for delivering care. A deeper discussion about the consequences of *de facto* splitting of the market into two categories according to different levels of quality might be worthwhile. It can happen that the state licenses facilities to deliver care that neither it nor institutions performing state functions will contract for because quality requirements for delivering care with public money are higher. Does this not imply that licensing practices are insufficient to warrant quality? Is it defensible to leave providers in a marketplace that the state itself will not purchase from because of limited quality? Could this be interpreted as a neglect of the state's stewardship function?

Note

1 In exceptional cases a licence might be withdrawn as a sanction and, after a given period, renewal might be required.

References

Berwick, D.M. (2001) Not again! Preventing errors lies in redesign, not exhortation. *British Medical Journal*, **322**: 247–248.

Burgers, J.S. *et al.* (2003) Characteristics of high quality guidelines: evaluation of 86 clinical guidelines developed in 10 European countries and Canada. *International journal for technology assessment in health care*, **19**: 148–157.

Busse, R. *et al.* (2002) Best practice in undertaking and reporting health technology assessments. *International journal for technology assessment in health care*, **18**: 361–422.

Campbell, D.T. (1975) Reforms as experiments. *In*: Guttentag, M. and Struening E.L., eds. *Handbook of evaluation research*. Beverly Hills, Sage.

Casalino, L.P. (1999) The unintended consequences of measuring quality on the quality of medical care. *New England journal of medicine*, **341**: 1147–1150.

Cerniauskas, G. and Marauskiene, L. (2000) *In* Tragakes, E., ed. *Health care systems in transition – Lithuania*. Copenhagen: European Observatory on Health Care Systems and Policies.

Council of Europe (1997) *Recommendation No. R (97) 17 on the development and implementation of quality improvement systems (QIS) in health care*. Strasbourg, Council of Europe.

Council of Europe (2001) *Developing a methodology for drawing up guidelines on best medical practices* (Recommendation (2001) 13 and explanatory memorandum). Strasbourg, Council of Europe.

Cubanski, J. and Kline, J. (2002) *Improving health care quality: can federal efforts lead the way?* Issue Brief No. 539. New York, The Commonwealth Fund.

Donabedian, A. (1988) The quality of care – how can it be assessed. *Journal of the American Medical Association*, **260**: 1743–1748.

Donatini, A. (forthcoming) Case study on Italy. *In*: Figueras, J., Robinson, R. and Jakubowski, E., eds. *Purchasing to improve health systems performance: Case studies in European countries*. Copenhagen, European Observatory on Health Systems and Policies, World Health Organization.

Donatini, A. *et al.* (2001) *In*: Rico, A. and Cetani, T., eds. *Health care systems in transition – Italy*. Copenhagen: European Observatory on Health Care Systems and Policies.

Federal Ministry of Labour, Health and Social Affairs (1998) *Quality in health care: conference report of the meeting of European health ministries on quality in health care*. Vienna: Federal Ministry of Labour, Health and Social Affairs.

Federal Ministry of Social Security and Generations (2001) *Quality policy in the health care systems of the EU accession candidates: status quo and perspectives*. Vienna, Federal Ministry of Social Security and Generations.

Hafez Afifi, N., Busse, R. and Harding, A. (2003) Regulation of health services. *In*: Harding, A. and Preker, A.S., eds. *Private participation in health services*. Washington, D.C., The World Bank.

Halm, E.A., Lee, C. and Chassin, M.R. (2002) Is volume related to outcome in health care?

A systematic review and methodologic critique of the literature. *Annals of internal medicine* **137**: 511–520.

Heaton, C. (2000) External peer review in Europe: an overview from the ExPeRT Project. *International journal of quality in health care*, **12**: 177–182.

Hughes, D. (1993) General practitioners and the new contract: promoting better health through financial incentives. *Health policy*, **25**: 39–50.

NHS Confederation (2003) *GMS contract negotiations*. URL: www.nhsconfed.org/gmscontract/ (accessed 20 September).

Øvretveit, J. and Gustafson, D. (2003) Using research to improve quality programmes. *BMJ*, **326**: 759–761.

Pellegrini, L. (2002) Le quattro fasi dell'accreditamento: perchè il sistema stenta a decollare? [The four phases of accreditation: why does the system have trouble taking off?] *Monitor*, **1**(2): 2–6 (http://www.assr.it/monitor/Monitor_02.pdf).

Polton, D. (2001) *Purchasing questionnaire: France*. Copenhagen, European Observatory.

Polton, D. (forthcoming) Case study on France. In: Figueras, J., Robinson, R. and Jakubowski, E., eds. *Purchasing to improve health systems performance: Case studies in European countries*. Copenhagen, European Observatory on Health Systems and Policies, World Health Organization.

Scrivens, E. (2002) Accreditation and the regulation of quality in health services. In: Saltman, R.B., Busse, R. and Mossialos, E., eds. *Regulating entrepreneurial behaviour in European health care systems*. Buckingham, Open University Press.

Shaw, C.D. (2003) *How can hospital performance be measured and monitored?* Health Evidence Network synthesis report on hospital performance. Copenhagen, WHO.

Shaw, C.D. and Kalo, I. (2002) *A background for national quality policies in health systems*. Copenhagen, WHO.

Shekelle, P. (2003) New contract for general practitioners: a bold initiative to improve quality of care, but implementation will be difficult. *BMJ*, **326**: 457–458.

Sowden, A.J., Grilli, R. and Rice, N. (1997) The relationship between hospital volume and quality of health outcomes. *CRD Report 8 (Part 1)*. York, NHS Centre for Reviews and Dissemination.

Tiesberg, P. *et al.* (2001) Pasientvolum og behandlingskvalitet. [Patient volumes and quality of care] *SMM-Rapport 2/2001*. Oslo, SINTEF.

Velasco-Garrido, M. and Busse, R. (2004) Förderung der Qualität in deutschen Krankenhäusern? Eine kritische Diskussion der ersten Mindestmengenvereinbarung [Quality promotion in German hospitals? A critical view on the first minimum volumes agreement] *Gesundheits- und Sozialpolitik* **58**(5/6): 10–20.

Vermeire, P.A., *et al.* (2002) Asthma control and differences in management practices across seven European countries. *Respiratory medicine*, **96**: 142–149.

eleven

Purchasing and paying providers

John C. Langenbrunner, Eva Orosz,
Joe Kutzin and Miriam M. Wiley

Why focus on rewarding providers?

In a perfect market, patients express their willingness/ability to pay through consumer demand. Suppliers compete in a full market and prices are the equilibrium point between the expressed demand and supply. The advantage of direct payment by the patient is that it sends a clearer signal to the consumer about the price of the service used. It also makes the provider aware of demands. The major disadvantage is that poor patients or patients receiving expensive care for major illnesses may not have the disposable income needed to bridge the period between paying for the service and receiving a full or partial reimbursement.

The high cost and uncertain demand leads to the need for *insurance* – public or private. This introduces a third party, which pools funds. Payment to providers is then typically mediated through a pooling arrangement. Once funds are pooled, funds then must be allocated in some fashion. The form of allocation is the purchasing arrangement. The equilibrium point may be considerably altered by subsidies and copayments/informal charges in the case of demand, and restrictions in production and monopolies on the supply side. The net effect of these distortions on market prices will also depend on the provider reimbursement or reward mechanism used. The mechanism used rather than prices and demand often creates the incentive environment for suppliers of services.

Due to information asymmetry neither consumers nor producers have full information about preferences, prices or the market in which they operate. The level, mix and quality of care for consumers can be ascertained only *ex post* and good health depends on factors other than the health services consumed.

Although physicians act as agents for their patients (Arrow, 1963), even they often do not know the full impact of the interventions they are recommending. Both consumer and provider behaviour is therefore important. Pricing and payment mechanisms provide an opportunity to shape the behaviour of both through incentives. So-called 'strategic' purchasing connotes an active approach to addressing these various market failures that affect consumers, providers, and social citizenry generally. For providers in particular, it represents an important factor, although it is only one of many, along with better knowledge about clinical outcomes, cultural factors, and the professional ethics of providers.

This chapter examines provider reward or payment patterns and their effects in the European region. It examines the methods of payment and the set of incentives as tools for the purchaser to achieve one or more of its objectives. While the focus is cross-national, there are also distinct patterns over time. It focuses on remuneration of individual physicians and facilities. The chapter splits the discussion into Western European countries where a variety of mechanisms have been utilized for at least two decades, and Central and Eastern Europe (CEE)/Commonwealth of Independent States (CIS) countries where emergence of new forms of payment is roughly a decade old, and still maturing.

Payment methods: typology and historic use

A simple typology for thinking about reimbursing health care institutions and workers relates to whether payment is time based, service based or population based (Ensor & Langenbrunner, 2002). With time-based payment, providers are paid according to the length of time spent providing the service irrespective of the number served. Service-based remuneration is where payment depends on the number of services provided or patients treated. Population-based remuneration is payment according to the size of population served by the facility irrespective of the numbers of patients actually attending. Most types of payment can be categorized under one of these groups (Table 11.1).

Historically, in both Eastern and Western Europe, provider remuneration has been mainly time- and population-based. In countries in Western Europe such as the United Kingdom, and especially in countries of the Eastern bloc and Soviet Union countries prior to the 1990s, most staff were paid a time-based salary that was fixed irrespective of the level of work or size of the population catchments area. Time-based payments were typically based on input characteristics such as past qualifications and years of experience for individual providers and beds and staff for facilities.[1]

But the input-based approach allowed no flexibility to respond to local needs or changes in technology or treatment patterns. Basic population norms encouraged a certain degree of input-dominated equity, but the actual distribution was influenced both by the initial distribution of facilities and political, social and economic factors. Areas that generated more revenue had greater influence over their share than those with a smaller revenue base.

Table 11.1 One typology of provider payments

	Individual practitioner	*Medical institution*
Time based	salary	fixed budget (based usually on historic allocations)
Service based	fee-for-service	fee-for-service
	fee for patient episode (e.g., admission)	fee per hospital day (*per diem*)
	target payments	fee for patient episode
		budget based on case mix/ utilization
Population based	per capita payment, territorial payment	block contract

Source: Ensor & Langenbrunner (2002).

Moving to performance-based payment systems

Under these circumstances, it is not surprising that many countries in the region have moved away from these input-based budgets and salaries for providers. There has been an interest to reorient the system of payment towards services or activities, as measured by outputs or even outcomes. This is reinforced by the early experience in the 1980s of many health insurance systems in Western Europe/ North America that were developing or utilizing service-based systems of payment. Today, more sophisticated purchasers increasingly attempt to link payment with performance, outputs, and ultimately, outcomes (although the latter is still not employed much). They may also couple these 'performance-based' mechanisms with demand-side mechanisms such as copayments or deductibles.

These service-based approaches can be categorized on the basis of unit of service, and payment is typically made by the purchaser on a retrospective basis (that is, after the service is rendered). So-called fee-for-service (FFS) pays for basic units of services to individual providers, such as office visits, X-rays or laboratory services. Importantly, the level of remuneration under FFS can be determined either retrospectively or prospectively. Popular with providers, the traditional type of FFS is an open-ended fee charged by the doctor according to the market. The experience in industrial countries, and increasingly in other parts of the world, is that FFS correlates with a pronounced increase in volume and overall health expenditure. One short-term response to expenditure growth under fee-for-service has been to cap overall spending on the supply side, and to encourage some patient cost sharing to minimize moral hazard. One variant, the negotiated fee schedule, allows purchasers to negotiate with providers or provider associations a set of standard charges for the items of services. In general, FFS systems promote providers' internal efficiency but work against social efficiency from the consumer's point of view.

For facilities, purchasers often use *per diem* payment as the basic mode of payment. Like FFS, *per diem* methods are administratively straightforward but can encourage increases in volumes (overproduction) of services.

During the last couple of decades, new and more sophisticated payment systems have evolved with units of payment becoming broader, and prices for these 'bundles' of services set mostly on a prospective basis. Purchasers have adopted a fixed-price payment for definable products that mimic entire clinical episodes, such as an ambulatory surgery, and more often, for inpatient stays. These fixed-price payments, if administered correctly, control costs and improve internal efficiency. The general approach removes economic incentives for the hospital to overprovide services (Figure 11.1). Diagnosis-related groups (DRGs) are the best known example of these mechanisms.

There are also examples of prospective budget setting related to service outputs. Global budgets fix price as well as volume for, say, all inpatient services or outpatient services. In some EU countries the relative size of these budgets is related to information on case mix, cost and expected volume. Some countries also use capitation payments which provide a fixed amount per capita for some defined mix of services over a defined period of time (Langenbrunner & Wiley, 2002). Hence, even these prospectively oriented methods can be related to data from earlier periods on service mix and cost. As unit of service becomes broader, providers have greater incentives to contain the overprovision of services under the fee-for-service, and have the incentive to provide cost-effective care including preventive services. The provider is motivated to innovate in cost-reducing technology, use of lower-cost alternative treatment settings, and deliver cost-effective care. At the same time, providers have a new incentive for cutting down on necessary care. Providers may attempt to select low-risk clients and then cut quality of care to reduce provider costs and risk. Finally, if referrals are outside the unit of service, a patient is more likely to be sent to a specialist or a hospital while the referral is not necessary.

Table 11.2 summarizes payment methods and the incentives for provider behaviour.[2] Optimal payment systems for providers should induce providers to perform high-quality, effective treatments, while promoting a rational allocation

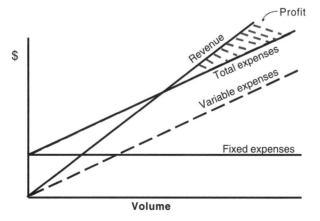

Figure 11.1   The economics of per case payment.
Source: Lyles & Palumbo (1999).

Table 11.2 Provider payment methods and indicative incentives for provider behaviour

Mechanisms	Incentives for provider behaviour		
	Prevention	Delivery/production of services	Cost containment
Line item budget	+/−	−	+++
Fee-for-service (FFS)	+/−	+++	−−−
Per diem	+/−	+++	−−−
Per case (e.g., DRGs)	+/−	++	++
Global budget	++	−−	+++
Capitation	+++	−−	+++

Sources: Adapted from WHO (2000); Jegers *et al.* (2002).

of resources within the health sector. As suggested by Table 11.2, international experience and the asymmetry of information discussed in the literature reflect tensions across these multiple objectives. Several objectives may be equally desirable, but mutually irreconcilable, in the sense that payment systems that can achieve each individual objective are not the same, and these may be in conflict with each other. Among the tensions illustrated by the existing literature on provider payments are:

- quality enhancement and cost containment (Ellis & McGuire, 1990);
- provider risk and production efficiency;
- risk-selection and production efficiency (Newhouse, 1998);
- 'fairness' in levels of payment and optimal levels of service (Jencks *et al.*, 1984).

To reach equilibrium among conflicting objectives, a mixed reimbursement system may be necessary to optimally balance multiple objectives such as cost containment and quality (Dranove & Satterthwaite, 2000).

Developments in Western Europe

Tables 11.3 and 11.4 present an overview of approaches to paying for physician and hospital services in selected Western European countries. As in other OECD countries, payment systems have been utilized to contain costs as well as redistribute increasing shares of expenditures to less expensive primary and outpatient care.

Physician services

Three models have dominated payment for physician services historically: salary, capitation and fee-for-service or some combination. In general, physicians in private practice are paid on a fee-for-service basis while salary or

Table 11.3 Payment of physicians in Western Europe

Country	Salary	Capitation	Fee-for-service	Combination
Northern 'NHS' model/tax-based health systems				
Denmark				X (capitation + FFS)
England	X (hospital-based)	X (public)	X (private)	
Finland	X			
Ireland	X (hospital consultants in public practice)	X (public patients)	X (private patients)	
Norway			X	
Sweden	X (public)		X (private)	
Southern 'NHS' model/tax-based health systems				
Italy		X		
Portugal	X			
Spain				X (salary + capitation)
Social health insurance-based health systems				
Austria				X (flat rate + FFS)
Belgium			X (private)	
France			X	
Germany			X (free practising)	

Table 11.4 Payment of hospitals in Western Europe

Country	Line item	Per case	Global budget	Combination global budget with DRGs/ case-mix adjuster
Northern 'NHS' model/tax-based health systems				
Denmark		X	X	
England				X
Finland		X		
Ireland				X
Norway				X
Sweden				X
Southern 'NHS' model/tax-based health systems				
Italy				X
Portugal				X
Spain				X
Social health insurance-based health systems				
Austria				X
Belgium				X
France				X
Germany				X

capitation or some combination tend to dominate as payment methods for service provision in the public sector, though countries such as France and Germany also pay on a fee-for-service basis for all patients.

Some models have been undergoing almost constant change and evolution. In England, some purchasing responsibility in the early 1990s was allocated to selected general practice (GP) fundholders with at least 11 000 patients registered with them. Their budgets typically covered up to 20% of the total per capita allocation for each patient; the remainder rested with the health authority. Initially, 306 practices joined; by 1998 there were 3500 GP fundholding practices, covering 60% of the population.

The new Labour government abolished fundholding in 1997 and established a nationwide system of primary care groups (PCGs)/primary care trusts (PCTs). Unlike fundholding – which was voluntary – membership of a PCG was compulsory for all GP practices. The average PCG covered a population of 100 000, although there were variations ranging from approximately 50 000 to over 250 000. Over time, PCGs have been converted into PCTs. These are freestanding bodies with a budget for commissioning care, covering average populations of 170 000 and controlling about 50% of the overall national budget for health; by 2004, it is intended that they control approximately 75% of the budget.

Hospital services

Within the hospital sector, most countries in Western Europe have moved to a performance-based approach, using some combination of case-mix adjusted diagnosis-related groups (DRGs) and/or global budgets. Within this general framework, some diversity of approaches to payment for inpatient services is in evidence. Most have developed to meet cost-containment objectives.

The shift to a performance-related payment scheme for inpatient hospital services in Austria in the early 1990s was very much driven by cost-containment objectives. The allocation of funding for health system support is, in the first instance, based on fixed-term statutory agreements between the federal government and the *Länder*. The *Länder*, in turn, negotiate budgets with the hospitals (Hofmarcher & Riedel, 2003). While the distribution may vary, the largest component of the hospital budget is now determined on the basis of the Austrian DRG system known as the LKF (*Leistungsorientierte Krankenanstaltenfinanzierung*). Within the LKF-model, costs on a case-mix basis may be determined at the hospital level so hospital funding may be directly related to performance. Recent research suggests an initial reduction in the rate of growth of hospital costs though costs have begun to accelerate again (Hofmarcher & Riedel, 2003).

In Belgium, DRGs are applied within a prospective budgeting framework for funding acute inpatient services. Unlike Austria, the case-mix adjustment depends upon the length-of-stay level. Specifically, where length of stay for a hospital differs significantly from the national average for a DRG category, a positive or negative adjustment may be applied depending on the direction of the observed difference. The redistribution of funding from hospitals with excessively long lengths of stay to those with shorter average stays is intended as a reward to those hospitals considered to be performing well (Roger France *et al.*, 2001).

Scandinavian countries are characterized by very decentralized systems, but activity-based reimbursement is increasingly being used, and in place of the capped global-budget approach (Pedersen, 2002: 14). They have developed the Nord-DRG system. Although based on the DRGs, it allows for local adaptation.

In 1997, activity-based financing (ABF) was introduced for Norwegian hospitals with a key objective of encouraging counties and hospitals to increase the number of hospital treatments without reducing hospital efficiency. Within this system, a proportion of the block grant from the central government to the county councils was replaced by a matching grant determined on a DRG-basis. Bjorn *et al.* (2002) found that ABF did increase productivity. Poor information systems did not allow for a good measure in change of cost structure and the cost of increasing the number of patients treated remained uncertain.

Responsibility for health-system organization in Finland rests with the municipalities. Hospitals are increasingly using DRGs as the basis for billing municipalities for services delivered (Pedersen, 2002: 14). A number of pilot tests are under way to test different models including the purchaser–provider model, models based on virtual and real integrated primary–secondary providers as well as those based on contracting-out primary care to external providers (Rico & Wisbaum, 2002).

In Sweden, in the early 1990s, many county councils implemented reforms broadly based on the model of purchaser–provider split. These reforms generally involved the separation of the purchaser and the providers; allocation of funds based on DRGs; competition between private and public caregivers and increased choice for patients (Lofgren, 2002). Bruce and Jonsson (1996) found that county councils that had implemented the purchaser–provider split had higher levels of productivity compared with those counties that had continued to implement the traditional global budgeting approach. However, the latter group of counties seemed to be more successful at containing costs.

In Denmark, global budgets are used to fund hospitals that are owned, financed and run by the county councils. While not mandatory, the so-called 90/10 model has become increasingly used for funding hospitals. Within this model 90% of the budget requirements estimated for a projected level of activity are allocated to the hospital, whereas 10% of the funding is earned by grants per treated patients (Hansen & Nielsen, 2001). As patients can now choose to receive treatment in any hospital of their choice, cross-county, free-choice patients are now funded by DRG-based payment.

Regional hospital agencies (*Agence Régionale de l'Hospitalisation* (ARH)) in France have some functions in relation to planning, contracting and funding for public and private hospitals within their jurisdiction. While this agency may come closest to playing the purchaser role, the extent to which this happens in practice is questionable. The potential for purchasing-type functions to be applied may arise in relation to contracting and funding rather than planning. The ARH is supposed to sign a contract with each hospital agreeing on the range of activities over a defined time period. While this facility would be expected to provide an opportunity for the introduction of tools to improve efficiency, in practice it seems that the realization of such objectives is limited. The problem of deficiencies in information systems was partially addressed with the requirement from the early 1990s of hospital participation in the *Programme de Médicalisation du Système d'Information* (PMSI), which collects data on activity for analysis by the French DRG-type system, *Groupes Homogènes de Malades* (GHM).

Since the late 1990s, budget determination for hospitals has been partially based on the GHM system with the objective being that all hospitals will be funded on a GHM basis for services related to acute care from 2004 (Rodrigues & Trombert-Paviot, 2001: 61). While in theory this would be expected to provide the ARH with the tools and the information to facilitate the development of a more informed purchasing role, in practice this does not seem to have developed. This has been partially explained by a range of factors, including being engaged in multi-annual contractual arrangements and an annual budget cycle. These may actually constrain the power of the ARH, if there is a contractual agreement to deliver a service, it seems to be difficult to make changes even where inefficiencies occur. An additional factor relates to the finding that, while the thrust of policy development is to increase local and regional autonomy in the hospital sector, in reality responsibility for many significant decisions (like wage rates) remains at the national level and therefore may result in *a priori* constraints for more innovative practices at the regional or local level.

With the Reform Act of Social Health Insurance (SHI) 2000, the German federal government has committed itself to the introduction of a DRG-based payment system for hospital patients on a voluntary basis from January 2003 and on a mandatory basis from 2004. It has been proposed that this system will be introduced on a budget neutral basis and will be based on a German adaptation of the Australian DRG system (AR-DRGs). The main objectives proposed for this reform of the hospital payment system is 'the establishment of an adequate (efficient) reimbursement, a greater transparency and a better comparability of inpatient services' (Schellschmidt, 2001: 72).

With the regionalization of the Spanish NHS in the 1980s, the autonomous regions gained responsibility for the organization and development of their own health care system. In general, regional health care purchasers and the hospitals and primary care centres agree on annual contracts called *contrato-programa* (Costa & Rico, 2001). These contracts established the basis for prospective payments due to hospitals subject to the fulfilment of the contractual conditions. With the shift to contracting, some form of activity measure was needed to establish the specification and costing of hospital services (Casas & Illa, 2001). Over time, the DRG system has come to be the accepted measure of case mix in use in Spain. The general approach to hospital funding has evolved to a prospective basis, which may be product based or budget based or a combination depending on local circumstances. In Catalonia, for example, hospital inpatient activity is funded by prospective global budgets adjusted for case mix whereby 30% of the budget is determined on a DRG basis and the remaining 70% determined by an agreed assessment of hospital structural characteristics (Casas & Illa, 2001). Evidence of the implications of the different approaches pursued is limited and may vary between regions but there is some support for the belief that hospital efficiency in the public sector has improved, although mainly as a result of the homogenization of efficiency levels across hospitals (Costa & Rico, 2001).

A case-mix adjustment has been applied within a global budgeting framework for acute hospital services in Ireland and Portugal since the early 1990s (Wiley, 1999). In both systems, an agreed proportion of the budget, determined in advance, was estimated on a DRG basis with the objective of providing incentives for increased efficiency in the provision of hospital services. In Ireland currently, about 20% of the acute hospital budget is determined on a DRG basis and this level of adjustment is projected to increase over the coming years (Wiley, 2001).

In England, a DRG-type system called Healthcare Resource Groups (HRGs) has been developed. To date, this system has been most frequently used for determining contracts for the commissioning of hospital services. It is now proposed, however, to move towards commissioning at a specialty level based on volumes adjusted for case mix using HRGs (Department of Health, 2002). Initially, the focus will be on commissioning of elective care between PCTs and NHS trusts, to be extended later to all services. Output efficiency showed some improvement following on the 1991 NHS reforms, but now seems to be 'disimproving' (Oliver *et al.*, 2002). In contrast, the responsiveness of the system is considered to be improving as indicated by reductions in long-term waiting times for hospital services.

Developments in CEE and CIS

Until the break-up of the Eastern bloc the overall budget was dominated by the hospital. Activity was supply driven. At the core was low status, low training standards, and poor capability of primary care and outpatient providers. The budget then reinforced an emphasis on the inpatient sector. Large hospitals led to more patients, in turn increasing the budget for non-staff items and even 'justifying' greater investment in inpatient infrastructure (Ensor, 1993; Preker & Feachem, 1993). This allocation process at a macro level, combined with a lack of competition, choice and efficiency incentives at the micro level, encouraged a divergence in care and utilization patterns in the CIS countries relative to Western European countries. Referral rates to hospitals ran as high as 25% to 30% of first visits to clinics in CIS countries in the early 1990s (Sheiman, 1993), relative to less than 8.6% in the United Kingdom. Hospital admission rates, as a percentage of population, were 18% to 24% for these countries relative to 16% on average for all OECD countries. Average lengths of stay were two to three times as high as OECD countries. Approximately 65% to 85% of state health budgets were allocated to inpatient care (WHO, 1998), compared with around 45% to 50% in OECD countries (OECD, 1997). Thus, one objective of new payment methods was to improve efficiency, both technical and allocative.

A second issue was the perceived underpayment to physicians and nurses, which affected productivity of providers but also hurt both quality and access of care. Informal payments and gratuities were a way to supplement income and ration access to limited services. By the late 1980s, the flow of resources began to be more unpredictable with providers often missing payments or going without salary for long periods of time (Langenbrunner & Wiley, 2002). New payment mechanisms might be used to improve resource flows and improve productivity.

As early as 1987, many Eastern European countries began testing new organizational and financing models to improve efficiency. Later, the 'new economic mechanism' (NEM) in the CIS, for example, picked a number of geographic demonstration areas, reorganized the polyclinics into family practice groups and initiated fundholding arrangements. There were early successes, with drops in admissions (Sheiman, 1993; Langenbrunner *et al.*, 1994) and expenditure shifts from approximately 70:30 inpatient to outpatient spending to levels closer to 50:50 (Schieber, 1993). Samara, a region in the Russian Federation, reported closures of 5500 beds (*Meditsinskaya Gazete*, 1996).

With the break-up of the Soviet Union in the late 1980s and early 1990s, a number of CEE and CIS countries moved almost immediately to new insurance arrangements (Czech Republic, Hungary, the Russian Federation) and new resource allocation methods. Not all countries have changed, and payment systems in Ukraine, Moldova, Belarus and Turkmenistan, for example, resemble the ones in place more than a decade earlier. In some countries, particularly in the Caucasus (Armenia, Azerbaijan and Georgia) and Tajikistan in Central Asia, tax revenues collapsed in the early transition period to such an extent that out-of-pocket spending has dominated all other forms of payment.

Primary and outpatient care

Health insurance funds and even ministries of health now more typically purchase services in a strategic way, rather than just passively allocating salaries or line item budgets on a formulaic basis, and encourage improved internal efficiency through improved service payment systems (Saltman & Figueras, 1998). New primary care payment systems most often being developed are primary care capitation as seen in Figure 11.2. The countries utilizing some variant of this approach include Armenia, each of the Baltic states, Bulgaria, Croatia, the Czech Republic, Georgia, Hungary, Kyrgyzstan, Poland, Romania, Slovakia, Slovenia and Uzbekistan. Some of these models pay the physician directly; in other cases payment has gone to the facility. Some of these models extend the traditional mix of services (for example, minor surgeries) or 'carve out' priority services such as immunizations and pay fee-for-service for these services (Czech Republic, Estonia, Romania, Slovenia), or pay a bonus for rural placement (Estonia, Georgia, Lithuania). This fee-for-service and bonus add-on to the capitation model is important because some capitation models have been shown to decrease utilization of preventive services (for example, Kazakhstan) (Langenbrunner *et al.*, 1994).

Some countries have changed incentive structures more than once. Slovakia went from a fee-for-service point system in 1993 with an additional adjustment for private doctors. This adjustment had its desired effect in facilitating the start of private practices, but FFS led to cost increases, and Slovakia then quickly moved to capitation in 1994, then a 60:40 capitation/FFS mix in 1998.

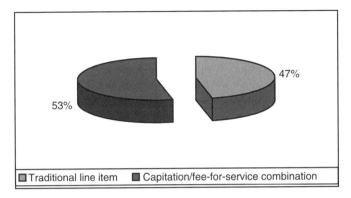

Figure 11.2 Percentage of countries in CEE/CIS with traditional line item budgets and capitation-fee combination in paying for primary care.
Source: European Observatory, HiT Reports (www.observatory.dk) 1998–2002.

Changes in payment incentives have effected behaviour change, especially if these have been accompanied by other reforms or institutional changes at the provider level. An important adjunct reform has been education and retraining of providers to improve quality and introduce new protocols. This coordination of reforms can increase impact, even in low-income countries. For example, Uzbekistan began implementation of a new rural primary care model in 1998 in three pilot regions. The basic elements of the model included formation of new, independent rural physician posts (or 'SVP's in the the Russian Federation vernacular), upgrading clinical skills and training in general practice, new information systems, pooling of funds for primary care at regional (*oblast*) level, and a new capitated rate payment system driven by consumer choice of SVP. Among other things, the increased autonomy of the providers to allocate their capitation payments led to changes in the cost structure of SVPs. In one of the three pilot *oblasts* for example, the share of SVP expenditures devoted to drugs increased by 44% from 1999 to 2001. Between 1998 and 2001, average annual visits to SVPs increased by 224%, while referrals from SVPs decreased by 33% (World Bank, 2002).

Similarly, pilot projects in consumer choice-driven capitated rate payment systems for primary care have been in place in pilot areas of Kazakhstan's Karaganda region since 1995. Whereas Uzbekistan appears to have been able to provide the needed provider flexibility through increased autonomy within the public sector, in Kazakhstan the primary care practices were privatized, and they compete for enrolees. There is an open enrolment period each year, and data indicate that the percentage of the population that changes providers ranged from 3.2% in 1999 to 11.1% in 2002. This suggests that the payment system combined with provider-level changes has increased the active involvement of the population and encouraged providers to be more responsive to consumers (O'Dougherty, 2003).

Primary care fundholding arrangements are emerging. In Estonia, family practitioners have undertaken a very limited form of fundholding since 1998. In 2002 they received a virtual budget representing just fewer than 20% of the total capitation fee with which they can provide and/or purchase selected clinical and diagnostic services. These include minor surgery and physiotherapy, common endoscopic procedures, X-rays and biochemical tests. In Latvia, the general practitioner receives a capitation payment adjusted for age of enrolled patients. The per capita amount covers salary, a nurse in low density areas, and specialist referrals. Specialists receive payment according to a per episode price list. Some specialists (for example, endocrinologists, psychiatrists, tuberculosis specialists) have separate accounts. In Hungary, a managed care pilot of about half a million enrolees was enacted in 1999. It provides an age-adjusted capitation payment to groups of family physicians, which in turn contract with secondary service providers. Provider groups have a separate account managed through the insurance fund.

Kyrgyzstan introduced an outpatient drug benefit programme called the Additional Drug Package (ADP) on a pilot basis in mid-2000 and is currently in the process of extending this nationally. The ADP is funded out of the primary care physician capitation payment, and thus is a virtual partial fundholding arrangement, with the Kyrgyz HIF managing the programme on behalf of each primary care practice. The ADP targets important causes of ill health and hospitalization, particularly hypertension, iron-deficiency anaemia, bronchial asthma and stomach/duodenal ulcers. The choice of these conditions was driven by purchaser data on hospitalizations, which showed many admissions related to these conditions for which good primary care, including appropriate medicines, could enable effective outpatient treatment. The ADP was also linked to the dissemination of new clinical practice guidelines for these conditions.

The payment method used under the ADP sets a 'basis price' for reimbursement of contracted pharmacies according to standard defined daily dosages for each covered drug. It functions as a reference price system similar to that used in Germany and the Netherlands, under which patients pay the difference between the reimbursement amount and the retail price (Kadyrova & Kutzin, 2002; Kutzin *et al.*, 2002). The ADP led to demonstrable gains in the efficiency of service delivery with reduced admissions and increased outpatient care. Pilot site data are presented in Table 11.5.

Many countries have enacted changes in the way outpatient specialists are paid. Some variant of fee-for-service points-based system, with an overall cap, is now utilized in the Czech Republic, Estonia, Hungary, Romania and other countries. The approach is not uniform. Armenia, for example, reports capitation; the Russian Federation still uses a mix of mechanisms depending upon region.

Finally, unofficial, out-of-pocket payment for specialist care is increasingly common in lower-income countries. While there may be some limited budget funding, providers can effectively demand some extra payment for either routine care or for 'queue jumping' or for access to limited diagnostic services. (This is discussed in more detail below.)

Table 11.5 Percentage of cases referred for hospitalization in ADP: pilot sites

Polyclinic	Hypertension		Stomach/ duodenal ulcer		Bronchial asthma		Anaemia	
	2000 %	2001 %	2000 %	2001 %	2000 %	2001 %	2000 %	2001 %
Bishkek #1	10.8	2.9	9.6	7.8	22.0	17.0	11.3	1.8
Bishkek #6	1.0	0.4	2.4	2.6	8.0	2.8	1.0	0.4
Alamudin	17.0	15.0	23.6	9.6	40.6	25.6	17.2	4.3

Source: Kyrgyzstan Ministry of Health data (first nine months of each year). 2000 data mainly reflect the situation prior to the introduction of the ADP in August 2000. 2001 data show the situation for a comparable period the following year.

Inpatient services

Many of these countries have or are developing new hospital payment systems which pay for a defined unit of hospital output. The Czech Republic, in the early 1990s, used a purely fee-for-service schedule for 4500 inpatient and outpatient procedures. The FFS system led to a cost explosion, with expenditures increasing 46% from 1992 to 1995, when expenditures were capped. Expenditure increases then slowed to less than 5% from 1995 to 2000 (Hava, 2001; OECD, 2003).

The most popular approaches in the early years of transition were the *per diem* and per case based payment systems, which can be viewed as linked. *Per diem* and simple per case were most often developed both because they required little data or capacity to design and implement but these were also seen as methods to promote greater productivity by providers and also generate increased revenues for them. Individual countries started at different levels of expertise and interest and have progressed differently. However, most combined different levels of *per diem* and simple case-mix (for example, department in a facility) measures, and typically included only recurrent costs not capital costs or depreciation. Nevertheless, these steps serve as a developmental framework for examining these countries in terms of alternative hospital payment models. Later, countries have refined these general models. For example, they adjust levels of payment for categories of facilities as a proxy for overall case severity, or pay a higher rate for statistical outlier cases as measured by standard deviations from the mean for measures such as costs or lengths of stay. A summary of *per diem* and per case systems is provided in Tables 11.6 and 11.7.

Providers have responded to these incentives, but not always as purchasers may have wished. These *per diem* and case-mix systems have driven up volume of cases admitted to hospitals, and have put fiscal pressures on the purchasing organization (for example, in Croatia, the Czech Republic, Hungary, the Russian Federation). A relative reduction in numbers of beds and reduced average lengths of stay (Figure 11.3) increased allocative efficiency. But these trends were offset by increasing admissions (Figure 11.4) in the 1990s – a trend that started in the mid-1990s in Eastern Europe and the late 1990s in former Soviet countries when these began using new payment methods. Average lengths of

Table 11.6 Features across countries of *per diem* payment systems for hospital services

Country	Case-mix adjuster	Facility adjuster	Overall expenditure cap	Other features
Croatia		X	X (1999)	Points system for providers
Slovakia		X	X	
Slovenia	X (bed-days and adjuster for high-cost cases)		X	
Estonia	X		X	Fee-for-service for some procedures

Source: Langenbrunner & Wiley (2002); updated by authors.

Table 11.7 Features across countries of per case payment systems for hospital services

Country	Payment categories	Payment rate calculation basis	Facility adjusters	Outlier payment feature	Overall spending cap
Latvia	64	Historic level of bed-days	X		
Lithuania	160	Historic level of bed-days		X	X
Poland	9–29	Estimated payroll, tax revenues			
the Russian Federation	From 50 000 to 55 000	Varies	X		
Georgia	30	Historic budget and productivity standards			
Kazakhstan	147	Step-down costing[3] to departmental level, further breakdown by relative ALOS within department	X		
Kyrgyzstan	139	Step-down costing to departmental level, further breakdown by relative ALOS within department			X
Hungary	758	Historic costs	X	X	X

Source: Langenbrunner & Wiley (2002); updated by authors.

stay fell by over 20% in countries such as the Czech Republic, Hungary, Poland, Slovenia and Romania (Orosz, 2001). Poland, where the volume of admissions jumped 30% in one year with the advent of per case payment, was typical. The Czech Republic with its fee-for-service policies of the early 1990s is the most blatant example of overutilization and expenditure increases. Was this a response to unmet need, or provider 'gaming' in response to incentives? If the latter, most purchasers had little capacity or experience in the way of quality or administrative mechanisms to stem the rapid increases in volume encouraged by the underlying incentives in these new systems (Healy & McKee, 2002).

At the same time, these incentive systems were not necessarily the only driver for reducing beds or admissions. In Bulgaria, for example, most public hospitals suffered from chronic shortages of financial resources due to economic crisis and contraction of government spending for health care (Delcheva & Balabanova, 2001). The number of beds was reduced through lack of funding rather than through new purchasing incentives. Figure 11.5 shows that some of the largest drops occurred in countries without new payment systems in the last decade. Figures 11.4 and 11.5 reveal that the poorer countries of the region were most likely to experience declines (particularly large declines) in admissions and beds. This may reflect demand-side factors, with the need to pay on an out-of-pocket basis (formally or informally) posing a financial barrier to hospital care.

At the same time, a number of countries in Eastern Europe have shifted or are now shifting policy objectives, from revenue enhancement and increasing provider income, to more cost containment and efficiency. With that shift in policy objective, purchasers see hospital global budgets and capitation as 'next generation' beyond *per diem* and per case systems, and have begun by instituting simple caps on hospital expenditures. Global budgets are being developed in several countries (see Table 11.8), with capitation pilots in a number of countries such as Hungary, Poland and the Russian Federation. Much of this activity is in response to volume problems under *per diem* and per admission payment systems (Langenbrunner & Wiley, 2001). Some countries (Croatia, Hungary and Lithuania) cannot wait for sophisticated risk-adjusted payment systems, and instead volume limits are being established and subsectors (for example, primary care, hospital care) are being capped as a first step to stopping the current haemorrhaging of expenditures.

Implementation of new payment systems: an unfinished agenda

While the number and types of new payment systems in the region show a clear change over the previous decade, results have been mixed to date, especially in CEE and CIS countries due to a number of issues in the region discussed above, as well as other specific issues that await future policy leadership, including the discussion below.

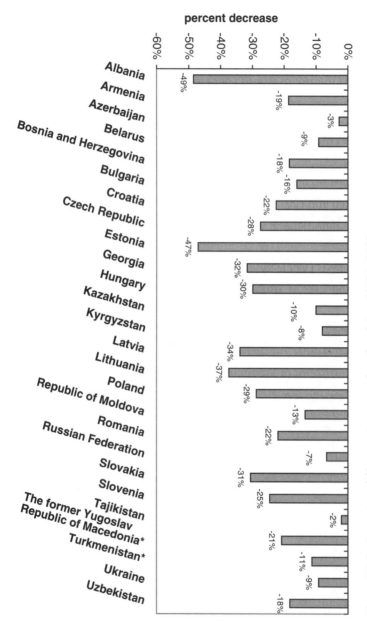

Figure 11.3 Percentage differences in average lengths of stay: 1990 to 2000.

Source: WHO, *Health for all database*, 2004.

* For The former Yugoslav Republic of Macedonia and Turkmenistan, the last available data is for 1997.

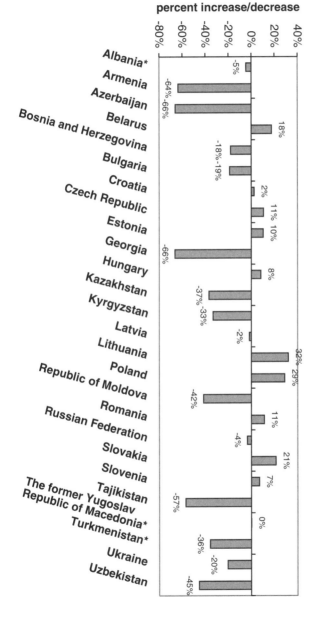

percent increase/decrease

Figure 11.4 Percentage differences in admissions per 1000 of population: 1990 to 2000.

Source: WHO, *Health for all database*, 2004.

* For The former Yugoslav Republic of Macedonia and Turkmenistan, the last available data is for 1997. For Albania, the first available year is 1993.

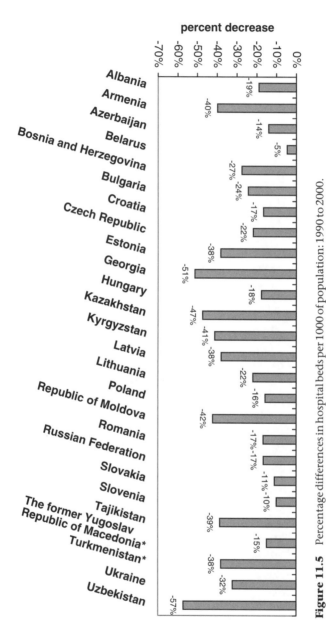

Figure 11.5 Percentage differences in hospital beds per 1000 of population: 1990 to 2000.

Source: WHO, *Health for all database*, 2004.

* For The former Yugoslav Republic of Macedonia and Turkmenistan, the last available data is for 1997.

Table 11.8 CEE and CIS countries: hospital payment systems

	Line item	Per diem	Per case	Global budget
Albania				X
Armenia			X	
Azerbaijan	X			
Bosnia and Herzegovina				Developing
Bulgaria			X	Developing
Croatia		X		Developing
Czech Rep.			X	X
Estonia		X	Partially implemented	
Georgia			X	X
Hungary			X	
Kazakhstan			Partially implemented	
Kyrgyzstan			X	
Latvia		X	Developing	
Lithuania			X	
The former Yugoslav Republic of Macedonia	X			Developing
Moldova	X			
Poland			X	
Romania			X	X
The Russian Federation		X	X	X
Slovakia		X		Developing
Slovenia			X	
Tajikistan	X			
Turkmenistan	X		X	Developing
Turkey	X			
Ukraine	X			Developing
Uzbekistan	X		Developing	

Source: Dixon *et al.* (2004).

Fragmented public sector pooling and purchasing

The scope for payment incentives changing behaviour is limited by disintegration of health finance pooling. Newly emerging insurance systems have often coexisted with the old financing mechanisms (often already fragmented by level of government administration) through direct (non-contractual) allocation of government resources to providers. In many countries too many actors have begun allocating funds (insurance, central and local treasuries and health authorities, sometimes commercial insurers), each trying to control its portion of the money.

In the Baltic states, the Czech Republic, Hungary, Slovakia, Slovenia and Kyrgyzstan, insurers control most (>70%) of public funds, irrespective of the source of funds. Purchasing is increasingly integrated, which facilitates financial planning and planning of medical services delivery (both strategic and operational) with the focus on efficiency gain and predictability of flows of funds. The most recent positive example is Kyrgyzstan, which has started the shift to a single purchaser model through integrating all general budget revenues at regional level and coordinating the use of these with SHI contributions (Kutzin *et al.*, 2002). Early effects of this in terms of reduced fixed costs in the service delivery system in the two *oblasts* that implemented the reform in 2001 are seen in Figure 11.6.

In the Russian Federation, the bulk of funding is not allocated by health insurers but mostly by local governments, with little coordination between them. Literally thousands of health pools of funds exist. Insurance covers less than one-third of public health expenditures. Similarly, purchasing reforms are now being considered in Armenia, Kazakhstan and Moldova, without concurrent plans to address the fragmentation problem. In such instances, payment reforms could include only selected recurrent costs, not capital costs or other types of costs such as utilities (for example, in the Russian Federation and Kazakhstan) or even salaries. This focus only on selected recurrent costs, dilutes incentives, and also dilutes the need to downsize and restructure facilities or provider organizations.

Poor complementarity of design

Payment reforms across settings often do not complement one another, hurting allocative efficiency. In Croatia, primary care capitation for physicians was 'matched' with fee-for-service payments at the specialist referral and inpatient settings. That meant that both primary care physicians and upper end providers had the incentive of referring up the delivery structure, instead of managing more patients at the primary care level. As a result, the share of inpatient spending (Figure 11.7) and hospital admissions increased in Croatia from

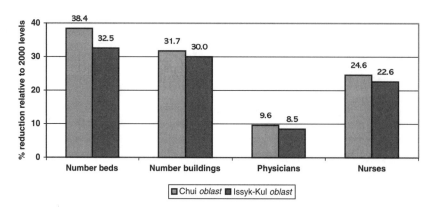

Figure 11.6 Kyrgyzstan: reductions in fixed inputs in the first year of the single pooling and purchaser model.

Source: Socium Consult (2002).

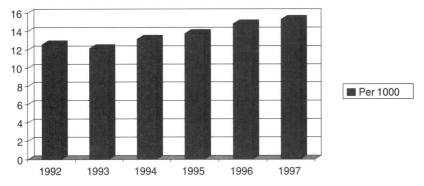

Figure 11.7 Croatia: increasing hospital admissions during years of primary care reform.

1993 to 1997, even as the World Bank's loan financing of nearly $50 million was targeted on primary care reforms.

Similarly, closed sub-budgets (of the primary care, outpatient specialized care and inpatient care) are now being applied in countries such as Hungary, Czech Republic, Slovakia and Slovenia. These are important tools for cost containment, but will they generate adverse incentives for purchasers? Are patients being 'dumped' from other subsectors? Are there adequate risk-sharing mechanisms? And if not, will this cap only result in a complete shift of all risk onto the providers, which is both inequitable and inefficient?

Institutional impediments

These remain the most serious obstacle to fundamental change. There have been a number of quite extensive experiments in innovative payment mechanisms but experiments are often blocked or prevented from having maximal impact because of legal or administrative impediments, such as civil service reform. Significant vested interests resist reform. Another institutional weakness is the system of property rights, which often impedes the development of greater facility autonomy over the use of funding.

Out-of-pocket payments (OOP)

One of the major changes in health systems in Eastern Europe over the last decade is the increased reliance on out-of-pocket payments (Preker *et al.*, 2001). The significant drops in output and the accompanying fiscal reductions during the initial stages of the transition put additional pressure on social sector budgets, particularly in the health sector which evidenced a significant over-supply of resources. Figure 11.8 provides an overview of revenues from pooled channels of funding versus individual out-of-pocket payments at the point of service. Because these payments are large for the lower-income countries in the region, however, their impact on the supply side, as a form of fee-for-service provider payment, must be considered as well.

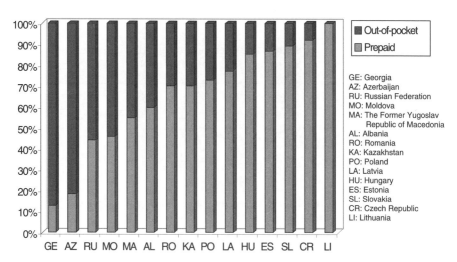

Figure 11.8 Prepaid versus out-of-pocket payments.
Source: Preker *et al.* (2001).

Out-of-pocket payments can influence treatment choice as patients tend to make larger payments for riskier interventions such as surgery. Increasingly, quality of care and waiting times are dependent upon a patient's ability to provide gratitude money (Lewis, 2000). In addition, indirect payments from medical equipment suppliers and pharmaceutical companies may also lead to distortion (Orosz & Hollo, 1999).

Informal payments by patients are pervasive in the poorer countries of the region, most extensively in the Caucasus and Tajikistan but also elsewhere in Central Asia, the CIS, and some countries of Central and Eastern Europe. Evidence from the 'single payer' reform in Kyrgyzstan indicates, however, that it is possible to reduce informal payments through a coherent set of incentives and purchasing arrangements. For inpatient care, there is an explicit inverse relationship between what the purchaser pays from pooled funds and what the patient is meant to pay as a copayment.[4] Patient survey data from 2001 suggest that the single payer reform worked in two important dimensions: (i) average spending by patients, where the copayment was implemented, was about the same after the policy as before, with the formal copayment largely replacing previous informal payments, particularly for drugs and medical supplies and payments to health workers; and (ii) being insured and being exempt in the single payer regions had significant negative effects on both total and informal out-of-pocket spending by patients. Prior to the implementation of the single payer (and in the other regions of the country), exemptions were not effective at reducing out-of-pocket spending (Falkingham, 2001; Kutzin, 2003; Kutzin *et al.*, 2003). This evidence suggests that coordinated policies on provider payment and the benefits package can have an effect on reducing the out-of-pocket spending burden for targeted groups in the population.

Deficits

Persistent deficits have plagued the operation of health care systems in all these countries. The major cause of deficits in Western health care systems is usually that expenditure grows faster than revenue. In the post-socialist countries, only in the Czech health care system, in the first half of the 1990s, was such a pattern evident. In most CEE/CIS countries, however, the major cause of the deficit was that revenue decreased more than expenditure. A typical response of the public providers was to become indebted to their suppliers (by not paying for the goods purchased), and to appeal to the government for subsidies or bailouts.

In many of the former Soviet republics, debt has been almost constant, such that much spending occurs not on a cash basis but through a process of mutual debt settlement. The mutual debt settlement system helps to ensure that services can be provided even in cashless circumstances, but does lead to suboptimal allocation decisions and is administratively costly to operate.

Monitoring and quality

Each payment system design brings unintended consequences and opportunities for changing levels of quality of care, both better and worse. The monitoring capabilities by the purchaser are, however, too often underdeveloped. Future directions for purchasers in the region should include providing support to ensure that quality is safeguarded and optimized. Data, techniques and the applications are at a very early stage of development in all health systems around the world, and not only in this region. Still, the integration of some form of quality benchmarks would seem an essential management mechanism in ensuring that quality was not compromised due to the application of a particular approach to funding.

While many of these problems also arise in Western European countries, particularly those relating to monitoring, quality, poor complementarity of design and institutional impediments to reform, the context is, of course, quite different so the implications for system performance may also differ. Western Europe is not faced with the same challenges of economic development as those arising in most of the countries to the east. Perhaps the single biggest challenge faced in the development of payment systems is ensuring that the inherent incentive structure is conducive to facilitating equity of access together with efficiency of performance. Countries vary in the extent to which these objectives are achieved. In particular, for those countries within the NHS/tax-based funding grouping, differentiation of payment systems according to the public/private status of patients may result in inequity in accessing services. This, in turn, translates into the lengthening of waiting lists for services, which is a feature of most of these countries. Where payment systems differ for the treatment of public and private patients, as for example in England, Ireland and Sweden, the resulting incentive systems also differ with potentially damaging consequences for the performance of the health system as a whole.

Discussion

Purchasing systems and payment incentive systems are only contributory factors needed to cope effectively with the undoubted inefficiency within the health sector, whether in the Eastern or Western European environment. The intertwined problems of health care reform demand a well conceived and long-ranging health care sector reform strategy, with specific programmes, a clear governance framework, skilled and committed health care management and administration, and support from health care professionals and the public for the aims and goals of the reforms. Unfortunately, none or few of these elements have been assembled so far in many of the countries to the extent needed. These are but a few of the challenges that lay ahead for the region in the next 10 years, and perhaps beyond.

It seems a reasonable postulate that the issues dominating improvements in performance of payment systems in Eastern European countries are largely influenced by development issues, for example the problems of out-of-pocket payments and fragmentation of public sector pooling, while the dominant influences for countries in the West are the refinement of incentive structures consistent with achievement of equity and efficiency. These objectives are, of course, important for all health care systems; the prioritization of objectives will vary depending on local circumstances.

The Western European countries clearly provide a leadership role for other countries in the region. Western Europe provides an interesting example of convergence towards a mixed payment system, with a majority using fee-for-service for 'priority services' such as preventive care and selected primary care services. At the same time, the majority currently use some form of case-mix system, whether the original or an adaptation of the DRG system, for funding hospital services, often with a global budget cap. Each system has adapted the specifics of the case-mix measure and/or the application to fit within the local funding framework and to address the objectives prioritized within the local hospital environment. Ashton (2002: 103) in a review of lessons to be learned from a decade of health reform in New Zealand noted that

> the effect of introducing market-like incentives into a health system depends upon the particular institutional arrangements that are in place. As long as governments place high priority on ensuring access to services for those in need, incentives for efficiency will inevitably be blunted.

From the overview presented here, it would seem that purchasing in its pure form is rarely in evidence within the health systems of Western European countries. The factors identified as being critical to so-called pure purchasing include the specification of a price for an agreed quantum of product of a specified standard. What is more frequently in evidence is the application of funding systems based on some form of cost or expenditure platform, combined with some form of utilization measure like number of visits, number of patient stays, number of bed-days and so forth. The differentiation of services according to resource requirements based on severity/complexity measures, together with adjustment for risk or quality/outcome indicators are increasingly in evidence in reforms of health funding systems. Nevertheless, these applications and techniques are still at an early stage of development. Quantification of resource requirements for services adjusted for morbidity, risk and quality continues to be a challenging objective.

Adding to the challenge are issues of chronic care and long-term care, fast arising in the countries of Western Europe, and emergent in places like Hungary and Poland. Hungary has already instituted payment systems for long-term care with hospital-based *per diem* payments, adjusted for types of chronic care, with an overall cap on expenditures. This area generally is clearly cause for concern given the growing importance of each of these factors in the development of funding frameworks.

The Eastern European experience lags slightly behind Western Europe but is one of increasing diversity, both at a macroeconomic level (for example, levels of GDP) and in terms of capacity for taxation and for governance of new institutions and payment systems. Full implementation of more complex incentive arrangements will be a challenge over the next several years. One clear lesson that has emerged is that, in many of these hierarchical public systems, payment reform is only one of several instruments, and should be utilized with parallel and coordinated reforms such as increased facility autonomy. In low-income countries, out-of-pocket payments now dominate the incentive structure. The public finance context in these countries means extensive reliance on private payments. Supply- and demand-side effects must be considered. New payment systems need to explicitly account for this reality of private spending.

Notes

1   For some observers, 'time based' may be a catch-all for 'budgets' and may not be useful as a conceptual framework. Nearly all payment methods are time based in the sense that there are time limits. There is overlap between time-based and population-based methods in the table as well. Other observers prefer the distinction of 'retrospective' versus 'prospective' payments indicating whether payment is made by the purchaser subsequent to or prior to the delivery of services.
2   This table provides indicative impacts for 'pure systems'. However, it should be noted that most systems use a mix of different mechanisms and hence incentives, yielding somewhat unique results.
3   'Step-down costing' is an accounting method for allocating costs per case by successively allocating costs across all departments, and from indirect costs (for example, administration), to direct costs (drugs and supplies) to reach an estimated amount overall.
4   More specifically, the amount paid per case is least for uninsured patients, higher for insured patients, and highest for patients meant to be exempt from copayment. Conversely, the copayment level is highest for the uninsured, lower for the insured, and zero for exempt persons.

References

Arrow, K.J. (1963) Uncertainty and the welfare economics of medical care. *The American economic review,* **53**: 941–973.

Ashton, T. (2002) Running on the spot: lessons from a decade of health reform in New Zealand. *Applied health economics and health policy,* **1**(2): 97–106.

Bjorn, E. *et al.* (2002) The effect of activity-based financing on hospital efficiency: a panel data analysis of DEA efficiency scores 1992–2000 (Working Paper 8). Oslo, Health Economics Research Programme, University of Oslo.

Bruce, A. and Jonsson, E. (1996) *Competition in the provision of health care: the experience of the United States, Sweden and Britain.* Arena, Ashgate Publishing Limited.

Casas, M. and Illa, C. (2001) Case mix in Spain: financial and clinical management. *In:* Roger France, F.H. *et al.*, eds. *Case mix: global views, local actions, evolution in twenty countries.* Amsterdam, IOS Press.

Costa, J. and Rico, A. (2001) *Consolidating the NHS model in a devolved state.* Presentation to the European Health Care Systems Discussion Group, London School of Economics and Political Science.

Delcheva, E. and Balabanova, D. (2001) Hospital sector reform in Bulgaria: first steps. *Euro health*, **7**(3): 42–46.

Department of Health (2002) *Reforming NHS financial flows, introducing payment by results.* London, National Health Service.

Dixon, A., Langenbrunner, J. and Mossialos, E. (2004) Facing the challenges of health care financing. *In:* Figueras, J., McKee, M., Cain, J. and Lessof, S., eds. *Health systems in transition: learning from experience.* European Observatory on Health Systems and Policies. Copenhagen. World Health Organization.

Dranove, D. and Satterthwaite, M. (2000) The industrial organization of health care markets. *In:* Culher, A.J. and Newhouse, J.P., eds. *Handbook of health economics.* Amsterdam, North-Holland.

Ellis, R. and McGuire, T. (1990) Optimal payment systems for health services. *Journal of health economics*, **9**.

Ensor, T. (1993) Health system reform in the former Socialist countries of Europe. *International journal of health planning and management*, **8**(3): 169–178.

Ensor, T. and Langenbrunner, J. (2002) Financing health care. *In:* Healy, J. and McKee, M., eds. *Health care in Central Asia.* Buckingham, Open University Press.

Falkingham, J. (2001) *Health, health seeking behaviour and out of pocket expenditures in Kyrgyzstan 2001* (DFID-funded Kyrgyz Household Health Finance Survey Final Report.) London, London School of Economics and Political Science.

Hansen, P.E. and Nielsen, S.W. (2001) Case mix in Denmark: status on the development and use of the Nord Dk DRG. *In:* Roger France, F.H. *et al.*, eds. *Case mix: global views, local actions, evolution in twenty countries.* Amsterdam, IOS Press.

Hava, P. (2001) Comparative institutional reform in social policy: the case of health care reforms in the Czech Republic. Unpublished manuscript.

Healy, J. and McKee, M. (2002) The evolution of hospital systems. *In:* McKee, M. and Healy, J., eds. *Hospitals in a changing Europe.* Buckingham, Open University Press.

Hofmarcher, M.M. and Riedel, M. (2003) *Impact of case-mix hospital payment reforms on health systems.* Report commissioned by the World Bank, Europe and Central Asia (ECA) Human Development Unit.

Jegers, M.K. *et al.* (2002) A typology for provider payment systems in health care. *Health policy*, **60**(3): 255–273.

Jencks, S.A. *et al.* (1984) Evaluating and improving the measurement of hospital case mix. *Health care financing review*, annual supplement.

Kadyrova, N. and Kutzin, J. (2002) *Purchasing case study – Kyrgyzstan.* Report produced for European Observatory on Health Systems and Policies.

Kutzin, J. (2003) Health expenditures, reforms and policy priorities, for the Kyrgyz Republic. (Manas Health Policy Analysis Project, Policy Research Paper 24.) Bishkek, Kyrgyzstan, World Health Organization and Ministry of Health.

Kutzin, J. *et al.* (2002) Innovations in resource allocation, pooling and purchasing in the

Kyrgyz health care system. (Health, Nutrition and Population Discussion Paper.) Washington, D.C., World Bank, Human Development Network.

Kutzin, J. *et al.* (2003) Formalizing informal payments in Kyrgyz hospitals: evidence from phased implementation of financing reforms. Presentation to Fourth World Conference of the International Health Economics Association. San Francisco, 15–18 June.

Langenbrunner, J. and Wiley, M. (2002) Hospital payment mechanisms: theory and practice in transition economies. *In*: McKee, M. and Healy, J., eds. *Hospitals in a changing Europe*, Buckingham, Open University Press.

Langenbrunner, J. *et al.* (1994) Evaluation of health insurance demonstrations in Kazakhstan: Dzheskasgan and South Kazakhstan Oblasts. Bethesda, Maryland, Abt Associates.

Lewis, M. (2000) *Who is paying for health care in eastern Europe and central Asia?* Washington, D.C., World Bank.

Lofgren, R. (2002) The Swedish health care system: recent reforms, problems and opportunities (Public Policy Sources Number 59). Vancouver, Fraser Institute.

Lyles, A. and Palumbo, F.B. (1999) The effect of managed care on prescription drug costs and benefits. *Pharmocoeconomics*, **15**(2): 129–140.

Newhouse, J.P. (1998) Risk adjustment: where are we now? *Inquiry*, **35**: 122–131.

O'Dougherty, S. (2003) Personal communication. Bishkek, Kyrgyzstan.

Organisation for Economic Co-operation and Development (1997) *Health systems and comparative statistics: facts and trends, I and II*, Paris, OECD.

Organisation for Economic Co-operation and Development (2003) *Health systems and comparative statistics: facts and trends*. 5th edition. Paris, OECD.

Oliver, A.E., Mossialos, A. and Maynard, A. (2002) The English National Health Service: analysing the impact of reform. Draft paper for IMPACT project.

Orosz, É. (2001) *Félúton vagy tévúton? Egészségügyünk félmúltja és az egészségpolitika alternatívái* (*On halfway or wrong way? The near past of our health care system and the options for health policy*). Budapest, Egészséges Magyarországért Egyesület.

Orosz, E. and Hollo, I. (1999) Hospital sector in Hungary: the story of unsuccessful reforms. London, European Observatory on Health Systems and Policies Case Study.

Pedersen, K.M. (2002) Reforming decentralized integrated health care systems: theory and the case of the Norwegian reform (Working Paper 7). University of Oslo, Health Economics Research Programme.

Preker, A. and Feachem, R. (1993) Market forces in the health sector: the experience of the former socialist states, central and eastern Europe. Presented at EDI Senior Policy Seminar, Beijing, 28–30 July.

Preker, A., Jakab, M. and Schneider, M. (2001) Health financing reforms in eastern Europe and central Asia. *In*: Mossialos E. and Saltman, R., eds. *Financing health care in Europe*. London, European Observatory on Health Systems and Policies.

Richter, K. (1998) The Social sector in Tajikstan. Some recent developments. Report to the World Bank, London, London School of Economics.

Rico, A. and Wisbaum, W. (2002) Radical devolution in Finnish health care. *Euro observer*, **4**(2).

Rodrigues, J.M. and Trombert-Paviot, B. (2001) Case mix in France: is there a French way from problem to paradigm in health care? The DRG/PMSI saga. *In*: Roger France, F.H. *et al.*, eds. *Case mix: global views, local actions, evolution in twenty countries*. Amsterdam, IOS Press.

Roger France, F.H. and Mertens, I. (2001) Case mix in Belgium: a rapid coverage and a progressive AP-DRG use. *In*: Roger France, F.H. *et al.*, eds. *Case mix: global views, local actions, evolution in twenty countries*. Amsterdam, IOS Press.

Saltman, R. and Figueras, J. (1998) Analyzing the evidence on European health care reforms. *In: Health affairs*, **17**(2): 85–108.

Schellschmidt, H. (2001) Case mix in Germany: DRG-based hospital payment in Germany. *In*: Roger France F.H. *et al.*, eds. *Case mix: global views, local actions, evolution in twenty countries*. Amsterdam, IOS Press.

Schieber, G. (1993) Health care financing reform in the Russian Federation and Ukraine. *Health affairs*, Supplement.

Sheiman, I. (1993) New methods of finance and management of health care in the Russian Federation. Health Sector Reform in Developing Countries Conference, Durham, New Hampshire.

Socium Consult. (2002) Funding of the health sector: improvements of health indicators and health sector reform. (Background paper for the World Bank Public Expenditure Review for the Kyrgyz Republic.) Bishkek, Kyrgyzstan.

Wiley, M.M. (1999) Development and localisation of case mix applications for inpatient hospital activity in EU member states. *Australian health review*, **22**(2): 69–85.

Wiley, M.M. (2001) Ireland: budgeting basis for acute hospital services. *In*: Roger France, F.H. *et al.*, eds. *Case mix: global views, local actions, evolution in twenty countries*. Amsterdam, IOS Press.

World Bank (2002) *Uzbekistan health project mid-term evaluation report*, Washington, D.C., World Bank.

World Health Organization (2000) *World health report 2000*, Geneva, WHO.

World Health Organization (2003) *Health for all database*, Copenhagen, WHO.

chapter twelve

Responding to purchasing: provider perspectives

Hans Maarse, Thomas A. Rathwell,
Tamas Evetovits, Alexander S. Preker
and Elke Jakubowski

Introduction

The subject of this book is purchasing health care. However, one of the key factors in determining whether purchasing will improve health system performance will be the way that providers respond to purchasers. Put another way: how well will the provider as agent follow the wishes of the purchaser as principal? This is the focus of this chapter.

The introduction of purchasing in health care raises a number of new aspects from the perspective of the provider, which are subject of this chapter. Following this introduction, the second section will introduce a typology of provider functions and organizations as a conceptual framework for analysing provider responses. The third section deals with types of responses and the fourth with factors and determinants influencing provider responses to purchasing. Finally, the chapter addresses the impact of purchasing upon the behaviour of providers. This chapter focuses mainly upon the response to purchasing of provider organizations such as hospitals, nursing homes or organizations for community care. We will not investigate how individual providers such as dentists and doctors respond to purchasing.

Purchaser–provider separation creates a new relationship between a purchaser of health services on the one hand and the provider of health services on the other. According to the theory of purchasing, and as outlined in Chapter 9, the purchaser and provider negotiate a contract outlining the nature and scope of the delivery of health services. For instance, when a health insurer or regional government purchasing agency contracts with a hospital, the contract may specify an agreement on the volume, price and quality of health services of the provider over a certain period of time, include maximum allowable waiting times, as well as measures of efficiency and effectiveness. Purchasing through contracting should motivate the purchaser to search for value for money and the provider to produce value for money. Purchasing refers to a shift from the traditional input-based and mostly incremental type of funding to a new policy-driven type of funding, and aims at shaping a more businesslike relationship between the purchaser and the provider.

From the provider's perspective, purchasing can be conceptualized as a change in its external environment that requires adaptive strategies such as greater and different accountability. Whereas this chapter deals with providers' adaptive strategies in reacting to changes in the external environment, Chapter 10 focused on primarily internal governance structures such as clinical pathways and quality management and assurance strategies.

Who is the purchaser?

An investigation of the response of providers to purchasing must take account of the question 'Who is the purchaser?' Here, a distinction can be made among the three different models described in Chapter 2. When purchasing is organized at the national or macro level in the health care system, a government purchaser or national health insurance agency negotiates a framework contract with different groups of providers, for instance acute hospitals, nursing homes, community care delivery organizations, general practitioners, medical specialists and so on. Typically, this model relies upon collective bargaining between purchasers and groups of providers to reach an agreement. In the second model, meso-level purchasing, a regional purchaser or a health insurance company negotiates a contract for the delivery of health care with different groups of providers in its service area. Contracting may be the result of collective bargaining or bilateral bargaining. Where purchasing is organized at the micro level, the purchaser may be a general practitioner who contracts with a hospital for the treatment of its patients (GP fundholding) or a small-scale organization such as a local health council which purchases health services for a defined local population, as is the case in some of the Nordic countries.

Conceptualizing provider responses

A typology of provider functions and organizations

An empirical investigation of the response of providers to purchasing must take into account that providers form quite a heterogeneous category (McKee & Healy, 2001). This may have important implications for their response to purchasing. For instance, a hospital with multiple medical functions may respond differently from a hospital performing only a few medical functions. A large tertiary or regional hospital will have a strong market position that a purchaser cannot easily ignore. In addition, hospital providers may have other functions beyond the interest of a purchaser organization, such as functions of teaching students and training staff in teaching hospitals. Another argument for taking the variety of providers into account is that there are great differences in the points of departure for providers when responding to purchasing. For instance, whereas some hospitals are accustomed to substantial autonomy or are familiar with market exposure, others are still monopolistic entities with little or no autonomy. These differences will influence their response to purchasing initiatives.

What is required is an analytical classification of provider organizations that sets the framework for investigating their response to purchasing. Such a classification has been developed by Preker & Harding (2003). Their typology, based on 'the economics of organizations', denotes five critical functions of provider behaviour. The functions that play a key role in health care reform are:

- *Decision rights.* The introduction of purchasing in health care presumes that the providers' decision rights are extended in order to enable them to respond appropriately to purchasing. Critical decision rights transferred to management from a hierarchical unit or an outside supervisory agency to the provider include control over input, labour, scope of activities, financial management, clinical management, market strategy, production process, and so on. In concrete terms, these mechanisms may be reflected in the rights to hire and fire, to determine skill mix, and the level of health care services supply, to decide to outsource health care provision and to provide supplementary services.

- *Residual claims.* The additional autonomy for providers and their managers does not automatically motivate them to increase their productivity. A complementary arrangement is that 'leftover' resources remain with the providers. As Wilson once put it: 'Why scrimp and save if you cannot keep the results of your frugality?' Therefore, a distinctive feature of purchasing reforms is the degree to which the public purse ceases to be the residual claimant on revenue flows. The other side of the coin is the extent to which hospitals are placed at financial risk (Kirkman-Liff *et al.*, 1997).

- *Market exposure.* Modern health reform is directed at the introduction of some form of market competition in order to give providers an incentive to improve their performance, for instance in terms of quality of care, productivity, unit costs, waiting times or patient satisfaction. According to the theory of purchasing, the purchaser will reward providers that perform well and punish providers with a poor performance.

- *Accountability.* A key element of market competition and purchasing is that strong emphasis is placed upon the accountability of the provider for its performance. Moreover, the methods of control have changed from directly hierarchical to indirect, through rules, contracts, monitoring of activities and the like. Purchasing also increases the need for greater accountability to the general public; providers must communicate with the general public on their performance level.

- *Social functions.* Social functions of health care put limits to the autonomy of providers. For instance, it would be unacceptable for managers to freely decide to decrease their activity in certain health areas or services for vulnerable groups simply because they are considered unattractive or financially inefficient. Therefore, it is important to introduce mechanisms to ensure the performance of social functions. This can be done by imposing rules upon the providers or by including specific agreements on social functions in the contract.

Harding and Preker have developed a fourfold hierarchical classification of hospitals based on these five critical determinants of the providers' behaviour:

- *Budgetary organizations* are government owned and usually work within the existing political and administrative structures and cultures. They are typically associated with command-and-control systems, and/or integrated systems. Senior officials are often appointed on a political basis and subject to hierarchical control on input and financial matters. They have few or no decision rights. The provider budget is set by the state agency, following bureaucratic procedures, and is mostly very detailed and inflexible. Any surplus is returned to the public sector and any deficit covered by the public purse. Accountability is underdeveloped. Social functions are often not specified or funded separately.
- *Autonomized organizations* are also government owned but managers are given some autonomy for day-to-day decisions. Management's decision rights are still limited because the government is not willing to transfer control over essential input factors, such as labour, recruitment of staff or staff mix. Autonomized organizations have some scope for generating revenue tied to service delivery by moving towards funding via performance-related payments. Hospital managers may even be given an opportunity for gaining additional resources, for instance through the introduction of the delivery of care to patients who pay privately. A surplus may be retained. Furthermore, the manager's autonomy is increased by replacing a line-item budget with a global budget, whereby savings in one service or budget area can be shifted to another. Such an arrangement can be understood as a partial residual claimant arrangement. Accountability arrangements still generally come from hierarchical supervision but with more clearly specified and narrowed objectives. An agreement between the government and provider management may specify monitorable performance targets and responsibilities for performing social functions.
- *Corporatized organizations* can probably best be understood as public organizations operating as private companies. Provisions for managerial autonomy are stronger than under autonomization. Similarly, corporatized providers are more exposed to the vagaries of the market than their autonomized counterparts. Their revenues are related to performance, with providers operating as residual claimants; in case of poor performance they may go bankrupt. Management is accountable to the responsible minister, but the arrangements for accountability are different from those of the autonomized provider, and include binding contracts and performance targets, as well as benchmarking, whereby hospitals are classified according to predetermined criteria. The results of benchmarking may be made public so that consumers are also informed about the provider performance. Social functions are

ensured through public ownership, public regulation and/or agreements with the purchaser on specific social objectives to be achieved.

• *Privatized organizations* may operate on either a for-profit or a not-for-profit basis. They have many decision rights but usually the government retains some regulatory control. They are subject to strong market exposure. Supervision is different from that of corporatized organizations. Privatized hospitals are owned by private organizations that install a board of directors to which hospital management is accountable for its performance. Social functions are ensured through public regulations and/or agreements with purchasers on specific social objectives. Providers may also declare social goals voluntarily, to strengthen their position in the community.

The variety of hospital providers in Europe

Table 12.1 gives an illustration of the classification of hospitals in a number of European countries. It illustrates the complexity of using the typology as a framework to describe and analyse provider responses to purchasers for a number of reasons. First, the classic distinction between public and private hospitals is too simple. The category of public hospitals masks quite different types of hospitals. These differences are important when investigating the response of providers to purchasing. Second, it is important to note that the range of provider organizations in many countries is heterogeneous. For instance, public hospitals of the autonomized and corporatized type often co-exist with privatized hospitals. Whereas curative or acute medicine is delivered in public hospitals of whatever type, long-term nursing care or community care may be mainly provided by privatized organizations. Third, the typological character of the classification must be stressed. Clear demarcation lines between each of the four categories do not exist. It is often difficult to place a provider in precisely one category, for example in the Netherlands and Canada where all hospitals are privately owned and operate on a not-for-profit basis. Yet, they do not fit well into the category of privatized hospitals because market exposure is still very limited and the governments have retained considerable control rights over their behaviour (hospital planning, price regulations and so on). In essence, the hospitals in both countries are hybrids – they contain aspects of both corporate and privatized organizations. The call in the Netherlands for more market competition and less government regulation illustrates the difficulty of classifying these hospitals as privatized provider organizations.

Table 12.1 demonstrates a great variety in provider organizations. In the following, we will seek to identify clusters of common trends in the main groups of Western European and Central and Eastern European countries.

In Western Europe many providers are public entities of the autonomized or corporatized type. But interesting new developments are taking place – for instance full or partial privatization of provider organizations. In the latter case, a hospital may remain in public hands while its management is fully contracted out to a private company. In the countries with a mixture of public (often corporatized) and private hospitals, the willingness to opt for privatization seems to be increasing. For instance, in the Netherlands and Canada there is

Table 12.1 Features of hospital provider organizations in selected European countries

Country	Hospital numbers and sizes	Private/public ownership of hospitals	Private/public ownership of hospital beds	Classification of hospitals according to predominant form	Decision rights of hospital managers	Recent changes
Albania	Twenty hospitals of 100 to 400 beds and 22 of below 100 beds.	All hospitals public.	All hospital beds publicly owned.	Regional and district hospitals budgeted; pilot of the Durres regional hospital as a semi-autonomous, funded directly by the health insurance fund.	No autonomy over skill mix, ward organization and utilizing budgets.	Closure of small hospitals; change of 6 to 12 district hospitals to regional.
Austria	Seventy hospitals with fewer than 200 beds; 21 hospitals with between 200 and 500 beds; six hospitals with between 500 and 999 and three with more than 1000 beds (1998).	In 1998, 49 private hospitals – 37 not-for-profit; 142 public hospitals.	Two-thirds of hospital beds public (about 50 000 beds) and one-third private, of which about 5600 private not-for-profit.	In 1998, 147 hospitals (45%) with about 52 000 beds (75%) were budgeted (fund hospitals).	Full autonomy over hiring, firing, skill mix, ward organization but limited autonomy in utilizing budgets.	Introduction of performance financing; introduction of a hospital plan, including high capital intensive technology.

Belgium	Two-hundred and twenty-seven hospitals (2001)	Sixty per cent not-for-profit private institutions (191 in 1995); 40% publicly owned by municipal welfare centres, provinces, the state or inter-municipal associations (91 in 1995); 5% owned by mutualités.	Sixty-four per cent of private hospital beds (1998)	A mixture of autonomized, corporatized and privatized hospitals.	Public hospitals: full autonomy over hiring, firing, skill mix, ward organization but limited autonomy in utilizing budgets. Private hospitals: full autonomy over hiring, firing, skill mix, wards and in utilizing budgets.	
Denmark	Eighty hospitals (1995).	Majority of hospitals county owned.	Less than 1% private beds.	Budgetary hospitals predominate.	Autonomy over hiring and firing, but limited autonomy to determine skill mix and utilize budgets.	In 2003, there were governmental plans to create autonomous hospitals.

Table 12.1 (continued)

Country	Hospital numbers and sizes	Private/public ownership of hospitals	Private/public ownership of hospital beds	Classification of hospitals according to predominant form	Decision rights of hospital managers	Recent changes
Estonia	Fifty hospitals in 2002; 8 hospitals with more than 300 beds; 4 hospitals with 151–300 beds; 18 hospitals with 51–150 beds; 20 hospitals with 51 beds or fewer.	Majority of hospitals are publicly owned (state and municipality). Four hospitals are privately owned.	Majority of hospital beds are in publicly owned hospitals. Private beds account for less than 2% of the total.	All hospitals are corporatized institutions, operating as not-for-profit foundations or joint-stock companies.	Hospitals headed by a hospital manager and a supervisory board with state and/or municipality representation. Hospital managers are autonomous with respect to employment and staff salaries, subject to approval by the hospital supervisory boards. Hospitals can generate additional income by renting out space to private enterprises and providing health services to the private sector.	Hospital mergers in large urban settings during 2000–2003. In the capital Tallinn, 17 hospitals were merged into four networks in 2001. In North-Eastern Estonia, hospital mergers were carried out in 2003.

Finland	Five university hospitals, 15 central hospitals, 40 smaller specialized hospitals.	Majority of hospitals public, owned by federations of municipalities (i.e. hospital districts).	Thirty-eight thousand municipally owned hospital beds; 1400 private.	Majority of hospitals autonomized.	Decision rights limited; managers accountable to hospital districts; hospitals not allowed to generate profits; assets owned by hospital districts.	There are pilots of splitting the hospital to introduce a purchaser–provider split.
France	In 2002 there were 1000 public hospitals at three levels: 562 general hospitals, 29 regional hospitals, 349 local hospitals (160 beds on average).	Twenty-five per cent public hospitals (1000 out of 4000); 33% not-for-profit (1400); 40% private for-profit (1750).	Of 490 000 beds 65% are public; 15% not-for-profit beds; 20% for-profit.	Public hospitals are autonomous and manage their own budgets.	In public hospitals staffing decision rights limited by national rules; most public hospital employees are civil servants with tenure; director has no power determining wages.	Introduction of the regional hospital agencies for planning and financial resource allocation for private and public hospitals. Introduction of a system for hospital accreditation.
Germany	In 2001, 2240 hospitals.	Of 2030 general hospitals, around 790 were publicly owned; 820 private not-for-profit; 420 private for-profit. (2001)	In 1998, 55% public beds (295 382); 38% not-for-profit (202 270) and 7% for-profit (36 118). Still, 95% financed publicly.	Autonomous, corporatized and privatized hospitals.	Decision rights considerable on staff hiring and firing; hospitals can have deficits and profits; public hospital investment costs are covered by the *Länder*, running costs by the health insurance funds.	Introduction of a country wide DRG system.

Table 12.1 (*continued*)

Country	Hospital numbers and sizes	Private/public ownership of hospitals	Private/public ownership of hospital beds	Classification of hospitals according to predominant form	Decision rights of hospital managers	Recent changes
Italy	1381 hospitals (1998).	In 1998, 61% public hospitals (842); 39.5% private (539).	Eighty-one per cent public, 18.5% private.	By 2000, 98 autonomous hospital trusts.	Decision rights increased in hospital trusts, materializing power of managers to define hospital's mission and objectives in 3-year strategic plans.	Introduction of hospital trusts.
Netherlands	In 2000, a total of 208 hospitals.	More than 90% are private not-for-profit, the rest are public (University) hospitals.	Most private not-for-profit.	Formally privatized but with many characteristics of corporatized hospitals.	Only major planning decisions must be approved by government; all decision rights with respect to internal hospital management.	In 2004 start of the first tranche of case-based payment.

Portugal	In 1999, 205 hospitals.	Forty-one per cent private hospitals (84), half for-profit and half not-for-profit.	27 327 (77.2%) beds were public and 8077 (22.8) beds were private.	In 2002 a selective contracting system was introduced with a new performance-related payment system, and a new categorization of hospitals in four groups: public autonomous, public corporatized, public corporate with the state as exclusive shareholder, and private.	Hospital managers have little budgetary flexibility or autonomy in investment and human resources.	See under classification of hospitals.
Slovenia	In 2002, 26 general hospitals, including 9 regional and 3 local.	All general hospitals state owned.	Fewer than 50 private beds in 2002.	Majority of hospitals autonomized.		Introduction of DRG payment system.

presently more room than in the recent past for the creation of so-called private specialized clinics operating on a for-profit basis. Germany is another country where an increasing number of public hospitals are now being privatized (Busse & Wörz, 2004). This trend is not limited to the Western social health insurance systems but is also visible in a number of Nordic and southern NHS systems such as Portugal's. Proponents of greater privatization claim that these new providers will not only encourage market competition but also help to reduce waiting lists.

In many countries across Central and Eastern Europe most hospitals belong to the category of autonomized organizations, which are funded either directly by the state or by a centralized national health insurance scheme. The state also retains a considerable degree of hierarchical control over these providers. This observation suggests that in these countries the purchaser–provider split has only been partially realized; hospitals are still owned by governmental entities. Hospital reform has not yet led to substantial shifts from the left end of the spectrum – budgetary hospitals – to the right end of privatized hospitals. Reforms are difficult to implement due to many structural and cultural constraints in the system. In many countries, a strong reluctance to undertake large-scale reform can be observed. The common pattern seems to be that governments move in incremental steps. Hospitals with budgetary structures have been converted to autonomized hospitals, which have been in turn transformed into corporatized models. Many governments, it appears, remain convinced that hospitals should keep their public status and that privatization will undermine the public goals of cost control, equity and affordability (see Box 12.1).

Box 12.1 Public demands, private interests and hospital efficiency in Hungary

> In Hungary, decentralization of hospital ownership and privatization of provision for diagnostic services resulted in an oversupply of CT scanners, yet the Health Insurance Fund and ultimately the government has to pay for services that are performed using inefficiently utilized diagnostic equipment. For the private sector it is the profit motive that drives investment decisions; for the hospital-owning local councils, the politics of providing access drives decisions to invest in new equipment. In both cases the purchaser and the government find it difficult to turn away new applicants for service contracts funded by the Health Insurance Fund. The local population supports the introduction of new technologies in the hospitals even if this means inefficient use of scarce resources.

There is also serious concern about the efficiency of private hospitals relative to public hospitals. For these reasons governments are not willing to transfer their decision rights on essential aspects of management to hospitals. The strong ties between the purchaser and the provider organization suggests that one can hardly speak of a new relationship between them. The influence of the purchasing agency in affecting the behaviour of the provider is limited. Not contracting with a hospital or implementing a substantial budget cut to punish it for poor performance are not real options when the purchasing agency is still intricately involved in the operation of the hospital. Furthermore, the control that the purchasing agency has over the provider is still so strong that the latter does not have the essential decision rights it needs to respond effectively to purchasing.

Purchasing and provider accountability

The requirements of purchasing place a strong emphasis upon the autonomy and accountability of the provider. A provider that has many external constraints and limited decision rights cannot respond properly to purchaser demands. Here, a distinction must be made between two types of accountability: managerial and public (Stein, 2001). The emergence of greater managerial accountability is directly linked to the development of a new relationship between purchaser and provider. In countries with an integrated health care system, purchasing implies that the traditional hierarchical relationship between the funder and provider will be replaced by a contractual relationship in which specified performance targets on service delivery are agreed upon. Preker and Harding define such a contractual relationship as an important feature of transforming budgetary and autonomized provider organizations into corporatized and privatized organizations. Accountability is a crucial element of such a new relationship and tools for monitoring must be developed to assess whether the performance targets have been achieved. In countries where the funding and delivery of health care have traditionally been split, accountability will become equally more important. In these countries, purchasing implies that health insurers no longer act as passive payers for health services rendered to the patients they represent. They will be converted to active payers negotiating performance targets with the providers, monitoring the extent to which these targets have been achieved and amending or terminating contractual agreements if they have not been achieved.

Whereas managerial accountability is concerned with the relationship between the provider and a purchasing agency, public accountability concerns the relationship of the provider with the wider public. The quality and efficiency of health service providers are no longer being taken for granted. The public should have access to reliable information on the performance level of providers in order to make intelligent choices about medical care.

There is a growing emphasis upon a systematic and independent measurement of provider performance. For instance, in the Netherlands the government contracted with an external research agency in order to benchmark the performance of home care delivery providers. It is the government's intention to extend the scope of benchmarking in the near future. In the United Kingdom a new state-sponsored agency, the Commission on Health Improvement (CHI) was created in order to measure the performance of providers. The Commission has published the first NHS performance ratings, which are accessible to the general public. Experience indicates that performance measurement is complicated because of many conceptual and methodological problems. These problems are partly related to the heterogeneity of health services and partly to enormous differences in the severity of illness of the patients treated. For instance, it is misleading to use simple hospital mortality league tables as an indicator for the quality of hospital services as they are often not corrected for differences in severity of illness and say little or nothing about the quality of elective care or the treatment of chronic disease patients. Performance measurement should be based on a multidimensional approach, combining a variety of performance indicators. Another problem is the accuracy of measurement and the reliability of data. The measurement of the average waiting time in hospitals is a good illustration: there are various sorts of waiting lists, hospitals tend to follow their own measurement procedures, data often are inaccurate and the results depend on how waiting times are measured. Further problems are that providers may be tempted to avoid risky patients or to adapt their behaviour to the criteria used for measurement. There is also the methodological problem of regression to the mean, which may lead to false conclusions about the impact of interventions.

Types of responses

Providers may respond to purchasing in different ways. Several distinctions can be made. This section considers five distinctive groups of responses: positive and negative; structural and tactical; provider- and purchaser-driven; managerial, political and litigious; and collective and individual.

A first distinction is that between a positive and negative response. Whereas some providers develop a positive response because they perceive purchasing as a good opportunity for strategic change and to achieve their goals, other providers are more sceptical about the perceived benefits. Indeed, they may even opt for outright resistance when their strategic interests are considered under threat. The real meaning of this simple distinction is that a positive response to purchasing should not be taken for granted.

One can also differentiate between a structural and a tactical response to purchasing. The former is when the provider undertakes activity to strengthen its bargaining position in contracting with the purchaser. Merging with other providers to increase market power or collusion with other providers are well-known strategies in this respect. The intention is not to influence the outcome of a single contracting process but rather to set the scene for a whole series of contracting processes. Tactical responses, on the other hand, refer to a provider's actions in a specific contracting process.

In the third, purchaser-driven response model, the provider will adapt opportunistically to changes the purchaser seeks to implement. Thus, if the purchaser allocates resources to reduce long waiting periods, the provider will increase its activities in order not to miss its part of the extra resources. In the provider-driven model, the provider deploys initiatives to influence the purchaser, who is seen as a partner who can help the provider to realize its ambitions.

Examples of this strategy, among others, are contracting out, investments in human resources including hospital management, the creation of integrated health care delivery networks, initiatives to reduce waiting times, the design of innovative programmes to improve the quality and efficiency of health services. The provider responses can also create incentives for changes in purchasing health care services. For example, where hospitals opt for diversifying care, for example by substituting inpatient with ambulatory care, this by itself may stimulate purchasers to adapt contracts to purchase different packages of care.

Another example is the introduction of one-day surgery services, which may offer a better quality and lower-cost alternative to some traditional surgical procedures that require longer hospital stays.

In the case where individual patients act as the purchaser, the provider may respond by developing well-designed marketing strategies to attract patients. Marketing is a further example of a provider-driven response to purchasing. Box 12.2 illustrates some other examples of purchaser- and provider-driven responses and their interrelations.

Box 12.2   Purchaser- and provider-driven responses

In many instances purchaser-driven responses are correlated with provider-driven responses to the purchasing incentives. For example, the introduction of performance-related payment to providers resulted in reduced waiting times in Norway, and lower length of stay in Estonia and Hungary. The purchaser can alter providers' responses by adjusting the payment system or simply by changing the level of payment for selected services. A more complex approach is when purchasers use a mixture of instruments to obtain specific provider responses. When Hungary introduced fee-for-service payments for dialysis treatments and allowed private providers to enter the market and contract with the National Health Insurance Fund, this resulted in a growing capacity, mostly in the private sector, which ultimately relieved the effects of the previous underprovision of this particular service.

A fourth distinction is that among managerial, political and litigious responses. The key characteristic of a managerial response is that the provider makes a deliberate assessment of the costs and benefits of alternative contracts with the purchaser. The eventual agreement (or non-agreement) is the result of a rational bargaining process between purchaser and provider in which each agency seeks to maximize its net result. However, the provider may also mobilize political resources in the contracting process in order to increase pressure upon the purchasing agency. The political model is frequently used when the provider fundamentally disagrees with the purchaser. A well-known example is the plan of a purchaser to close a hospital or to downsize it considerably on the argument of local or regional overcapacity. The political activity of the provider is to mobilize the local social and political elites to resist the purchaser's initiative. Mobilization will often be easy to accomplish because the local population will not accept the closure or downsizing of 'their hospital'. Boxes 12.3 and 12.4

provide some examples of political interference in providers' responses to purchasers.

Box 12.3 Hospital rationalization in Estonia and Hungary

Estonia and Hungary inherited hospital overcapacities from Semashko-type health care systems. So far Hungary has failed in all its attempts to close hospitals due to the political resistance by an opportunistic coalition of providers and the communities they serve. Even mergers of hospitals to achieve economies of scale and other efficiency gains were unsuccessful in Budapest, where hospital overcapacity is most apparent. This failure is important even if the introduction of case-based payment for hospitals resulted in significant increases in efficiency within the individual provider organizations. Estonia, in contrast, designed a hospital master plan and successfully closed or merged hospitals in order to reduce overcapacity and to rationalize services. The reform, which involved corporatization of hospitals, provided a good basis for providers to react to purchasing incentives. Providers' reactions to using DRGs and fee-for-service techniques were structural and managerial in nature and resulted in restructuring the production process, changing the input mix and the reorganization of services (Pikani, 2003).

Box 12.4 Political regulation in the United Kingdom

The government sought to introduce a radical internal market in 1991. Many purchasers chose to reallocate their spending away from existing hospitals when free to do so, leading to falling revenues for some hospitals. This was particularly apparent in the case of the major, inner-London teaching hospitals, some of which lost up to 20% of their income. However, the prospect of these long-established hospitals failing threatened major political consequences. As a result, the government intervened to 'plan' reconfiguration rather than leave it to the market. More generally, regulation of the market took place nationwide to avoid purchaser-led destabilization.

Finally, the provider may challenge the legality of the purchaser's plan in court. This is the litigious type of response. There are indications that on both national and European Union levels court decisions will become ever more important in health care. Purchasing may provoke a further growth in the litigation in health care.

A common feature of the models discussed so far is that they presume an individual provider responding to a purchasing entity. One could speak here of an individual response. This type of response must be distinguished from a collective response. Providers may decide to act collectively in dealing with purchasers and organize themselves as an interest group to influence them (for example, the hospital associations across Europe). Depending upon their perception of purchasing and its perceived impact on their corporate goals, they may either support or resist health care reform and the further development of purchasing.

Thus far, we have provided a short exploration of some models to categorize the response of providers to purchasing. These models are not exclusive. In the real world, the provider will often use a combination of them to suit its particular purpose. For instance, a provider may respond negatively to purchasing, use political means, public disclosure or litigation to counteract the purchaser's decisions and seek wider political support to influence the course of health care reform and development of purchasing. Alternatively, a provider may adopt a positive attitude to purchasing, opt for a provider-driven approach and organize collective political action to remove obstacles to the further development of purchasing (Busse & Wörz, 2004).

Determinants of provider's response

Purchasing is not an end in itself but a tool for stimulating providers to improve the overall quality and efficiency of their health services and to become more client oriented. The key question to consider is to what extent purchasing operates as an effective incentive for providers to produce more value for money. There are several factors that influence the way providers respond to purchasing. This section will consecutively deal with: political stability and governmental consistency; the degree of providers' ambition; providers' perception of purchasers; the degree of decision rights; market exposure; incentives in the contract: and complexity of the provider organization.

The first factor is consistency in the government's health reform policy. In order to understand this factor one should realize that the development of purchasing and the provider's response to purchasing take time. They are not one-off operations but rather a time-consuming process. Under these circumstances, it is essential that the government pursues a consistent policy that enables the purchaser to develop a contracting policy and the provider organization to engage in strategic management as a response to purchasing. A frequent problem, however, is that a consistent government policy is often lacking. Experience in many countries demonstrates that health care reform is inconsistent. Reform decisions that were taken at one moment are cancelled later because of political pressure, impatience with delays of the expected results, emerging implementation problems or simply the rise of new political majorities that have different ideas about how to proceed with reform (Wlodarczyk, 2004).

The United Kingdom has witnessed a cascade of health reform programmes since the early 1990s, leading to much scepticism among purchasers and providers about the future of such reforms. In some Central and Eastern European countries, decentralization of purchasing to the meso level in the health care system was followed only a few years later by recentralization. For instance,

Poland centralized its insurance system in 2003 from a regionally based system. Recent research (Szócska *et al.*, 2003) on sources of failed implementation of health reforms suggests that providers are reluctant to react to new policies due to the frequent changes and the inconsistency of the different reform initiatives. Ministers come and go, and new ideas might not be consistent with previous reform attempts, leading to failure and further political change. This is illustrated in Central and Eastern European countries, which have witnessed a very high turnover of health ministers in the last ten years.

A second determinant is the provider's ambition. An ambitious provider in search of strategic change to create more value for money is expected to respond differently to purchasing from a provider with a strong interest in keeping the status quo. Not all providers are ambitious, however. A distinction can be made between pioneers, followers and conservatives. Pioneering providers are those who see the immediate benefits of exploring new opportunities associated with purchasing. On their way to change they are willing to take risks. Often, they form only a minority but that minority may play an essential role in the reform process. A second group consists of followers, who after some time begin to copy the pioneering initiatives. Conservatives, finally, are those providers who wish to maintain the status quo as long as possible. In fact, they are reluctant to change. An interesting illustration of the concept is the introduction of GP fundholding in the United Kingdom. It is usually seen as a purchasing innovation rather than a provider innovation but it obviously has a provider role as well. It was introduced in 1991–1992 with much fanfare by the then Conservative government. Initially, uptake was slow and to encourage more GPs to join the scheme additional incentives were introduced. By the time the scheme was abolished by the new Labour government, about half of the practices in England and Wales had become fundholders. A modified version of the GP fundholding concept was introduced in Hungary in 1999 (Gaál and Evetovits, 2002). In contrast to the United Kingdom implementation strategy, the government started to pilot the new scheme with a few participating providers. The pilot has been expanded every year since then and each year more providers are interested in joining this new care managing organization model than were allowed by the political decision. In 2004, 20% of the population is covered by this new arrangement.

A third determinant of the provider's response to purchasing is the way the provider perceives the impact of purchasing. This determinant is closely linked to the positive versus negative type of responses described in the previous section. Is purchasing viewed as an important step in the right direction or is it considered a threat? In this respect, it is a mistake to assume that all hospitals are strong believers in the model of market competition and purchasing. For instance, purchasing could result in strong interference by the purchaser in internal affairs or with the physician's professional autonomy in treating patients. Market exposure may lead to fundamental changes in the provision of care that conflict with the institutional interests of providers. Competitive bidding procedures may result in lost contracts that could have serious consequences for the financial sustainability of the provider organization. Providers may also have serious doubts about the potential of purchasing. It may lead to a new bureaucracy with little added value. Fair competition and fair purchasing may prove an illusion. For all these reasons providers may develop a sceptical attitude towards purchasing. Scepticism may turn into outright resistance should the purchaser announce steps that the provider perceives as threatening.

The issue of decision rights is a fourth key determinant of the provider's response to purchasing. In order to respond strategically to purchasing, the provider must have sufficient decision rights to enable it to change its behaviour. For instance, it must be able to control input factors and the scope of activities, to develop its financial and clinical management or to redesign its production process. Governments may abstain from conferring essential decision rights on the purchaser and provider resulting in growing tensions between central control and local decision making. From this perspective it is probably fair to conclude that hospitals in many countries still do not have the essential decision rights they require to change their behaviour drastically. This problem is particularly urgent for budgetary and autonomized provider organizations, which are characterized by strong organizational ties with the purchaser. The purchaser has many regulatory controls that restrict the scope for change. Corporatized and privatized hospitals have more decision rights but such hospitals still face various social or political constraints that restrict their possibilities for change. Provider organizations must comply with a multitude of public regulations that constrain their range of activities. For instance, state planning arrangements or quality criteria may reduce their options for establishing new service delivery units or for closing them. State wage regulations or collective bargaining arrangements may inhibit them from initiating schemes that link payment to performance. State price regulations may make it unattractive or even impossible for providers to make an offer to the purchaser. State regulations may reduce the possibility of increasing the number of physicians or nurses. Thus the response to purchasing depends upon how purchasing is shaped (Busse *et al.*, 2002).

A fifth determinant affecting the provider's response to purchasing can be described as market exposure. As market exposure increases, providers will have a stronger need for responding to purchasing. Compare, in this respect, a hospital in a rural or remote area, where the next hospital is at considerable distance, with an urban hospital among many others. It is evident that the pressure on the hospital in the remote area to change its behaviour will be less than that upon the hospital in a competitive urban setting. Market exposure is not only determined by the presence of other providers in the service area. Other important factors are the scarcity of hospital services, public regulations, the contestability of the provider market, and technological change. A scarcity of hospital services reduces the purchaser's options and gives the provider a strong position in contracting. Public regulations may protect providers against market exposure. For instance, in various countries with a Bismarckian type of health care system, the purchaser is forced by law to contract with all providers that have acquired a licence to deliver care to patients. It is either not possible or extremely difficult to deny a contract to a provider, even if it performs poorly. Postcode assignment of patients to providers gives them a monopolistic position. The concept of contestability draws attention to the fact that the market position of a provider is dependent not only upon the presence of competing providers but also upon the threat of new entrants and substitute products and services. The more contestable the market is, the more the negotiating power of the provider will decline. At the same time, the need for an adequate response to purchasing increases. The contestability of health care markets is quite heterogeneous, however. Generally speaking, one may say that the market for hospital care is less contestable than the market for community care or nursing home care because of greater sunk costs, the need for large investments and specialized resources. Nevertheless, due to technological advances, an increasing number of treatments that were once risky and expensive have become relatively cheap and routine. As a result, new specialist providers (for instance of cataract surgery) may arise offering these services as an attractive option to the purchaser, thus weakening the power base of the traditional hospital.

A sixth determinant is incentives or disincentives in the contract. The key question here is to what extent the provider can win or lose in contracting. If, for instance, a hospital can secure capital for its health service infrastructure, extend its volume of services or retain and reinvest operating surpluses as a result of contracting, purchasing will work as a powerful stimulus to respond strategically. The payment regime is of great importance in this respect. For instance, it makes a great difference whether revenues come from a global and input-based health budget or from performance-related schedules. A frequent problem, however, is that the purchaser has little incentive to offer providers because its decision rights are constrained by the public regulations with which it must comply.

A seventh determinant refers to the complexity of provider organizations (in particular, hospitals), and the quality of provider management. Many providers, especially hospitals, comprise quite complicated organizations, which are difficult to manage. They should not be thought of as monolithic entities with strong hierarchical structures. Instead, they should be described as professional bureaucracies populated by a variety of medical professionals with diverging interests who are in permanent internal competition with each other for scarce resources. Medical professionals also have great difficulty accepting strong management (unless they can directly benefit from it), which they mostly perceive as bureaucracy and an intrusion into their professional autonomy. Thus, provider organizations are difficult to manage effectively. An additional problem in this respect is that provider management in many European countries is often weakly developed and managers are often not particularly well trained. In various countries hospital management is still not considered as a full-time professional activity but only a part-time activity for a director-clinician who spends part of the time treating patients. However, there are also promising developments in part as a result of the introduction of purchasing reforms. Hungary provides a good example for this (Box 12.5).

Another determinant of a provider's behaviour is the degree of asymmetry of information between the purchaser and the provider. That is, to what extent do providers have greater knowledge about the needs and responses of their patients? The degree of monitoring of providers by the purchaser, and the attitude of purchasers, especially the degree of trust and the style of contracting (relational versus classical contracting), are further determinants.

Box 12.5   Management capacity building in Hungarian hospitals

---

The Hungarian hospital payment reform shows how providers react to changes in decision rights, market exposure and the issue of residual revenue. The introduction of case-based payment was part of the transformation process of budgetary units to more autonomous hospitals owned by the local councils, with revenues based on actual output using the DRG system of payment. The more services they provide, the more income they generate, and by reducing the unit cost of services the hospital's financial balance can be further improved. Hospitals are competing for patients and now have more decision rights over how they spend their revenue. The realization that the hospitals' financial viability depends on how they can increase output and reduce costs has led to more cost-conscious clinical behaviour and the professionalization of hospital management, which was neglected during the era of budgetary units. By now most of the hospital directors have participated in some form of postgraduate management training and it is now a standard requirement for a newly appointed hospital director to have a degree in health care management.

The impact of purchasing

Earlier we stated that, to our knowledge, no systematic comparative studies have been conducted examining the impact of purchasing upon the behaviour of providers. The main reason for this state of affairs is that purchasing is still in its infancy, not only in Eastern Europe but also in Western Europe. One country that has considerable experience with purchasing in health care is the United Kingdom. A recent evaluation concluded that the introduction of the internal market and purchasing (commissioning) brought only limited change. Le Grand *et al.* (1998) conclude 'the incentives were too weak and the constraints were too strong'. They point to a permanent and strong tension between the internal market on the one hand and central government control over health care on the other hand as a crucial determining factor. Another key factor for implementing fundamental reform in health care is policy stability. However, policy stability has not been a strong characteristic of health care policy making in the United Kingdom since the early 1980s, given the cascade of new reforms quickly succeeding and partly displacing each other.

The Netherlands is another country where purchasing is still in a developmental stage. There is a gap between the government's rhetoric of purchasing and its actual practice. Health insurers are handicapped in implementing a contracting policy of their own. Not only do public regulations constrain their decision rights but they must also struggle with market deficiencies on the provider side (for instance, regional monopolies, scarcity of health services, a culture of collective bargaining on contracting, resistance to bilateral purchasing). The same is true for providers who demand that their decision rights be enhanced and government control rights be reduced. Hospitals that want to operate as a kind of private entrepreneur with a public mission have to overcome substantial bureaucratic, political and cultural obstacles. Many directors of provider organizations are sceptical about concepts like market exposure, purchasing, selective contracting, competitive bidding and benchmarking. There is also fear about moving towards a two-tier health care system. Nevertheless, there are a number of pioneers seeking to enforce change. A fundamental step towards purchasing will be the introduction of case-based payments for hospital care. The situation in Germany resembles that of the Netherlands in many respects. As yet, in Europe, arrangements for managed care, for instance health maintenance organizations or preferred provider organizations, have hardly come into existence. Thus, the health care landscape is only slowly changing (Maarse *et al.*, 2002).

Conclusion

This chapter discussed some aspects of the response of provider organizations to purchasing. It is still difficult to draw firm conclusions about how providers respond and the implications of their response for the quality, efficiency and accessibility of health services. This conclusion is based upon the observation that the impact of purchasing is difficult to disentangle from other determinants of provider behaviour. Another observation is that it takes time for the impact of purchasing upon provider behaviour to materialize. In this respect, one should not ignore the fact that purchasing across the European continent is still in its infancy. Countries, purchasers and providers are all at the beginning of the learning curve.

An analysis of the providers' response to purchasing must contend with several conceptual difficulties. One is the question of who the purchaser is or, phrased differently, to which purchaser the provider must respond. Here, we considered the distinction between purchasing at the macro, meso and micro levels in the health care system.

Another difficulty concerns the great variety of providers. In this respect, we used the Harding and Preker model, which classifies provider organizations into four analytical categories: budgetary, autonomized, corporatized and privatized. The essence of their classification model is that each type of provider may be expected to respond differently to purchasing. We also observed that budgetary and autonomized provider organizations still prevail in the countries of Central and Eastern Europe. We warned against overstated expectations of purchasing upon provider behaviour in these countries. However, even in Western Europe, purchasing must be further developed in order for there to be a visible impact upon providers.

Providers can respond in different ways to purchasing. We explored several classifications for the modelling of provider responses. Distinctions were made between positive and negative responses; tactical and structural responses; managerial, political and litigious responses; purchaser-driven and provider-driven responses; bilateral and collective responses.

We were concerned with an exploration of key factors that influence the provider's response to purchasing. Several determinants were identified: the consistency of the government's reform policy; the provider's ambition; the provider's perception of the advantages and disadvantages of purchasing; the provider's decision rights; the extent of market exposure; the type of (dis)-incentives in the contract; and finally, the internal complexity of the provider organization and the professional quality of provider management.

References

Busse, R. and Wörz, M. (2004) The ambiguous experience with privatisation in German health care. *In*: Maarse, H., ed., *Privatisation in European health care*. Maarsen: Elsevier Gezondheidszorg.

Busse, R., van der Grinten, T. and Svensson, P. (2002) *Regulating entrepreneurial behaviour in hospitals: theory and practice. In*: Saltman, R., Busse, R. and Mossialos, E., eds. *Regulating entrepreneurial behaviour in European health care systems*. European Observatory on Health Systems and Policies Series. Buckingham, Open University Press.

Gaál, P. and Evetovits, T. (2002) The purchasing function in the Hungarian health care system. Case study prepared for the European Observatory on Health Care Systems and Policies.

Harding, A. and Preker, A., eds. (2003) *Private participation in health services*. Washington, D.C., World Bank.

Kirkman-Liff, B., Huijsman, R., van der Grinten, T. and Brink, G. (1997) Hospital adaptation to risk-bearing managerial implications of changes in purchaser–provider contracting, *Health Policy*, **39**(3): 207–223.

Le Grand, J., Mays, N. and Mulligan, J., eds. (1998) *Learning from the NHS internal market. A review of the evidence*. London: King's Fund.

Maarse, J. *et al.* (2002) *Marktwerking in de ziekenhuiszorg. Een analyse van de mogelijkheden en effecten (Market competition in hospital care. An analysis of opportunities and effects)*. Maastricht, Datawyse.

McKee, M. and Healy, J., eds. (2001) *Hospitals in a changing Europe*. European Observatory on Health Systems and Policies Series. Open University Press. Buckingham.

Pikani, J. (2003) Estonian hospital reform: case study of the reorganization of Tartu University Hospital. Presentation at the 5th Regional Flagship Course on Health Sector Reform and Sustainable Financing, Budapest, 1 July.

Preker, A. and Harding, A., eds. (2003) *Innovations in health service delivery. The corporatization of public hospitals*. Washington, D.C., World Bank.

Stein, J.G. (2001) *The cult of efficiency*. Toronto: Anansi.

Szócska, M., Réthelyi, J. and Normand, C. (2003) Why organizational realities block policy reforms – feasibility considerations for health politicians. *Health policy* (submitted for publication).

Wlodarczyk, C. (2004) The re-emergence of the private sector in Polish health care. *In*: Maarse, J., eds, *Privatisation in European health care*. Maarsen: Elsevier Gezondheidszorg.

Index